Healthcare in the Arabian Gulf and Greater Middle East

Healthcare in the Arabian Gulf and Greater Middle East

A GUIDE FOR HEALTHCARE PROFESSIONALS

EDITED BY

MAY MCCREADDIE, PhD, MEd, BA, PG Cert PE, RNT, RN

Lecturer
School of Nursing and Midwifery
University of Galway
Galway, Ireland

GARY E. DAY, DHSM, MHM, BNurs, DipAppSc
(Nursing Mgt), RN, EM, FCHSM, FGLF

Professor-Health Services Management and Academic Campus Manager
ECA College of Health Sciences and Asia-Pacific International College
Brisbane, Australia

JANE LEANNE GRIFFITHS, RN, COTM, Dip. NA, BAN, MHP

Ex-Chief Nursing Information Officer
Informatics
Dubai Health Authority
Dubai, United Arab Emirates

ELSEVIER

Notices

Practitioners and researchers must always rely on their own experience and knowledge in evaluating and using any information, methods, compounds or experiments described herein. Because of rapid advances in the medical sciences, in particular, independent verification of diagnoses and drug dosages should be made. To the fullest extent of the law, no responsibility is assumed by Elsevier, authors, editors or contributors for any injury and/or damage to persons or property as a matter of products liability, negligence or otherwise, or from any use or operation of any methods, products, instructions, or ideas contained in the material herein.

ISBN: 978-0-323-83356-1

Content Strategist: Robert Edwards
Content Project Manager: Tapajyoti Chaudhuri
Cover Design: Matthew Limbert
Marketing Manager: Deborah J. Watkins

Printed in India.

Last digit is the print number: 9 8 7 6 5 4 3 2 1

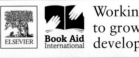

Working together to grow libraries in developing countries

www.elsevier.com • www.bookaid.org

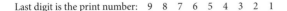

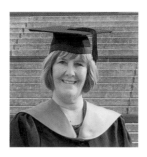

Sandra Goodwin, RGN, MSc (Public Health)
(27 December 1960–12 October 2020)
MKCC—Bahrain Defence Force

The best clinical practice coordinator in the Arabian Gulf and Greater Middle East—bar none.
Vibrant. Funny. Passionate.
A real loss.

CONTENTS

SECTION I

Specific Conditions, Specific Challenges

SECTION II

Key Healthcare Approaches

CONTRIBUTORS

EDITORS

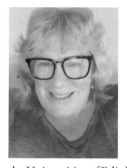

May McCreaddie, PhD, MEd, BA, PGCert PE, RNT, RN

She is a nurse academic with over 35 years' experience, with seven of those spent working in nurse education in the UAE and latterly Bahrain while she has also previously worked in Romania and India. She has held academic posts at the Universities of Edinburgh, Lancaster University and latterly, University of Stirling. She is an award-winning nurse (Most Inspiring Lecturer University of Stirling 2014, shortlisted Times Higher Education most innovative lecturer 2014, Excellence in Clinical Practice Award SGNA (Society for Gastroenterology Nursing Association) 2012, Robert Tiffany International Award 2001). She has obtained and led numerous research grants and has published widely in peer-reviewed journals. Her main area of interest is authentic interactions, specifically healthcare interactions—routine to problematic interactions. Her PhD reviewed humour in healthcare interactions from which she published widely and she retains an interest in that area.

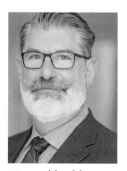

Gary E. Day, DHSM, MHM, BNurs, DipAppSc (Nursing Mgt), RN, EM, FCHSM, FGLF

He is an adjunct professor and a senior international healthcare executive with extensive operational, academic and consulting experience across Australia, South-east Asia and the Middle East. He has over 35 years' healthcare experience in health services management, public health, executive leadership, higher education and workforce development. He has taken lead roles in major hospital infrastructure projects, large-scale change management, executive manager development, medical education and organisational culture development. Over the last 4 years he has been the Director of Quality and Safety, and the Director of Clinical Education, Training and Research at Sheikh Khalifa Medical City, Ajman. He currently holds a visiting professorial position at Gulf Medical University, College of Health Management and Economics.

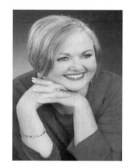

Jane Leanne Griffiths, RN, COTM, Dip. NA, BAN, MHP

She is a registered general nurse from Australia. She was based in the UAE from 2007 to 2020 working for the Dubai Health Authority. Her clinical experience and qualifications are in operating theatre techniques and management. Her experience has included both operational roles such as director of nursing and general manager positions in tertiary-level facilities as well as strategic roles in healthcare, facility planning, informatics and disaster management in Australia, Qatar and the UAE. She is currently a healthcare management consultant providing advice, mentoring and publications focussed on healthcare management and technology. She chaired the UAE Nursing and Midwifery Council Scientific Committees for Research and Excellence and participated in a number of UAE boards and councils. She also has extensive academic experience in teaching and research at universities in Australia, Ireland and the USA with over 25 scientific publications and is a Healthcare Information and Management Systems Society (HIMMS) Future50 Healthcare IT Leader.

AUTHORS

Hadya Abboud Abdel Fattah, PhD, MSc, BN, RN

She is a registered nurse and has a PhD from the British University in Dubai, UAE. Her PhD dissertation focussed on the impact of nursing education curriculum and workforce preparation on nursing students' critical thinking, moral reasoning and cultural sensitivity in the UAE. She has a master's degree in leadership education, from Abu Dhabi University and a bachelor's degree in nursing from the University of Jordan (Amman). She has a broad range of experience and interests over 26 years working in the GCC, previously working as an ICU, Operation and Recovery Room Manager and as the Head of Nursing Education in Saudi Arabia. Her research interest is in critical thinking, health promotion, cultural context and values, and contextualising the nursing curriculum.

Catherine Abou'zaid, EdD MSc, PGDip (Psychol, Coun, Micro, Pharm), RGN

She works in Mohamed Khalifa Cardiac Centre, Department of Training Development & Research in the Kingdom of Bahrain where she has been a resident for more than 23 years. Her research interests lie within health education, and she teaches within the centre itself as well as being Associate Lecturer with the Royal College of Surgeons in Ireland-MUB. Her aim is to facilitate the progress of new graduates, making them future leaders within healthcare settings by providing them with guidance and courses that encourage research and educational activities. She gained her doctorate degree in higher education from the University of Liverpool in 2018.

Ahmed Allaithy, BA, MA, PhD

He is Professor of Translation Studies at the Department of Arabic and Translation Studies, Australia. He has a PhD in comparative translation of the Holy Qur'an from the University of Durham, UK. He is the current President of Arabic Translators International (ATI), General Editor of ATI Academic Series and ATI literary Series (Arabic Literature Unveiled), and General Director of *Dragoman* journal of translation studies. He has taught courses in Arabic-Islamic heritage, translation and interpreting in universities across three continents. His research interests include linguistics, Arabic rhetoric, translation, intercultural communication and Islamic/Qur'anic studies.

Amina Al Marzouqi, Dip. Nursing, BSc, MHM, PhD

She is the Assistant Chancellor at the University of Sharjah. Her specialties include health economics, health services development and improvement, human resources development, quality management, risk management and leadership in healthcare sectors. She received her PhD from the High Institute of Public Health—Alexandria University, as well as a master's degree in health management—planning and policy from Leeds University. She completed her undergraduate degree in community health education from the University of South Carolina. Her research interests are in health economics and financing.

Nabeel Al Yateem, BSN, MSN, PhD

He earned his PhD in children and adolescent health nursing from the Galway University, Ireland. He is currently working as Associate Professor in the Department of Nursing, College of Health Sciences, the University of Sharjah in the city of Sharjah in the UAE. He is also an adjunct Associate Professor at Charles Sturt University, Faculty of Science and Health, Charles Sturt University in New South Wales in Australia; adjunct Professor at Binawan University in Indonesia; and Visiting Research Fellow at Trinity College Dublin in Ireland.

Stephanie Annett, BPharm, MPharm, PhD

She is Lecturer of Pharmacy in the School of Pharmacy and Bimolecular Sciences at RCSI University of Medicine and Health Sciences, Ireland. She obtained her Master of Pharmacy (MPharm) degree at Queen's University Belfast in 2012 and completed her preregistration pharmacist training in hospital and community pharmacy. She returned to Queen's University Belfast to complete a PhD in experimental therapeutics in 2017, investigating the role of FK506-binding protein like-based therapeutics to target ovarian and breast cancer. Following this she was appointed as a post doctorate researcher at RCSI University of Medicine and Health Sciences and investigated the role of FKBPL in inflammation and obesity and was appointed as a lecturer of pharmacy in 2021.

Stephen L. Atkin, BSc, MBBS, MRCP, FRCP, PhD

He is the Head of the School of Postgraduate Studies and Research at the Royal College of Surgeons of Ireland in Bahrain. Previously he was Professor of Medicine at the Weill Cornell Medical College in Qatar, and prior to that role he was Professor of Medicine and Head of Diabetes and Endocrinology at the Hull York Medical School, UK. He has an established international reputation in diabetes and obesity research, encompassing polycystic ovary syndrome and metabolic syndrome.

Sharon Brownie, RN, RM, BEd, MEdAdmin, MHSM, MAppMgt (Nursing), DBA, PhD

She has extensive educational, health management and policy development experience developed through her work in Australia, New Zealand, East Africa, Fiji and the Middle East. Her leadership roles have included significant capacity building, workforce development, business growth and change management mandates. Her initial doctorate evaluated New Zealand's partnership-based public policy model for local and regional economic development. Her nursing focus is strengthened by a second doctoral qualification, specifically, a PhD by published works entitled 'Nursing in Health Service Leadership'.

She spent several years in senior academic roles in the UAE as well as senior academic and research roles at Aga Khan University. She is currently the Campus Principal and Discipline Lead Nursing at the University of Canberra.

Alexandra E. Butler, MBBS, PhD

She is Senior Research Fellow, Royal College of Surgeons in Ireland and Medical University of Bahrain, Adliya, Bahrain. She is based at RCSI Bahrain where she is undertaking translational research related to islet cell biology. Previously, she served as Principal Investigator at the Qatar Biomedical Research Institute and as Professor of Medicine/Endocrinology at the University of California, Los Angeles. Her research has focussed on pancreatic islet biology and pathology as it relates to the study of Type 1 and Type 2 diabetes. Her more recent work has involved studying the regenerative capacity of human pancreas, as well as proteomic metabolomic analysis of diabetes and other insulin resistant states, such as polycystic ovary syndrome.

Sandra Goodwin[†], RGN MSc (Public Health)

She was a nursing supervisor in Mohamed Khalifa Cardiac Centre, Department of Nursing, specialised centre in the Kingdom of Bahrain. She was also the Clinical Placement Officer for the RCSI-MUB nursing students. Sandra was a passionate nurse and dedicated her life to the care of patients with cardiac disease. Sandra had a keen interest in health promotion and gained her MSc in public health from the University of Liverpool.

Ghufran Jassim, PhD, MD, MSc, MBBS, Dip. HPE

She is the Head of Department of Family Medicine and Associate Professor in Family Medicine at the Royal College of Surgeons in Ireland-Medical University of Bahrain. She is a strong advocate of women's health, has published many articles on women's health in peer-reviewed journals and set up the first women's health clinic at a public hospital in the Kingdom of Bahrain. Her research interests are women's health, breast cancer, menopause, cervical cancer.

Keith Johnston, MBChB, BMSc (Hons), FRCA

He is an Ulster man who studied at the University of Dundee, Scotland, before completing his postgraduate training in the Northern England. He has spent the past 8 years working as a consultant in anaesthesia and pain management at the King Hamad University Hospital. In addition, he lectures in anaesthesia, pain and palliative care at the Royal College of Surgeons of Ireland-Medical University Bahrain. He was previously the Head of Department of Anaesthesia and Critical Care in Muscat Private Hospital in Oman for 3 years. His interest in the region was peaked when he was a founding member of the Newcastle Gateshead Medical Volunteers Group, a charity providing orthopaedic, humanitarian and medical educational aid to post war Iraq and Kurdistan. He undertakes charitable work for Operation Childlife, providing both clinical anaesthesia for children with cancer as well as educational initiatives in Tanzania and Vietnam.

Noon Abubakr Adbelrahman Kamil, BPharm, PhD

She is an instructor at Fatima College of Health Sciences, UAE. She has a PhD in pharmaceutical chemistry from University of Khartoum, Sudan, in 2019. During that time, she managed to publish many articles and contextualise many pharmacy practice courses to the Middle East. She has about five publications in peer-reviewed journals with high-impact factor. Furthermore, she obtained the prize of the best academic performance in Pharmaceutics University of Khartoum in 2004. She gave two oral presentations at two international conferences. Her research interest includes pharmacy education, global health pharmacy, pharmaceutical chemistry, randomised control trials and drug analysis.

Wendy Maddison, MA (Social Science and Psychology), EdD, Dip. CBT, Cert. Online Teaching & Learning

She is Head of Student Development and Wellbeing at RCSI Bahrain. She has a doctorate in higher education from the University of Liverpool, UK, and is a qualified cognitive behavioural therapist. Her areas of expertise include the provision of support and wellbeing in different cultural contexts, in particular within transnational higher education, and transformational learning. She is active academically as the nominated MENA representative in the Kingdom of Bahrain for the qualitative research methodology of interpretative phenomenological analysis (IPA), through Birbeck University, UK. She has published in high-impact journals such as *Studies in Higher Education* and *International Journal of Learning and Development*, covering topics such as identity and professional transitions of local (female) Middle Eastern students. She has many years' experience working in international business and academic environments, in particular in the Middle East.

Hani Malik, MB, BCh, BAO, LRCP, SI, ABFM, PGDip, HPEd, MSc, LIH

He is Bahraini and a lecturer in family medicine at RCSI Medical University of Bahrain and a consultant family physician at both Royal Bahrain Hospital and Western Medical Center. He is Irish and Arab board certified in family medicine. He obtained a postgraduate diploma in health profession's education at RCSI Bahrain and a master's degree in leadership and innovation in healthcare at RCSI Dubai. He recently completed the certificate of learning and teaching in higher education from Advance HE in the United Kingdom. In a previous role as quality coordinator in 2019, Hani was an instrumental member of the quality enhancement team that achieved 'Diamond status' for primary health in Bahrain's Ministry of Health, awarded by the Canadian Qmentum International Accreditation Program.

Orla Merrigan, MSC, FFNMRCSI, BSC, PG Cert., RGN, RNT

She is Head of Learning & Development, Orpea Residences Ireland. She is a nurse with over 25 years' experience in clinical management, critical care, academia, nurse education, project management, research and healthcare digitalisation. She is a passionate healthcare expert with extensive experience in Ireland, the United Kingdom, Egypt and the Middle East. Orla was responsible for the first mass cardiopulmonary resuscitation (CPR) training project of the lay public in the Middle East, and the first Hands-only CPR advert in Arabic in the Gulf region which was launched as a public service awareness campaign on Gulf Air, the national airline in Bahrain. She has been an adjunct faculty member of John Hopkins School of Nursing Baltimore and is currently associated with University of Hewler, Iraq. Orla was a recipient of a Nursing & Midwifery Fellowship award from The Royal College of Surgeons in Ireland for her contribution to nursing (2014). She is currently completing an educational doctorate.

Maryam Jameel Naser, MBBS

Maryam is a graduate of the Royal College of Surgeons in Ireland-Medical University of Bahrain, 2019, and class of medicine valedictorian. She has been the recipient of numerous awards including the John Murphy Award of Medicine and the HH Stewart Award of Psychiatry from the National University of Ireland. She is Bahraini and is currently pursuing a medical residency in internal medicine at University of Massachusetts Medical School, Baystate. She is interested in academic medicine, health advocacy and research in medical oncology

James O'Boyle, MBA, MSc (Biochemistry), Advanced Diploma in Personal, Leadership and Executive Coaching (Distinction), Innovations in eLearning

He has an MBA from University College Dublin and an MSc in biochemistry from King's College London. He is a Fellow of the Institute of Biomedical Science London and a leadership and executive coach, accredited by the European Mentoring and Coaching Council. For over 9 years, James directed operations at the Royal College of Surgeons in Ireland—Dubai campus and was a program director of the internationally accredited MSc in healthcare management for working healthcare professionals. As an independent consultant, James has worked with organisations such as the Mohammed Bin Rashid University of Medicine and Health Sciences, Murdoch University, DP World and Croydon University Hospital, all within a healthcare context.

Sheila Payne, BA(Hons), PhD, RN, DipN, CPsychol

She is Emeritus Professor, International Observatory on End of Life Care, Lancaster University, UK, and a health psychologist with a background in nursing. She led three research groups and was President of the European Association of Palliative Care (2011–2015). She has worked closely with the World Health Organization ad hoc Technical Advisory Group on implementation of palliative care. She has worked in collaboration with the WHO EMRO (Eastern Mediterranean Region Office) in supporting palliative care development in the Eastern Mediterranean Region, including assisting with the development of the first National Strategy for Palliative Care and Home Care in Jordan.

Diaa E. E. Rizk, MB, BCh (Hons), MSc (Hons), FRCOG, FRCS, MD, Dip. BA

He is a professor in the Department of Obstetrics and Gynaecology, College of Medicine and Medical Sciences, Arabian Gulf University, Manama, Bahrain. He is an obstetrician and gynaecologist who has published extensively in the subject area including 170 research articles, 170 research articles and two book chapters on reproductive and women's health, medical education, biomedical journalism and urogynaecology. He is a co-editor of *Insights into Incontinence and the Pelvic Floor*. He was the Editor for the *International Urogynecology Journal* and currently serves on the Editorial Board of Urogynecology. He has organised postgraduate multidisciplinary educational courses in urogynecology for the International Continence Society (ICS) and International Urogynecological Association (IUGA). He has contributed to urogynecology clinical service, development of residency training programmes, community care of female incontinence and public education on incontinence. He has been a member of regional and international committees for IUGA, ICS, FIGO and WHO, and he co-founded the Mediterranean Incontinence and Pelvic Floor Society and is the current president of the society.

Rachel Rossiter, RN, BHS, MC, MN, DHS

She is Associate Professor of Nursing and Associate Head of School (Research and Graduate Studies), School of Nursing, Paramedicine and Healthcare Sciences, Faculty of Science and Health, Charles Sturt University, New South Wales.

Beginning in 2015, Drs Al-Yateem and Rossiter have collaborated on research projects focussed on mental health literacy, and upskilling paediatric nurses and school nurses in the United Arab Emirates. Together, they have had more than 10 research papers published in high-impact journals.

Razan Shaheen, BA (Psychology), MA (Social Science Administration), Licensed Psychologist (National Health Regulatory Authority of Bahrain and National Register of Psychotherapists & Counsellors (UK))

She is a psychologist at Insights Therapy Center in the Kingdom of Bahrain. She earned her master's degree from Case Western Reserve University and has worked in several hospitals and clinics in the United States and Bahrain. Her experience and cultural awareness offer a unique perspective to her work in the Middle East.

Khatoon Husain Shubbar, MD, ABFM, PGDip Dermatology, MSHCM

She is Bahraini and a consultant family physician at the Ministry of Health in Bahrain. She is Irish and Arab board certified in family medicine. She obtained a postgraduate diploma in dermatology at the

University of South Wales and a master's in healthcare management at RCSI Bahrain. As head of the quality and risk management committee in all primary health governmental facilities, she led her team in achieving 'Diamond status', awarded by the Canadian Qmentum International Accreditation Program. She is a member of the national quality and clinical standards committee and part-time surveyor at the National Health Regulatory Authority. She is also a representative of the telehealth services for primary health and teaches part-time at RCSI Bahrain.

Eman Tawash, PhD, MSc, PG Dip., FFRNMCSI, RN

She is Senior Lecturer in the School of Nursing and Midwifery, RCSI Bahrain, with a PhD in Nursing and is Fellow of the Faculty of Nursing & Midwifery-RCSI with Certificate in Learning and Teaching in Higher Education, Master's in Health Professions Education, PG Dip. in Health Care Management from RCSI Bahrain. She is also a registered nurse and a member of the Bahrain Nursing Society.

She is interested in research related to nursing education, nursing practice, population health and quality improvement. She is the founder of Future Nurses Bahrain initiative which aims at promoting nursing as a positive career choice and contributing to the future development of the nursing workforce in Bahrain and the Arab region.

James Waterson, RN, BA (Hons), MMedEd, MHEc

He is Medical Affairs Manager, Middle East & Africa, Medication Management Solutions, Becton Dickinson Ltd, Dubai, UAE. His special interests are the development of real-world evidence of the impact of healthcare solutions, developing health-technology assessment tools and collaboration with healthcare facilities to create integrated medication safety systems. He has written and presented extensively on healthcare automation and closed-loop safety systems for medication compounding, administration and dispensing, on the use of robotics in health care and on the interaction of clinicians with technology. He is a reviewer for the *Journal of Pediatrics Pharmaceutical Therapeutics*, *The Journal of Applied Clinical Informatics* and *The Journal of Medical Internet Research: Human Factors*.

ABBREVIATIONS

ASHP	American Society Health System Pharmacists	FI	Faecal incontinence
ACHS	Australian Council on Healthcare Standards	GCC	Gulf Cooperation Council
ADA	American Diabetes Association	GP	General practitioner
AIDS	Acquired immune deficiency syndrome	HAS	Health savings account
APPT	Adolescent Pediatric Pain Tool	HDL	High density lipids
BMI	Body mass index	HRA	Health reimbursement arrangement
BSc	Bachelor of Science (degree)	HIV	Human immunodeficiency virus
CPOE	Computerised Provider Order Entry	HAI	Healthcare acquired infection
COCM	Crescent of Care Model	HDI	Human Development Index
CBT	Cognitive behavioural therapy	HIV	Human immunodeficiency virus
CHD	Coronary heart disease	ICD	International Classification of Diseases
CDHS	Consumer driven health care	IDU	Intravenous drug user
CCP	Container control program	ILO	International Labour Organisation
CAM	Complementary and alternative medicine	IMPACT	International taskforce on counterfeit medical products
COVID-19	Coronavirus disease	Interpol	International criminal police organization
CDC	Centers for Disease Control	IqPHVC	Iraqi pharmacovigilance centre
CFR	Case fatality rate	IPE	Interprofessional education
CAI	Community acquired infection	ISO	International Standards Organisation
CVD	Cardiovascular disease	INCB	International Narcotics Control Board
CPG	Clinical practice guidelines	IRP	Intramural Research Programme
CAP	Community acquired pneumonia	IF	Intermittent fasting
CF	Cystic fibrosis	JFDA	Jordan food and drink administration
COPD	Chronic obstructive pulmonary disease	JCI	Joint commission international
DSM-5	*Diagnostic and Statistical Manual of Mental Disorders*	KSA	Kingdom of Saudi Arabia
DNR	Do not resuscitate	LGBT	Lesbian, gay, bisexual and transgender
EoLC	End-of-life care	MetS	Metabolic syndrome
EMR	Electronic medical record	MhGAP	Mental health gap action program
EMR	Eastern Mediterranean Region	MOHAP	Ministry of health and prevention
EUIPO	European Union Intellectual Property Office	MENA	Middle East and Northern Africa
FAMCO	Department of Family and Community Medicine	MERS	Middle East respiratory syndrome
		MSM	Men who have sex with men
		MSc	Master of Science (postgraduate) degree
		MDG	Millennium Development Goals
FIP	International Pharmaceutical Federation	MMR	Measles, mumps, rubella
FPG	Fasting plasma glucose	MECC	Middle East Cancer Consortium

MoH	Ministry of Health	STST	Satir transformational systemic therapy
NCEP	National cholesterol education program	SBFM	Saudi board family medicine
NSAID	Non-steroidal anti-inflammatory drugs	SM	Self-medication
NGOs	Nongovernmental organisations	SFDA	Saudi Food and Drug Authority
OIC	Organisation of Islamic Cooperation	S/F	Substandard and falsified
OECD	Organisation for Economic Co-operation and Development	SDG	Sustainable Development Goals
OCD	Obsessive compulsive disorder	STIs	Sexually transmitted infections
OOP	Out of pocket	SA	Sleep apnoea
OPL	Order of Pharmacists Lebanon	SCD	Sickle cell disease
PCOS	Polycystic ovary syndrome	T2DM	Type 2 diabetes mellitus
PTSD	Post-traumatic stress disorder	TB	Tuberculosis
PHC	Primary health care	TRA	Telecommunications Regulatory Authority
PCC	Person-centred care	UAE	United Arab Emirates
POM	Prescription only medication	UK	United Kingdom of Great Britain and Northern Ireland
PPE	Personal protective equipment		
PBUH	Peace be upon him (an honorific phrase when referencing the Islamic Prophet Muhammad)	USA	United States of America
		UNDOC	United Nations Office of drugs and crime
		UNICEF	United Nations International Children's Emergency Fund
PSA	Physician-assisted suicide	UI	Urinary incontinence
ROI	Return on investment	WHO	World Health Organization
SARS	Severe acute respiratory syndrome	WONCA	World Organization of Family Doctors
SDG	Sustainable development goals	WCO	World Customs Office
SBAR	Situation, background, assessment and recommendations	WSMI	World self-medicating industry

PROLOGUE

MAY MCCREADDIE ■ GARY E. DAY ■ JANE LEANNE GRIFFITHS

Travelling—it leaves you speechless, then turns you into a storyteller.

Ibn Battuta

When I (MMcC) first experienced travelling or 'working abroad' in 1991–1992, I was an experienced staff nurse in my mid-20s. I left the safe environs of Scotland for the Eastern European country of Romania. Romania was then slowly emerging from the rule of the dictator Ceaușescu and was in the middle of an orphan scandal where HIV/AIDS was rife, especially around the Black Sea coast area of Constanta. It was a dark, dank, grey and black and white kind of a place where the temperatures could plummet to –40°C in the winter and nudge 30°C plus in the summer. People wore layers of clothing inside and out as there was often insufficient fuel for heating. People also spoke Romanian, with English speakers being few and far between and likely to be remnants of the Ceaușescu regime in any case. Our working environment was an infectious diseases hospital that housed children, often from poor or Gypsy families, several to a cot, with babies being prop fed. For a children's hospital ward, it was incredibly quiet. By the time we left, it was noisy and vibrant and the previously empty corridor was full to the brim with children at small dinner tables, happily eating and chatting away.

Leaving home in any circumstances is hard. Leaving home to go and work in a completely different culture and setting among western and local workers who all speak different languages is incredibly challenging. It demands a degree of resilience and a great deal of understanding. I had learned (colloquial) Romanian and had a distinct advantage over my colleagues—not least when exchanging money on the black market(!). Local people although private, sometimes dismissive and very wary, were enthralled by my Romanian—as most had never heard a foreigner speak their language before—but it gave them a window into my world and me into theirs. And it was incredibly important to engage with the local population and also to draw upon expatriate colleagues for support. In those days, there was no internet, no skype, Facebook, Instagram or WhatsApp, only the occasional telephone call home which required you to speak Romanian to the operator and wait anything up to 5 hours to place a relatively expensive call.

Today, through globalisation, the world is a much smaller place. It is commonplace in the region to see migrant workers going about their daily business whilst conducting a video call with their young family in Indonesia, Sri Lanka or the Philippines. And it is heartwarming to see—if, of course, they are not driving at the same time! Whether you are an indigenous local healthcare worker or a migrant worker seeking to provide remittances for your extended families at home, we are all travellers of some description. Some of your experiences will leave you speechless and others will become stories that will enrich you and others' understanding of a country or region with a different culture, language and values.

Unfortunately, people often assume that someone who is considered 'well-travelled' is knowledgeable, open and understanding when that is not necessarily the case. There will be people who have been working in this region for years who may, for example, know that you are seven times more likely to die in a road traffic accident in the United Arab Emirates (UAE) than in the United Kingdom (UK), but equally, do not know the five pillars of Islam, the true (etymological) meaning of the words Islam and Jihad and the five daily prayer times. Moreover, they may be at a loss to tell you the native language of the Philippines or the differences between North and South India, be they cultural, language, religion and food tastes. While this book cannot provide all the answers, it will hopefully enhance your understanding of multicultural working and motivate you to learn more about things you do not know or understand. Indeed, the fact you have picked the book up in the first place is a good start. We hope you find it as fascinating to read as we did to write.

BACKGROUND

So, welcome to the first edition textbook *Healthcare in the Arabian Gulf and Greater Middle East: a guide for healthcare professionals*. This is a unique social and cultural text and, as far as we know, the only book of its kind. We have 'cherrypicked' the most relevant conditions and interventions to provide the reader with a broad overview of health care in the region and the most appropriate approaches given the region's diversity. The key challenges of the conditions within the regional context are highlighted in conjunction with the fundamental aspects of healthcare interventions and treatment. These topics are then addressed through key strategic, local and individual healthcare approaches, providing the reader with an overview of the main challenges and methods, with thinking grids or case studies to merge theory with practice.

This text is eminently suitable for a range of prospective readers including, but not limited to: students of health care in the region and their qualified and practicing counterparts (nurses, doctors, paramedics, pharmacists, physiotherapists, radiologists), for all associated industries, agencies and educational entities (recruitment agencies, medical companies, hospitals, clinics, higher education institutions/tertiary level), or those considering working in the region that may want a deeper understanding of local health issues. In short, this book is for those practicing health care, developing health care or leading health care in the region and beyond. This is the first textbook that is specific to their needs and written by a diverse range of well-qualified academics and practitioners who have current credible knowledge and experience of health care in the region.

The idea for this text was first mooted in the early, dark days of the COVID-19 pandemic in 2020. As people who had worked in the region for a number of years at that juncture, we were dismayed by the lack of a culturally competent text that was specific to the region and drew together the unsaid aspects of working in such diverse working environments with an equally diverse workforce and patient populations. Given the hundreds of generic textbooks on health care, the emergence of medical tourism in the region and the continuing insatiable demand for more healthcare workers, it seemed strange that no one had thought to develop a text specific to their needs. As McCreaddie points out in Chapter 11, while outlining the difficulties of communication *per se*, the predominant ethnicities amongst healthcare staff in the Arabian Gulf and Greater Middle East are Indians and Filipinos with Arabs and western expatriates being relative minorities in comparison. Thus, most healthcare workers in the region are expatriates from a host of different countries across the world who work with local staff to greater or lesser degrees; for example, 90% of healthcare workers in Dubai are expatriates, whilst 61% of nurses in Bahrain are Bahrainis. In turn, these healthcare workers provide healthcare services for the local population, expatriates and (medical) tourists from a host of other countries. Consequently, health care provision in the Arabian Gulf is a cultural mosaic drawn from across the globe but practiced in a distinctly Islamic setting with English as the preferred means of communication. Thus, this is a unique, diverse and vibrant culture in which to practice modern health care—unlike any other on the planet.

While the emergence of COVID-19 prompted the idea that this might be an opportunity to bring together the necessary expertise to produce such a distinct social and cultural textbook, we failed to reckon with the considerable fall-out from the pandemic and the personal cost it would have on potential contributors. While COVID-19 helped the idea to germinate, it was not quite the short hiatus we initially thought it was going to be and like many others, we were faced with ongoing illness and repeated withdrawals as our colleagues tried to combat the vagaries of the pandemic.

In addition to the pandemic, we also faced some challenges that are very specific to the region and despite being experienced healthcare workers, academics and writers, we perhaps underestimated those somewhat. For example, the Arabian Gulf and Greater

Middle East is—for some people—merely a staging post in their lives before they move on, while for others it may be a short-term contract to generate much needed funds or a lifetime in service. The workforce is transient and some people elect to leave the region quickly once their employment is curtailed. English, although the predominant language used in clinical areas, is not the first language of most healthcare workers and academics. Moreover, contributing to a major textbook is not the kind of opportunity that some of our contributors might have previously been afforded and thus there was a need to recognise this and provide appropriate support to the writers. In addition, as an evidence-based textbook, we and many of our contributors experienced challenges in accessing appropriate and local evidence in a region that is often at the mercy of predatory journals. Finally, we have also tried to provide an evidence-based text that is constructive and culturally competent but also one that adheres to the publication rules of the region and Islamic values.

Now, let us introduce ourselves.

THE EDITORS

It will not have gone unnoticed that the three editors comprise one Scot (Scotland, UK) and two Australians. We tried hard to include a local colleague as a co-editor, but we were regrettably unsuccessful. However, as indicated previously, this region relies on expatriate, migrant workers who comprise about 40%–95% of the healthcare workforce. Consequently, it follows that the people with the greatest experience of working in the region are not necessarily indigenous. The region relies on being able to recruit experienced, well-qualified individuals from abroad who can take their healthcare industry forward and this is likely to be the case for some time yet. Accordingly, the more senior positions in health care and education in the region tend to be filled by expatriates. However, we sincerely hope and expect that subsequent editions of the text will have local co-editors and more local evidence-based contributions. That said, we have still managed to draw upon a wealth of knowledge, experience and local writers where at all possible and believe there is a diverse mix of contributors (ethnicities, disciplines, experience) across the chapters. We have contributions from Bahrain, UAE, Jordan, Palestine, Sudan, Egypt,

UK, Australia, New Zealand and Ireland, thereby representing the diverse ethnicities that work in the region. Moreover, they comprise a number of esteemed professors, academics and clinicians, with all having worked in the region for some considerable time.

Whilst the biographies of the co-editors are outlined in full in 'Contributors', let us briefly introduce ourselves:

- Dr May McCreaddie is a nurse academic with over 35 years' experience, with 7 of those as a Senior Lecturer in the UAE and Bahrain. She has also worked in Romania and India, has published widely and specialises in communication/interactions.
- Associate Professor Jane Leanne Griffiths is also a nurse with extensive academic experience at Universities in Australia, Ireland and the USA and has numerous scientific publications. Jane has worked in Qatar and was latterly the Chief Nursing Information Officer (CNIO) of the Dubai Healthcare Authority, working in the UAE for over 14 years.
- Adjunct Professor Gary E. Day is a senior healthcare executive as well as a clinician and researcher. His research interests lie in healthcare bureaucracies, work values and resilience in health care and health workforces. Gary has also published widely and has undertaken a number of consultancies in Australia, Vietnam, Saudi Arabia and China. More recently, he has been a senior health executive in a Medical City in the UAE. He has also been a visiting Professor in the School of Health Management and Economics in a University in the Northern Emirates.

THE CHAPTERS

This text is broadly organised across four sections: context, non-communicable diseases, communicable diseases and interventions. In addition to this prologue, we provide three key chapters to help the reader understand the broader context. In Chapter 1, Dr Ahmed Allaithy from the American University of Sharjah in the United Arab Emirates provides us with an overview of *Islamic beliefs about healthcare*, thereby setting the scene by outlining the importance of the specific cultural and religious aspects and how Islam shapes current healthcare beliefs and practices. The concept of health care in the Islamic Sharia is discussed as well as the relevant teachings of the Prophet Muhammad (PBUH), the theological basis for the treatment of Muslim patients, Islam's proposed 'cures' for physical and psychological ailments—all of which are discussed within the context of Arab world culture. These specific aspects are important as they provide the context for subsequent actions or inactions such as those discussed in Chapter 16 on *end-of-life care* and Chapter 15 on *pain management*.

We are particularly indebted to Dr Allaithy for keeping oversight of the book and ensuring it is congruent with Islamic values and beliefs.

Building upon Chapter 1, Chapter 2 discusses the constituent role of family members and how they relate to health and health care and the importance of being aware of '*the family*' as context in health care. Given the dominant role of the male gender in the family, we have elected to include a section on men's health in this chapter rather than as a separate section.

This chapter brings together a Bahraini medic, an Australian professor with a wealth of offshore experience in the Middle East and North Africa (MENA) and an Irish academic with considerable experience in, and knowledge of, healthcare leadership in the region. This eclectic triumvirate of authors arguably epitomises the workforce and experience you tend to come across in the region and ably provides an engrossing discussion of the pre-eminent role of the family in the Arab world including family structure and function.

Chapter 3 further extends the specific healthcare aspects of the region by providing an overview of *consumer-driven healthcare*. Adjunct Professor Gary E. Day and Professor Amina Al Marzouqi review the importance for patients/consumers having control or input into the care they are receiving including the financial implications, but also highlight the differences in the demographics across the various countries that make up this region as well as how each country funds health care.

In the following section, we review the role of non-communicable diseases and the impact these have in the region. In Chapter 4, Professor Steve Atkin and Dr Alexandra Butler provide an intriguing and technical journey through *metabolic syndromes and type 2 diabetes mellitus* highlighting the prevalence and challenges faced. Whilst this chapter may be very technical, it also exemplifies the wealth of work and expertise that is available in the region. Continuing the metabolic theme, Dr Eman Tawash then guides us through the challenges of *obesity* and being overweight in Chapter 5 and how this significant problem has the potential to lead to numerous other life-threatening conditions. The region's climate along with rapid urbanization, wealth and changes in lifestyles over a relatively short timeframe have all contributed to this epidemic and is something that needs to be addressed in a proactive and culturally competent way. Thereafter, Dr Ghufran Jassim provides a comprehensive account of *women's health* (part one) in Chapter 6 and the relevance of gender and culture in healthcare access, provision and concordance, whilst Professor Diaa Rizk highlights the very important but relatively hidden problems of urinary and faecal incontinence in women in Chapter 7 on *women's health* (part two). In Chapter 8, Associate Professor Jane Leanne Griffiths, Professor Rachel Rossiter and Dr Nabeel Al Yateem discuss the importance of *mental health and well-being*. This chapter explores the cultural, religious and historic approaches to mental health. It identifies the stigmas and shame associated with mental health diseases and the approaches and changes that need to be implemented to provide safe, effective and culturally appropriate psychiatric care.

Our communicable diseases section provides two chapters which broadly address *infection*. Associate Professor Jane Leanne Griffiths contributes to Chapter 9 on *infection* which outlines the region's impressive response to COVID-19. The geographic challenges caused by infectious diseases are highlighted especially as the region acts as a hub or portal to the rest of the world while the importance of effective infection control is discussed. In Chapter 10, Orla Merrigan reviews *upper and lower respiratory disorders* and ably demonstrates the particular challenges of climate and environment in a largely sedentary population.

As we progress to the interventions section, Dr May McCreaddie, Sandra Goodwin [RIP] and Dr Catherine Abou'zaid—a Scottish triumvirate—provide us with an important overview of *communication, care and diversity* in Chapter 11. This very practical chapter provides readers with an overview of the challenges of communicating effectively in health care in a high context culture with some examples of good and bad communication. In turn, two Bahraini family medicine practitioners (Dr Hani Malik, Dr Khatoon Husain Shubbar) provide us with Chapter 12 on *family medicine*, ably outlining the challenges of providing a 'general practice' approach in this context and culture. Chapter 13 on *psychosocial support* (Dr Wendy Maddison and Ms Razan Shaheen) follows on seamlessly building upon Chapter 8 (*mental health and well-being*) by discussing the myriad difficulties patients may face within a specific culture. This chapter also provides insights/tips into how psychosocial support can be provided in a culturally appropriate manner. Chapter 14 on *pharmacy* brings together two scholars and practitioners from Ireland and the Sudan (Dr Stephanie Annett and Dr Noon Kamil) providing a thorough understanding of the kinds of problems that can emerge in the region including overprescribing, self-medication, the challenges of introducing antimicrobial stewardship and the varying quality of medications (substandard and falsified), in addition to the provision of local complementary and alternative medicine.

As we move toward the end of the broad spectrum of care, Dr Keith Johnston—a Northern Irishman with a wealth of experience in the region as a consultant anaesthetist *and* a part time news anchor for Bahrain TV (!)—takes us through the challenges of *pain management* (Chapter 15) in an Islamic culture including opiophobia, sedation, addiction and prescribing protocols. This chapter tailors nicely with Chapter 16 on *end-of-life care* contributed by Dr Hadya Abboud—a Jordanian working in the UAE—and the esteemed Emeritus Professor Sheila Payne—formerly Director of the International Observatory on End of Life Care at Lancaster University and Past President of the European Association for Palliative Care. Both chapters tackle culturally sensitive issues that highlight the importance of being fully congruent with the context and values of the region to ensure respect and optimal health care and treatment.

Last, but not least, we finish with a 'hot' topic given the emergence of COVID-19–*technology-enhanced learning and leadership*. Chapter 17 therefore explores the impact technology has and is having on healthcare delivery in the region including the use of remote technology and the reliance on electronic medical records to provide nationwide data. The diversity of staffing cultures is outlined as well as the techniques used to educate and support staff. The epilogue concludes the text with a summary and the book-end appendix provides a helpful guide for expatriate healthcare workers to be considered prior to working in the region. It includes information on pre-onboarding, onboarding, on spending time in the region and equally importantly, what to consider when preparing to leave.

Given the numerous challenges in bringing this text to publication over the past few years, there are patently some chapters that have either been totally omitted or briefly included as part of another chapter. Consequently, 'Working with Migrant Workers' 'Paediatrics and Adolescents' and 'Accident, Emergency and Trauma' are specific areas of interest we have, regrettably, been unable to fully include in this edition. Nonetheless, we are confident that these areas will be included in full in future editions. Moreover, if you think you can add to future editions or contribute to a specific chapter, please feel free to contact Elsevier directly who will put you in contact with the Editors.

SUMMARY

We trust that the introduction to date has fully whetted your appetite for the rest of the book. What should be strikingly evident already is the diversity of the contributors in terms of discipline, ethnicity, experience and qualifications. This is an international book, albeit firmly rooted in the Arabian Gulf and Greater Middle East. As the editors of this text, we have had some frank and fearless exchanges—indicative of natives from a low context culture. We have suffered IT failures, seen valued contributors having to withdraw due to personal circumstances, mourned the passing of a colleague and finally, disembarked. It has been an odyssey of sorts. But then again, we are all travellers. We hope you enjoy the journey and come back and revisit it time and again. Bon Voyage!

FURTHER READING

The Daily Tribune—News of Bahrain, 2022. 61% of Government Nurses in Bahrain Are Citizens: Health Ministry. 18 January. Available at https://www.newsofbahrain.com/bah-rain/78074.html. Accessed 10 June 2023.

Section I

SPECIFIC CONDITIONS, SPECIFIC CHALLENGES

This section presents the conditions specific to the Middle East, the particular challenges these conditions present and the existing evidence base in the area, highlighting commonalities and differences.

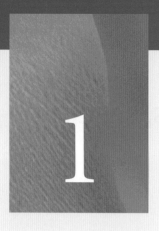

1

HEALTHCARE IN ISLAM

AHMED ALLAITHY

CHAPTER OUTLINE

OVERVIEW

This chapter deals with healthcare in Islam. It discusses the objectives of the Sharia in the area of health in general and outlines the steps advanced by the Holy Qur'an and Sunnah of the Prophet Muhammad (peace be upon him) in this regard. It also looks into the expectations of the recipients of medical care as well as what is Islamically required from the medical practitioners in terms of providing a Sharia-compliant medical service within the context of the culture of the Arab world. The chapter shows how Islam shapes current healthcare beliefs and practices.

The topics included are as follows:

- Providing medical professionals who may not be familiar with Islam with a brief idea about its meaning, basic tenets and practices

- The objectives of the Islamic Sharia as based on the teachings of the Qur'an and *Sunnah* and how they relate to healthcare
- The Islamic healthcare system including prevention and related matters such as seeking treatment in the light of what is permissible and impermissible in Islam
- The Islamic beliefs regarding health and sickness and how to deal with medical afflictions, be those physical or spiritual
- Some of the methods of handling health issues through fasting and dieting as well as the handling of afflictions that require un-Islamic means of treatment
- The instructions of the Prophet Muhammad in the area of healthcare

- The Islamic rulings regarding modern issues such as do not resuscitate (DNR), palliative care, physician-assisted suicide (PSA), euthanasia, suicide, removal of life support equipment, and blood and organ donation

INTRODUCTION

Recognised as the fastest growing religion in today's world, Islam seems to be gaining more ground day by day. It currently enjoys a population of approximately 1.91 billion according to *The World Population Review* (worldpopulationreview.com). This means that in a world of almost 8 billion people, one in every four is a Muslim. In our global age, encounters with Muslims seem to be inevitable in almost all walks of life. It is therefore, important—and for some essential—to have at least a basic understanding of the faith that has a direct impact on shaping the physical and spiritual life of a quarter of the world's population.

Islam: Linguistically

Linguistically, the word '*islām*' is a verbal noun derived from the root 's-l-m'. This root acts as the carrier of the core meanings of concepts and values such as: submission and obedience /*istislām*/, peace and being free from imperfections /*salām*/, safety /*salāmah*/, reconciliation /*musālamah*/, acceptance and reception /*istilām*/, to name but a few. Other meanings such as tolerance, coexistence, inflicting no harm on others, leading an upright life, all share the same root 's-l-m', and Islam as a religion is believed to incorporate all these meanings. It is established that Islam means total submission to the Will of God in all aspects of life. The Arabic word for God is Allah and Muslims believe that Allah is the *name* of God. In other words, it is not just a word that means God. In the Arabic translations of such divine revelation as the Torah of Moses, and Injīl of Jesus, the word used for God is no other than *Allah*.

As Islam denotes complete submission to Allah, Muslims believe that all God's prophets—124,000 of them (Ibn Ḥanbal, v.5, p. 265, no. 22342)—including Noah, Abraham, Jacob, David, Moses, Jesus and Muhammad (peace be upon them all), have preached one religion, Islam, and are consequently, called Muslim (Q22:78). Muslims therefore believe in and have the utmost love and respect for all the Prophets and Messengers sent by Allah to humankind from the

days of Adam to the last of them, namely, the Prophet Muhammad (peace be upon them). According to the Qur'an, which is the holy book of Islam, no distinction of any kind is made between any of those mighty messengers (Q2:285).

Islam: Technically

Technically, Islam is the religion that has been given to the Prophet Muhammad (c.570–632 CE), an Arab from Mecca, to convey by himself or via his followers, to the whole of humankind. The teachings of Islam are mainly extracted from two primary and indispensable sources: the Holy Qur'an and the Sunnah/Hadith of the Prophet. The Qur'an is Muslims' holy scripture and is believed to be the exact word of Allah (Q15:9), while the term Hadith refers to what the Prophet Muhammad said, did and/or approved. *Sunnah* means the *way* of the Prophet Muhammad, and following various Qur'anic instructions, Muslims are commanded to follow the example of the Prophet Muhammad as best they can (see for example, Q33:21 and Q59:7).

BASIC ISLAMIC BELIEFS

In terms of belief, Islam has five pillars (Buḵārī, 2002, Book of Īmān, p. 12, no. 8) and six articles of faith or *Īmān* (Buḵārī, 2002, Book of Īmān, p. 23, no. 50). The pillars are: first, the testimony of faith, that is, to bear witness that there is no god but Allah, and to bear witness that Muhammad is His Servant and Messenger; second, to perform the five obligatory daily prayers; third, to pay the annual *zakah* which is prescribed for eight categories of recipients as specified in the Qur'an; fourth, to perform Hajj (pilgrimage to Mecca) at least once in one's lifetime for those who are able to do so; and fifth, to fast during the month of Ramadan (the 9th month in the lunar calendar) from dawn to sunset.

The articles of faith are: to believe in Allah, His angels, His Books, His Messengers, the Last Day (of Judgment) and Fate (good and bad). The belief in *fate* is in the sense that 'whatever befalls you is not predestined to miss you; and whatever misses you is not predestined to befall you' (Al-Albānī, 1997, no. 62). It is with this understanding that Muslims accept all afflictions, including medical ones, as being the decision of Allah and therefore, they submit to His Will in total acceptance. This provides many with the inner strength to cope well and try to overcome the indisposition, which is also believed to be one of the many tests encountered in life (see Q29:1-2).

THE SHARIA

The Holy Qur'an and the Prophet's Hadiths are the backbone of the Islamic Sharia, which revolves round a core concept that aims, according to the consensus of Muslim scholars as extracted from the Holy Qur'an and the Sunnah of the Prophet Muhammad, at the preservation and protection of five elements. These are referred to in Islam as '*the five necessities*'. The absence or mere degradation of any one of them is bound to have a drastically negative—and sometimes immeasurable—impact on the human condition. Those elements as loosely translated from Arabic are: the *dīn*: Faith (religion), *nafs*: Life, *nasl*: Lineage, *mal*: Property and *ɛaql*: Intellect (Al-Ŝātibī, v.1, p. 38). Muslim jurists differ in opinion concerning which of these elements should have priority over the others in terms of protection and in cases of conflict. Without disregarding the validity of some of the well-articulated arguments as put forward by some Sharia scholars (Al-Jaknī, 1993, p. 349; Al-Āmidī, v.4, p. 275), it suffices for the purpose of this research to put *life* first since the other four elements seem, as far as we are concerned, to be dependent on its existence and continuation. With death, one is unable to engage in any fathomable pursuit related to the rest. To this end, Islam has gone to great lengths to ensure a reasonably acceptable continuation of one's life during the various stages of the human cycle. This by default includes one's health. Islam has indeed a healthcare system that begins with prevention and goes all the way to complete recovery in cases of illness or similar/related health afflictions. While Islam does not provide an all-in-one healthcare manual, the primary sources (i.e., the Qur'an and Sunnah) provide ample instructions, guidelines and various other information that are worthy of consideration and merit much more rigorous investigation than has been conducted in the last 14 centuries. The scholars of Hadith, however, have dedicated specific sections in their collections that deal directly with health-related matters covering a wide range of topics including personal hygiene, prevention measures, permissible and impermissible types of foods and drinks, treatment of specific ailments, etc. Such collections contain an unprecedented wealth of

information of great relevance to this day. This fact is not a surprise to Muslims owing to the belief that Islam is for the guidance the whole of humankind until the Last Day on earth.

THE MUSLIM COMMUNITY AND HEALTHCARE

Muslims naturally belong to various ethnicities, demographics and geographical locations, and have different educational and cultural backgrounds including customs and traditions. They also live under different political and religious regimes, which come with their own challenges. All these factors, among many others, significantly influence their perception, reception and expectations of what healthcare the Muslim way involves. Based on the regional distribution of Muslims in 2010, the 2017 report of the Pew Research Center states 'nearly two thirds (62%) of Muslims live in the Asia-Pacific region… In fact, more Muslims live in India and Pakistan (344 million combined) than in the entire Middle East-North Africa region (317 million)' (DeSilver & Masci, 2017). The sheer number of 1.91 billion and distribution of Muslims in the present age means that medical professionals all over the world cannot avoid dealing with Muslim patients at some point in their careers. The Arabian Gulf States, for example, have for decades been a magnet for people from all over the globe seeking employment and investment opportunities. As a result, millions of Muslims (and non-Muslims) belonging to different cultural and socioeconomic backgrounds have moved either temporarily or permanently to this region, which has become much more than a meeting point of different cultures. Contact with Muslims there is inevitable. One fantastic thing about Islam is that it aims at bridging the gap(s) between its followers and replacing specific untoward values with new Islamic ones. While this does not make the burden of the medical professionals any less demanding when caring for Muslim patients, having a basic understanding of Muslims' special and shared health requirements and expectations helps care providers be better equipped and certainly goes a long way when providing medical care to Muslims of various backgrounds. In fact, one would be justified in assuming the existence of similar *shared* values by the great majority of Muslim patients. Saying this, the Islamic healthcare system is by no means restricted to the treatment of Muslims. The benefits transcend faith affiliation.

PREVENTION

Islam considers illness as an affliction that is ultimately ascribed to God and as a result, Muslims believe that healing and recovery come directly from God. Consequently, prayers and supplications are always offered by and for the sick (Buḱārī, 2002, p. 1439, no. 5675 and p. 1436, no. 5662) as will be elaborated on shortly under 'Sickness is a Test'. Psychological support is encouraged as the Prophet Muhammad instructs that there is a great reward for visiting the sick (Buḱārī, 2002, v.1, p. 1432, no. 5649, 5650). Such practices provide significant psychological support to the afflicted. Seeking medical treatment and taking prescribed medications are also in accordance with Islamic teachings in the understanding that they are no more than a means which Allah has made available for all, Muslims and non-Muslims alike. In other words, Muslims believe that Allah has created both the illness and the cure and instructed that one has to seek the means and follow proper steps leading to complete recovery.

Healthcare in Islam includes instructions that are aimed at prevention for the maintenance of good health. Two examples to clarify this point should suffice for our purpose here. First, personal hygiene is of paramount importance and is considered part of faith. In fact, to perform any of the five daily obligatory prayers, for example, one needs to be in a state of Ṭahārah (ritual purification) (Muslim, 2006, v.1, p. 121, no. 224, 225) which is obtained through the washing of various parts of the body, namely the hands, mouth, nose, face, arms to the elbows, hair, ears and feet (Ibid, no. 226). This is known as *wuḍūᶜ*, which is prescribed before prayers as well as various other religious duties. In one report regarding *wuḍūᶜ*, both Buḱāri and Muslim narrate that the Prophet also instructs that upon waking up from sleep, one needs to wash one's hands first. The Prophet states: 'One does not know where one's hand has been during one's sleep' (Buḱāri, no. 162; Muslim no. 237). The exact instruction is given in relation to coming into contact with anything consumable that is placed in a container such as water, food or any kind of drink as one wakes up after sleep (Ibn al-Mulaqqin, 1425AH, v.1, p. 504, no.14 and v.2, p. 97, no. 20).

Muslim additionally reports the Prophet as saying: 'When one wakes up, let one wash one's hands three times (first)' (Muslim no. 278). There are many other teachings regarding toilet etiquettes, such as methods of cleanliness, which are prescribed by the Prophet Muhammad. The scholars of Hadith also dedicate entire sections in their compilations for such topics, as they do for other topics.

A weekly wash of the entire body for men and women is also a Muslim obligation, as is washing after any sexual act or sexual intercourse. Other important practices in terms of personal hygiene are stated in the hadith: 'Five things are part of *Fitrah*: circumcision, shaving the pubes, clipping the nails, plucking the armpit hair and trimming the moustache' (Ibid., p.133, no. 257–258), with the two last acts 'not to be left for more than 40 days' (Ibid., p. 134, no. 258). Regular flossing (Al-Albānī, 1988, no. 2567) and teeth brushing with the *siwāk* is also emphasised in many Prophetic statements (Ibid., pp. 132–133, no. 252–256).

Second, in cases of affliction with a contagious disease (e.g., plague, pandemic), the Prophet Muhammad instructed that the sick and healthy should not unnecessarily mix. He stated, 'a sick person should not be taken to one who is healthy' (Muslim, v.40, no. 5923; Buḱāri, 76, p. 1461, no. 5771, 5774). He also instructed that uncalled-for contact with individuals afflicted with leprosy should be avoided as best as one could. He stated, 'one should run away from the leper as one runs away from a lion' (Buḱāri, book 76, p. 1447, no. 5707). Additionally, according to Buḱāri and Muslim, the Prophet stated, 'if you get wind of the outbreak of plague in a land, you should not enter it; but if it spreads in the land where you are, you should not depart from it' (Nawawī, 2007, pp. 497–498, no. 1791, 1792). Social distancing is also found in the hadith: 'Do not stare at lepers, and if you speak to them, let there be a distance of a spear between you and them' (Ibn Ḥanbal, book II, no. 581, Shamela). A courteous etiquette such as covering the mouth with one's sleeve or any other item when sneezing for the prevention of the spread of germs is also stated in a Prophetic hadith (Al-Albānī, 1998, no. 5029).

Such Prophetic health teachings become particularly important to adhere to when dealing with mega events such as Umrah and Hajj (annual pilgrimage) where hundreds of thousands of people happen to be in the same place at the same time creating the largest mass gathering in the world. The precautionary prevention measures stated earlier are also of great relevance in cases of pandemics, which necessitate the imposition of various levels of restrictions as stated in various hadiths in terms of travel, contact with the sick, gatherings of all kinds, quarantine, self-isolation, etc., until a cure is found or the pandemic is somehow lifted. Managing the current COVID-19 pandemic can benefit tremendously from the teachings of Islam, especially given that Islamic records include, in addition to Prophetic statements, references to historical pandemics occurring at different times; starting from what is known as 'The Plague of Amwas' in Palestine in the year 640 CE and many others afterwards in various parts of the Islamic territories and how the physicians of the time explained and dealt with the resulting situations.

SICKNESS IS A TEST

As Muslims believe that all maladies are from Allah, and so are healing and recovery, afflictions are described in Islam as tests of faith (see Q29:2) and/ or expiation for one's sins. (Buкārī, 2002, book 75, p. 1431–1435, no. 5640, 5641, 5642, 5648, 5660, 5667). Medicines are believed to be no more than a means, a step that one is encouraged to take. However, they have in themselves no power to cure. It is only with the will of Allah that a person is cured. It is because of this conviction that many Muslim patients accept their ill health conditions with submission to the will of Allah and hope that they would be cured regardless of how terminal their conditions may be. Muslims also believe in the power of prayer and that sincere $due\bar{a}^c$ (prayers and supplication to Allah) are a great source of relief as Allah makes the promise in the Qur'an, 'Your Lord has said: Pray to Me and I will answer your prayers' (Q40:60). The Qur'an also states: 'Who else (is there but He, Allah) who answers the distressed one when he calls upon Him, and removes the suffering?' (Q27:62). Recitation of the Qur'an, being the exact word of Allah, is also believed to be a powerful means of healing. Q17:82 reads 'And We send down of the Quran that which is a healing (a cure) and a mercy for the believers.' In the Islamic belief system, therefore, a Muslim is instructed not to neglect the seeking of treatment. A balance is created between what Allah wills to happen

and the fact that He himself has directed the believers to seek medical assistance.

SEEKING MEDICAL TREATMENT

In addition to $due\bar{a}^c$ (prayers) and Qur'an recitation, Muslims are instructed to seek medical advice. The Prophet's companion, Jābir, reports that the Prophet said 'Every illness has a cure; when the cure is applied to the illness, it is cured with the will of Allah, the Almighty' (Muslim, p. 1050, no. 2204). Knowledge of the effects of medicines, be it beneficial or harmful, may only be obtained from qualified professionals. Islam warns against seeking advice from imposters and warns imposters against assuming a medical role that is not theirs. In _Sahīh Sunan Abu Dāwūd_, the Prophet Muhammad is reported to have said 'Anyone who practices medicine but is not known to be a (genuine) practitioner, and kills a human being or inflicts harm on him, will be held accountable' (Al-Albānī, 1998, no. 4587).

Moreover, Umm Salamah, wife of the Prophet Muhammad, reports that the Prophet said 'Truly, Allah did not make your healing through the use of what He had made _harām_ (impermissible) for you' (Al-Bayhaqī, 2011, v.19, p. 591, no. 19711). Islam accordingly provides a guarantee that since all illnesses have a cure and that there is no cure which can only be derived from something prohibited, there is no immediate reason to resort to a _harām_ means of treatment. This topic will be discussed in some detail shortly under 'The Permissible and the Impermissible'. For all it is worth, this also opens the gate for medical investigations as to finding permissible means and cures that are compatible with the Islamic Sharia and Muslim requirements. The only two afflictions Islam states as having no cure are: old age and death. The Prophet was asked, 'Is it inappropriate for us if we seek treatment?' He responded, 'Seek treatment, O, servants of Allah, for Allah—Glorified be He—did not create an illness except that he created with it a cure for it, but not for old age' (Al-Albānī, 1997, v. 3, p. 158, no. 2789).

THE PHYSICAL AND THE SPIRITUAL

Islam directs its followers to endeavour towards the achievement of a balance between the physical and the spiritual making a clear link between the two. While the Qur'an instructs in Q7:31 that one should eat and drink, but not to excess 'for Allah does not love those who are excessive,' one has to be mindful of both the quality and quantity of what one consumes. An important stipulation, though, is found in Q7:32 which continues to state: 'Say: who has forbidden the adornment of Allah which He has brought forth for His servants, and the *Tayyibāt* (good, lawful, pure and clean provisions) from among the means of sustenance?' It is therefore clear that eating healthily and in moderation is what is being prescribed. The concept of excessiveness in Islam is understood to refer to the two extremes of consuming too much or too little. The harmful effects of both malnutrition as well as obesity are too well-known to merit recounting here. The same goes for the benefits of following a balanced healthy diet. In Islam, this is not only a matter of 'universal' commonsense, rather it is an Islamic obligation. To elaborate, in the most authentic book of Hadith (*Traditions of the Prophet Muhammad*), Imām Buḱārī (2002, p. 1292, no. 5063) reports that Anas ibn Mālik, a companion of the Prophet, narrated that a group of three men came to the houses of the wives of the Prophet to inquire about the Prophet's daily routine in terms of his acts of worship. When they were informed about that, they realised that there was nothing out of the ordinary in the actions of the Prophet. Therefore, they reasoned that since the past and future sins of the Prophet's had been forgiven by Allah (see Q48:2; Buḱārī, 2002, p. 1221, no. 4837), he did not have to do more than what he was doing. They further reasoned that since they could not in any way be compared with the Prophet, it was in their best interest before Allah if they offered more. Accordingly, one of them said, 'I will offer the prayer throughout the night forever.' The other said, 'I will fast throughout the year and will not break my fast.' The third said, 'I will keep away from the women and will not marry forever.' Allah's Messenger came to them and said, 'Are you the same people who said so-and-so? By Allah, I am more submissive to Allah and more afraid of Him than you are; yet I fast and break my fast, I do sleep and I also marry women. So he who does not follow my *Sunnah* (way) is not from me (not one of my followers).'

Voluntary and Obligatory Fasting

It is clear from this hadith that constant fasting is not only frowned upon but also impermissible. The hadith also addresses the issues of lack of sleep and abstention from marriage. While all these acts may be considered by some as enhancing one's spirituality, they are indeed physical, with serious health implications as well. In fact, these two latter aspects can hardly stand independently from each other if we consider the entire body of the instructions given by the Prophet Muhammad. The Prophet has guided those men, and in turn everybody else, to the importance of sleep, fasting and marriage. The hadith is indicative of the lifestyle one should lead. While Islam as a religion does not require outside validation of its teachings in the belief that they are all from Allah, the One with absolute knowledge and power, the Qur'an and the *Sunnah* of the Prophet encourage investigation and verification for the satisfaction of one's curious mind and heart (see Q2:260). In their study titled '*Effects of intermittent fasting on health, aging, and disease*', Rafael de Cabo, of NIA's Intramural Research Program (IRP), and Mark P. Mattson, a neuroscientist at the Johns Hopkins University School of Medicine, (2019) found that 'Hundreds of animal studies and scores of human clinical trials have shown that intermittent fasting can lead to improvements in health conditions such as obesity, diabetes, cardiovascular disease, cancers and neurological disorders' (National Institute on Aging, 2020; nia.nih.gov). In addition to the obligatory fasting in the lunar month of Ramadan, Islam encourages voluntary fasting as well and recommends in most cases that it never exceeds every other day. This is known as *Siyām Dāwūd* or David's Fasting (i.e., the fasting of the Prophet David) (Buḱārī, 2002, p. 274, no. 1131). When Abdullāh ibn Amr told the Prophet Muhammad that he was able to fast more days in the year than every other day, the Prophet stated that there was nothing better than the David's Fasting (Muslim, 2006, p. 514, no. 1159).

This point is of great significance for health in general since the same hadith prescribes various number patterns of fasting days and ends with the ultimate David's Fasting. While some medical professionals may prescribe different ways for intermittent fasting (IF) in terms of the number of hours and duration, Islam is very specific regarding what should *not* be exceeded. In her Harvard Health Publishing article of June 2018, titled *Intermittent fasting: Surprising update*, Monique Tello states 'Studies in humans, almost across the board, have shown that IF is safe and incredibly effective, *but really no more effective than any other* diet.' [emphasis added] (Harvard Health Publishing, 2021). Tello emphasises the importance of timing as she states that 'a growing body of research suggests that the timing of the fast is key, and can make IF a more realistic, sustainable, and effective approach for weight loss, as well as for diabetes prevention.' While Muslim fasting does not seem to have been a consideration in the studies referred to by Tello, she states 'An in-depth review of the science of IF recently published in *New England Journal of Medicine* sheds some light. Fasting is evolutionarily embedded within our physiology, triggering several essential cellular functions. Flipping the switch from a fed to fasting state does more than help us burn calories and lose weight. The researchers combed through dozens of animal and human studies to explain how simple fasting improves metabolism, lowering blood sugar; lessens inflammation, which improves a range of health issues from arthritic pain to asthma; and even helps clear out toxins and damaged cells, which lowers risk for cancer and enhances brain function' (Harvard Health Publishing, 2021).

In addition to voluntary fasting, the prescribed Muslim fasting starts at dawn and ends at sunset and involves complete abstention from drinking, eating and sexual intercourse (see Q2:183-187). This takes place for a whole month, Ramadan, the 9th month of the lunar calendar. The physical and spiritual benefits are undeniable. Perhaps more research on the way Islam prescribes fasting is meritorious. It seems obvious that fasting is a measure for good health when dealing with some cases of ill health, and it is also a means of prevention. This is in conformity with Islam's health system that starts with prevention all the way to complete recovery.

Dieting

Another hadith warns against the harms of having a full stomach. The Prophet Muhammad states 'There is no worse vessel for the son of Adam (human being) to fill than his stomach. It should suffice for the son of Adam to eat a few mouthfuls to straighten his back, but if he must (fill his stomach), then one-third for his food, one-third for his drink, and one-third for his breath (air)' (Al-Tirmiżī, p. 390, no. 2380; Ibn Mājah, v.4, p. 1111, no. 3349). According to al-Ḥarith ibn Kaladah (d. 635 CE), a renowned Arab *muḳadram* physician who lived in the pre-Islamic and early Islamic period,

'The stomach is the house of disease, and the key to healing is *al-Ḥimyah* (a balanced diet; reducing food intake)' (Ibn Al-Qayyim, v.4, p. 108). He also advises getting one's body used to hunger. He states 'Hunger is medicine' (Ibid.). His statements seem to be in agreement with what the Prophet had stated previously.

According to the three-men hadith, getting enough sleep is also important for maintaining good health. However, while primary Islamic sources do not specify a number of hours of sleeping, the bulk of literature in this area does not seem to support the commonly advised 8 hours of sleep daily for an adult. In fact, sleep patterns according to the multitudes of Islamic records regarding the actual practice of sleep was to sleep around two-thirds of the night and to have a short siesta just after midday (Al-Albānī, 1997, no. 909, 911; Al-Albānī, 1998, no. 997). It is undeniable, however, that this may vary depending on age and other given factors and circumstances. However, for the most part, the voluntary prayers of *Qiyām al-Layl*, that is, praying at night especially in the last third of the night just before dawn, is highly praised and encouraged (Buḳārī, 2002, pp. 227–279, no. 1120–1152, 1157; Al-Ājurrī, 1417AH; Al-Zahrānī, 2020; Ibn Abi al-Dunyā, 1998). Many hadiths mention sleeping for only the first half or two-thirds of the night (Buḳārī, 2002, p. 274, no. 1131; Al-ᶜAṣbīlī, 1994, pp. 160–161). In the praise of the Qur'an of the righteous and God-fearing, one major action of theirs is clearly specified, namely 'they used to sleep but little at night' (Q51:17). The siesta practice is also mentioned in the Qur'an, (see Q25:14 and Q7:4) and recommended by the Prophet Muhammad (Al-Albānī, 1988, p. 815, no. 4431; Buḳārī, 2002, p. 714, no. 2894). This is also another important area for modern medical research on sleep patterns to investigate.

THE PERMISSIBLE AND THE IMPERMISSIBLE

In Islam's endeavour to maintain a healthy lifestyle, it tightly links the protection of the five necessities to another important concept whose parameters are also defined by the Sharia, that is: the *Ḥalāl* (permissible/lawful) and the *Ḥarām* (impermissible/unlawful). This is clarified in the Qur'an in (7:157) which states: 'and make lawful for them the *Ṭayyibāt* (good, wholesome and pure things) and prohibit for them the *Ќabāᶜiĥ* (the bad, foul, impure and evil things).' For example, Islam considers alcohol, pork, dead animals (not Islamically slaughtered) together with all products extracted from them to be among the *ќabāᶜiĥ*, and therefore *ĥarām* (forbidden) to consume directly or indirectly either as food or medicine.

In addition, it is an Islamic maxim that the pursuit of the permissible following impermissible means is forbidden. In other words, while seeking treatment is allowed (*ĥalāl*) in Islam (Al-Albānī, 1997, v.3, p. 158, no. 2789), it is not allowed to use anything that falls under the category of *ĥarām* in the process. For example, the Qur'an forbids the consumption of *ќamr* (alcohol, intoxicants and similar substances) (see Q2:219 and 5:90-91). The Prophet Muhammad clearly states—as reported by 16 of his companions— that all intoxicants are *ќamr* and therefore, *haram* to consume (Abu Dāwūd, 1999, p. 528, no. 3679; Al-Albānī, 1988, v.2, p. 1225, no. 7336), use or to have any dealings with it at all (Al-Albānī, 1988, v.3, p. 142, no. 2741, 2742). Described further as the key to all evils (Al-Albānī, 1988, v.2, p. 1225, no. 7334; Al-Albānī, 1997, v.3, p. 142, no. 2733) and the mother of all sins (Al-Albānī, 1988, v.1, p. 631, no. 3344), any treatment of an ailment with the use of *ќamr* under any name as well as in any form, shape or quantity is not permissible. The Prophet Muhammad states 'What intoxicates in large quantities is not allowed (even) in small quantities' (Al-Albānī, 1998, v.3, p. 503, no. 5623, 5624). Umar ibn al-Ќattāb, the renowned companion of the Prophet Muhammad, provides a defining clarification as he states, 'All that befogs the mind is *ќamr*' (Ibn Ĥajar, 1987, v.8, p. 126, no. 4619). As a result, the consensus of the Muslim scholars is that anything that has a similar effect on the human being to *ќamr* has the same ruling as *ќamr* does. In other words, the use of narcotics and all substances of similar nature is incontestably forbidden in Islam. The impermissibility of the use of *ќamr* by way of treatment is further explicitly emphasised in another hadith where the Prophet Muhammad says: 'Seek treatment, but do not do so using what is *ĥarām*' (Ŝaraful-Ĥaq, n.d., p. 1652, no. 3874). The Prophet is also reported to have said to one of his companions, Ŧāriq ibn Suwayd, when Ŧāriq had said that he made alcohol only to use it for medicinal purposes and not for drinking: 'It is not a medicine; it is a sickness' (Al-Albānī, 1998, v.2, p. 465, no. 3874; Muslim, 2006, p. 955, no. 1984). Accordingly, the consumption of *ќamr* is categorically prohibited and cannot be used as a medicine or in the making of a medicine. Such absolute prohibition is the consensus of the Muslim scholars (Al-ᶜaynī, 2000, v.1, p. 447; Ibn Mufliĥ, 2000, p. 195).

THE PRACTICALITY OF ISLAM

Islam is however a practical and realistic religion. It recognises the fact that in certain situations taking extreme measures may turn out to be the only solution for the preservation of human life. When this is the case, the Islamic maxim 'harm is to be removed' (Al-Suyūŧī, 1983, p. 83) becomes applicable and effective. If this is to be implemented, the use of something impermissible to remove the harm may sometimes be the only possibility. The practicality of Islam and its realistic world view has led to the renowned sub-category 'Necessities allow prohibitions' (Al-Suyūŧī, 1983, p. 84). This clearly means that where emergencies, dire need or special circumstances arise requiring the use of something *ĥarām* (impermissible) to save a human life at the absence of a Sharia-permissible means, the *ĥarām* is not considered as such in this specific situation. In the medical field for example, when it is necessary to decide a method of treatment or the use of a certain drug or procedure, such necessity has to be determined by a qualified and credible physician. Other situations may include, but are not limited to, exposing, touching and/or looking at certain parts of the human body during a medical examination. This maxim is derived from the Qur'anic *āyahs* (verses) 'But if one is forced by necessity, without wilful disobedience, nor transgressing due limits, no sin shall be upon him. Truly Allah is All-Forgiving, Most Merciful' (Q2:173) and 'He (Allah) has explained to you in detail what is forbidden to you - except (when) you are under compulsion of necessity' (Q6:119). Based on these Qur'anic statements in addition to other explanatory Prophetic reports (Ibn Ĥanbal, al-Musnad, v.36, p. 227, no. 21948), it is therefore established in Islam that for the impressible to be allowed, four conditions need to be met:

1. The existence of a necessity.
2. The absence of a permissible means to remove the harm.

3. The absence of any doubt that the use of the impermissible will remove the harm.
4. The removal of the harm incurred by that necessity is not going to lead to another harm of similar or greater magnitude.

In spite of this, Islam also preaches that every illness has a cure. The Arabic word for *illness* is dā^c, which incorporates any human condition or defect, visible or invisible, internal or external, physical or psychological, that results in ill health or discomfort (Ibn Manẓūr, 1999, v.4, p. 436, under d-w-^c). It is in this Arabic sense that the word illness is used here regardless of any differences in the technical definition(s) that may occur between English words such as disease, ailment, sickness, malady and illness. According to Imām Buḵārī, the Prophet Muhammad said 'Allah does not send down an illness unless He sends down a cure for it' (Buḵārī, 2002, p. 1441, no. 5678). Such statement is a tremendous source of hope for those with all kinds of health conditions to seek medical assistance, and a motivation for the medical professionals to seek actual cures for health problems.

THE PROPHET'S MEDICINE

Major books of hadiths have sections dedicated to the medicines and methods of treatment as instructed by the Prophet Muhammad (see for example, Buḵārī's *Saḥīḥ*, book of Medicine no. 76, where there are 104 hadiths listed, pp. 1363–1441). Such statements of the Prophet are believed to be divinely revealed since the Prophet was not a medical practitioner. Some practices of the time may also be found in many Muslim communities to the present day, such as: *hijāmah* (cupping and/or bloodletting), *kayy* (cauterisation) (Buḵārī, 2002, book 76, p. 1441, no. 5680, 5681, 5683) and *ḵitān* (male circumcision) (Muslim, p. 134, no. 257). While the Prophet Muhammad is reported to have used cupping for unilateral headache and other aches (Ibid., no. 5698–5699, 5700, 5701), he also stated 'I do not like to be cauterized' (Ibid., no. 5702, 5704) and in another 'I forbid my followers to use cauterization [branded with fire]' (Ibid., no. 5680). This Prophetic instruction is considered as a recommendation since a number of companions of the Prophet Muhammad are known to have been treated

by cauterisation owing to the unavailability of other successful methods in their conditions. The relevance of this point is based on the fact that some Muslims consider LASER treatment to be a form of cauterisation. Refusal of or strict abstention from using LASER treatment, albeit being permissible as a last resort, could be related to the desire of the abstaining person to be among the 70,000 people promised Paradise without reckoning, that is, being held accountable for their deeds. The relevant hadith states that one of their attributes is that they do not use cauterisation with fire (Buḵārī, 2002, no. 3247). It is therefore important for medical practitioners to explain to Muslim patients what is involved in LASER treatment in order for them to make an informed decision to balance the permissibility of the treatment and the patient's desire, which may lead to trying other alternative methods of treatment first.

In as much as the Qur'an states that bees honey is endowed with healing powers, a number of Prophetic hadiths state the same. Q16:68-69 says 'And your Lord inspired the bees, "Take up dwellings among the mountains and the trees and among that which they build, …. Then eat of every kind of fruit, and follow the ways of your Lord made easy. *From their bellies comes a drink of different colours in which there is healing for people. Truly in that is a sign for a people who reflect".'* In a number of hadiths, Buḵārī reports that bees honey is one of three things the use of which is a cure (Buḵārī, 2002, book 76, p. 1441, no. 5680, 5681, 5683, 5684).

Medicinal herbs are also prescribed for various illnesses and conditions. By way of examples, in one hadith, the Prophet Muhammad says, 'Truly, there is a cure in the *black seed* for all illnesses, except for death' (Buḵārī, 2002, p. 1443, no. 5687–5688; Muslim, 2006, p. 1053, no. 2215). This Prophetic hadith directs the attention to a great medicine whose benefits are divinely revealed. The scientific name for the black seed is *Nigella sativa*. It is available in the markets under various names such as the blessed seed, black cumin, black caraway, black onion seeds and *kalonji*, among others. Other hadiths in the Buḵārī compilation mention the use of truffles' water for eye diseases and *kohl* for eye sores (no. 5708) and Indian and sea costus root for seven different diseases, mainly throat problems, tonsillitis and pleurisy (no. 5692 and 5696). The Prophetic medicine is clearly an area that modern medicine, based on Western traditions, has largely ignored.

DO NOT RESUSCITATE (DNR) IN ISLAM

Muslim countries in general and in the Arabian Gulf region in particular have different laws regarding DNR. Some of the rules governing DNR are ambiguous and make proper application more of a shot in the dark, opening the medical practitioner to charges of malpractice and negligence. It is therefore of extreme importance to familiarise oneself with the relevant laws in any given country. However, in their *fatwa* (religious ruling) on resuscitating a patient who is otherwise deemed dead, the Permanent Committee for Scholarly Research and Iftā in Saudi Arabia, Fatwa number 12086 for the year 1989 delineated 'six situations where a DNR is granted: if the patient arrives dead at the hospital, if the panel of (three) physicians determines that the condition is untreatable and death is imminent, if the patient's condition does not make him or her fit for resuscitation, if the patient is suffering from advanced heart or lung disease or repeated cardiac arrest, if the patient is in a vegetative state, and if resuscitation is considered futile' (Chamsi-Pasha & Albar, 2018, p. 10). This *fatwa* has had a significant impact on the standardisation and streamlining of palliative care practices in Saudi Arabia in particular and the Arab-Islamic world in general. In 2013 for example, Saudi Arabia witnessed the launch of the Saudi Society of Palliative Care. In 2011, Qatar launched its National Cancer Strategy with 62 recommendations to increase awareness and has been making significant developments in the area of palliative care (mdps. gov.qa). According to a 2018 study conducted by the Department of Medicine, University of Sharjah, 'current provision of effective and well-structured palliative care in developing countries including the United Arab Emirates (UAE) is at best very limited. … Cancer patients in the UAE are having major difficulties in accessing palliative care services due to the limited palliative care facilities and trained physicians and other palliative health support workers in this field. There is a general lack of national health policies that recognize palliative care as an essential component of the current healthcare system and there is inadequate training for both healthcare providers and the general public about palliative care.' Other countries of the Gulf Cooperation Council are not in a better position and the same may be said about other Middle Eastern countries owing to various domestic reasons. Advancing in this area requires concerted efforts as well as the introduction of clear regulations, in some countries more than others.

PHYSICIAN-ASSISTED SUICIDE, EUTHANASIA, SUICIDE AND REMOVAL OF LIFE-SUPPORT EQUIPMENT

Islam values human life tremendously and considers the taking of the life of one person unjustifiably to be equivalent to the killing of the whole of humankind. The Quran (Q5:32) states 'whoever kills a human being except as a punishment for murder or for spreading corruption in the land shall be regarded as having killed all humankind, and that whoever saves a human life shall be regarded as having saved all humankind.' Islam also instructs against a person wishing to die. The Prophet Muhammad states, 'None of you should wish for death because of a calamity befalling him; but if one has to wish for death, one should say "O Allah! Keep me alive as long as life is better for me, and let me die if death is better for me"' (Bukārī, no. 575). In spite of this, Islam does not encourage or commend any exercises in futility. Consequently, while Islam prohibits physician-assisted suicide (PSA) and euthanasia, it permits the withholding or withdrawal of any medical treatment that is considered futile.

After extensive discussions and professional explanations of all the intricate details of the various aspects of the issues in question in relation to the resuscitation equipment, the Islamic Fiqh Council meeting in Amman, Jordan, on 11–16 October 1986, concluded that 'In the Sharia, a person is considered to have died—and all the rulings that result from death come into effect—if one of the following two signs are proven: 1. If his heart and breathing have stopped completely and the doctors have determined that they cannot be restarted. 2. If all brain function has ceased completely, and the specialist, expert doctors have determined that this cessation is irreversible, and (the patient's) brain has started to disintegrate. In this case, removing resuscitation equipment that is connected to the person is permissible, even though some organs such as the heart may still be functioning artificially due to the action of (the) life support equipment.' In all the countries in the Arabian Gulf region, PSA and euthanasia are considered punishable crimes with severe penalties varying from one country to another. The relevant laws need to be checked to avoid unnecessary detrimental legal and social complications. As for suicide, it is considered a major sin in Islam and is thus totally forbidden (Buḵārī, 2002, no. 5442, 5700, 3276; Muslim, 2006, no. 109, 110, 113, 978).

BLOOD AND ORGAN DONATION

According to the ruling of the Council of Senior Scholars in Saudi Arabia, as long as no harm results from the blood donation, it is permissible (islamqa. info). Their ruling also permits the establishment of blood banks provided that no charges are levied on the patients or their families for the blood needed as treatment and that the banks do not use the donated blood for commercial purposes.

Muslim scholars, however, have differed regarding the permissibility of organ donation. Renowned scholars in the areas of Qur'an exegesis (*Tafsīr*) and Hadith, such as Imām al-Sha'rawi (youtube.com/watch?v=ixfJjx0wfsc) and Imām al-Albānī (youtube.com/watch?v=YarqGV7-NAQ), respectively, stated that organ donation is totally prohibited. In his commentary on Q10:31, al-Sha'rawi mentioned a number of considerations and concluded with the prohibition based on the fact that one may only donate what one possesses. Since human life is a gift from God and not something that any human being has earned, no one has true ownership of the human body except for its Creator. If the human had true ownership, God would not have prohibited suicide and one would not have incurred consequential punishment as stated in the Qur'an and Hadith. As the human body is also considered sacred even with death, violating this body is not allowed regardless of the consent of the person before his/her death.

However, the Islamic Fiqh Council of Saudi Arabia ruled in its fourth conference in Jeddah on 11 February 1988 that it is permitted to transplant 'organs from a deceased person to a living person if the life of the organ recipient depends on the organ to be received provided that consent is obtained from the donor before death, or from the deceased's guardians after death, or from the head of the Muslim community if the deceased cannot be identified or does not have any next of kin… This fatwa also (stresses) the prohibition of trading and smuggling of organs' (Ministry of Health, 2011, p. 25). This particular issue merits a dedicated study in its own right, and it is important that state regulations are taken into consideration before making any determination. This is owing to the fact that there are regulatory and statutory differences in the countries that are considered part of the Islamic world, and the Middle East is no exception. Additionally, donations of any kind are matters of choice and not obligatory. Therefore, the wishes of the deceased as stated in their will or expressed to family members need to be taken into consideration as long as such wishes are not in clear contradiction to Islamic rules. In many Arab and Muslim countries where organ donation is legal, the permission of the family of the deceased has to be sought first.

SUMMARY

Islam clearly influences both Muslims and their expectation of a Sharia-compliant healthcare system. It is therefore of paramount importance that medical and healthcare providers have at least a basic understanding of the requirements of Muslim patients as outlined in Islam's primary sources: the Holy Qur'an and Sunnah of the Prophet Muhammad. Understanding Islamic requirements helps a great deal in the decision-making process, especially when Sharia-compliant care becomes an impossibility. Additionally, Islamic teachings in healthcare is an understudied area of medical research in spite of the fact that the relevant information is found in abundance in thousands of credible references.

Medical practitioners need to familiarise themselves not only with the relevant Islamic teachings when dealing with Muslim patients but also with the state laws, statutes and regulations, as well as the cultural norms, in their given place of work. This will tremendously assist in balancing the risks involved and make their service provision experience a better-informed one.

Appendix—Transliteration System

Letter	Symbol	Ex.	Letter	Symbol	Ex.	Letter	Symbol	Ex.	Letter	Symbol	Ex.
ء	c postscript	an	د	d		ط	Ŧ ŧ		م	m	
ا	a		ذ	Ż ż	that	ظ	Ž ž		ن	n	
ب	b		ر	r		ع	ɛ ɛ		هـ	h	
ت	t		ز	z		غ	Ġ ġ	French /r/	و	w	
ث	Ħ	thank	س	s		ف	f		ي	y	
ج	J		ش	Ŝ ŝ	she	ق	q		ِ	a	
ح	Ħ ħ		ص	Ş ş		ك	k		ِ	i	
خ	Ҝ k	ch as in loch	ض	Đ đ		ل	l		ُ	u	
ج الجيم المصرية غير المعطشة				g	go						

| Long vowel /a/ للمد بالفتح Ā ā | | | | Long vowel /i/ للمد بالكسر Ī ī | | | | Long vowel /u/ للمد بالضم Ū ū | | | |

| ال | | /al/ whether the (l) is pronounced or not. Its pronunciation needs to follow Arabic rules. | | | | | | | | | |

Exceptions: Words with widespread common spelling are exempted, for example: Muhammad, not Muħammad; Abullah, not ɛabdullah; Ali, not ɛaliy; Abbās, not ɛabbās; Abū, not cAbū; Qur'an, not Qurcān; Hadith, not Ħadīħ.

The double adjectival /y/ at the end of names is reduced to the more common (ī); for example: Ibn Al-Rūmī not Ibn Al-Rūmiy.

REFERENCES

Abu Dāwūd, Sulaymān ibn al-AŝɛaŦ ibn Ishāq al-Azdi al-Sijistāni (d. 275 AH). (1999). *Sunan Abi Dāwūd*. Riyadh: Dar al-Salām.

Al-Ājurrī, Abu Bakr Muhammad ibn al-Ħusayn (d.360AH). (1417AH). *Kitāb Faḍl Qiyām al-Layl wa al-Tahajjud*. Taħqīq Abdul-Latif bin Muhammad al-Jilānī al-Āsifī. Medina: *Dār al-Ҝudayrī for Publishing and Distribution*.

Al-Albānī, Muhammad Nāsir al-Dīn. (1988). *Şahīħ al-Jamiɛ al-Saġīr wa Ziyādatuh (al-Fath al-Ҝabīr)* (3rd Edition). Beirut: al-Maktab al-Islāmi.

Al-Albānī, Muhammad Nāsir al-Dīn. (1997). *Şahīħ Sunan Ibn Mājah*. Riyadh: Maktabat al-Maɛārif.

Al-Albānī, Muhammad Nāsir al-Dīn. (1998). *Şahīħ Sunan Abu Dāwūd*. Riyadh: Maktabat al-Maɛārif.

Al-Āmidī, Ali ibn Ahmad. (1402 AH). *Al-Iħkām fī cUṣūl al-Aħkām*. Commentry: ɛafīfī, Abdul-Razzāq. (2nd ed.). Beirut: al-Maktab al-Islāmi.

Al-Bayhaqī, Abu Bakr Ahmad ibn al-ħusayn ibn Ali (d. 458AH). (2011). *Al-Sunan al-Kabīr*. Taħqīq: Al-Turki, Abdullāh ibn Abdul-Muhsin. (1st ed.). Cairo: Hajar Centre for Arabic and Islamic Research and Studies.

Buҝārī, Muhammad ibn cIsmāɛīl. (2002). *Şahīħ al-Buҝāri*. Damascuss and Beirut: Dār ibn KaŦīr.

Al-cAŝbīlī, Abu Muhammad Abdul-Haq ibn Abdul-Rahman (d.581AH). (1994). *Kitāb al-Tahajjud*. Beirut: Dār al-Kutub al-ɛilmiyyah.

Al-Jaknī, Muhammad Al-Amin. (1993). *Marāqi al-Sueūd ilā Marāqi al-Sueūd. Tahqiq: Muhammad al-Shanqītī*. Cairo: Maktabat Ibn Taymiyyah.

Al-Ŝāṭibī, Abu Ishāq Ibrahīm ibn Mūsā (d. 790AH). (n.d.). *Al-Muwāfaqāt fī cUṣūl al-Ŝarīɛah*. Commentary: Abdullah Dirāz. Cairo: al-Maktabah al-Tijāriyyah al-Kubrā.

Al-Suyūṭī, Jalālu-d-Dīn (d. 911AH). (1983). *Al-cAshbāh wa al-Naẓāᶜir*. Beirut: Dār al-Kutub al-ɛilmiyyah.

Al-Tirmiżī, Muhammad ibn ɛīsā ibn Sawrah (d. 279 AH). (n.d.). *Jāmiɛ al-Tirmiżī*. Amman and Riyadh: International Ideas Home Inc.

Al-Zahrānī, Hilāl ibn Abdul-Majīd. (2020). *Muҝtasar Kitāb al-Tahajjud min Saħīħ al-Buҝāri*. (no publisher's data).

Al-ɛaynī, Maḥmūd ibn Aḥmad ibn Mūsā (d.855AH). (2000). *Al-Bināyah fī Šarḥ al-Hidāyah*. Beirut: Dār al-Kutub al-ɛilmiyyah.

Chamsi-Pasha, H., & Albar, M. A. (2018). Do-not-resuscitate orders: Islamic viewpoint. *International Journal of Human and Health Sciences, Vol. 02*(No. 01), 8–12.

De Cabo, R., & Mattson, M. P. (2019). Effects of intermittent fasting on health, aging, and disease. *New England Journal of Medicine, 381*(26), 2541–2551. https://doi.org/10.1056/NEJMra1905136.

DeSilver, D, & Masci, D. (2017). World's Muslim population more widespread than you might think. Pew Research Center. Available at https://www.pewresearch.org/short-reads/2017/01/31/worlds-muslim-population-more-widespread-than-you-might-think/. Accessed 30 December 2020.

Harvard Health Publishing (2021). Intermittent fasting: The positive news continues. Available at https://www.health.harvard.edu/blog/intermittent-fasting-surprising-update-2018062914156. Accessed December 2020.

Ibn Abi al-Dunyā, Abu Bakr Abdullah ibn Muhammad ibn ɛubaid (d.281AH). (1998). *al-Tahajjud wa Qiyām al-Layl*. Taḥqīq: Musliḥ ibn Jazāᶜ al-Ḥārithī. Riyadh: Maktabat al-Rašīd.

Ibn al-Mulaqqin, ɛumar ibn Ali. (1425AH). Al-Badr al-Munīr fī Taᴋrīj al-ᶜAḥādīᵵ wal-Āᵵ̄ār al-Waqiɛati fī al-Šarḥ al-Kabīr. Taḥqīq: Mustafa Abul-Ġayt, et al. (1st ed.). Saudi: Dar al-Hijrah.

Ibn Al-Qayyim al-Jawziyyah, Muhammad ibn Abi Bakr al-Zarɛī (d.751AH). (1998). *Zād al-Miɛād fī Hadyi Ḱayri-l-ɛibād. Taḥqīq by al-ᶜArnāᵘūt* (3ʳᵈ Edition). Beirut: Risālah Publishing.

Ibn Ḥajar, Ahmad Ibn Ali (d. 852 AH). (1987). *Fatḥ al-Bārī bišarḥ Ṣaḥīḥ al-Buᴋari*. Cairo: Dār Al-Rayyan Lil-Turāᵵ̄.

Ibn Ḥanbal, Abu Abdullah Ahmad. (n.d.). Al-Musand of Imām Ahmad Ibn Ḥanbal. Cairo: Qurtoba Foundation.

Ibn Mājah, Muhammad ibn Yazīd Ar-Ribɛī al-Quzwīnī (d.275AH). (n.d.). *Sunan ibn Mājah*. Taḥqīq by Abdul-Bāqī, Muhammad Fuᶜād. Cairo: Dār ᶜIḥyāᶜ al-Kutub al-ɛarabiyyah.

Ibn Manẓūr, Jamāl al-Dīn Muhammad ibn Makram (d. 1311CE). (1999). *Lisān al-ɛarab* (3ʳᵈ Edition). Beirut: Dār ᶜIḥyāᶜ al-Turāth al-ɛarabī.

Ibn Mufliḥ, Burhān al-Dīn Ibrahīm Ibn Muhammad (d.884AH). (2000). *Al-Mubdiɛ Šarh al-Muqniɛ*. Riyadh: ɛālam al-Kutub.

Ministry of Health (Malaysia). (2011). *Organ transplantation from the Islamic perspective*. Malaysia: Transplantation Unit, Medical Development Division.

Muslim, Abul-Ḥusayn Muslim ibn al-Ḥajjāj al-Quŝayri al-Naysāburi (d. 261 AH). (2006). *Ṣaḥīḥ Muslim. (1426 AH)*. Riyadh: Dār Ṫaybah.

National Institute on Aging. (2020). Research on intermittent fasting shows health benefits. Available at https://www.nia.nih.gov/news/research-intermittent-fasting-shows-health-benefits. Accessed 11 September 2023.

Nawawī, Abu Zakariyyā Yaḥyā ibn Šaraf (d. 676 AH). (2007). *Riyāḍ al-Sālihīn. Taḥqīq Māhir al-Faḥl* (First Edition). Beirut and Damascus: Dār Ibn Kaᵵ̄īr.

Šaraful-Ḥaq, Abu ɛabd al-Raḥmān Muhammad Aŝhraf. (n.d). ɛawn al-Maɛbud ɛalā sunan Abi Dāwūd. Amman and Riyadh: International Ideas Home Inc.

Internet Sites

https://islamqa.info/ar/answers/307202/حفظ_الدين_على_حفظ_النفس_والضرورات_الخمس_والخلاف_في_تقديم. Accessed November 2020.

https://islamqa.info/ar/answers/2320/حكم_التبرع_بالدم. Accessed 1 January 2021.

https://www.mdps.gov.qa/en/nds1/pages/default.aspx. Accessed 1 January 2021.

https://www.nia.nih.gov/news/research-intermittent-fasting-shows-health-benefits. Accessed 19 April 2021.

https://www.youtube.com/watch?v=ixfJjx0wfsc. Accessed 1 January 2021.

https://www.youtube.com/watch?v=YarqGV7-NAQ. Accessed 1 January 2021.

https://worldpopulationreview.com/country-rankings/religion-by-country. Accessed 19 April 2021.

2

THE FAMILY IN HEALTHCARE IN THE ARABIAN GULF

JAMES O'BOYLE ▪ MARYAM JAMEEL NASER ▪ SHARON BROWNIE

CHAPTER OUTLINE

INTRODUCTION

The family is the basic social unit which is formed through bonds of kinship and marriage (Nasir & Abdul-Haq, 2008). Its role to provide companionship, security and protection to the constituent members is central to maintain and reinforce its functions. The nuclear family structure is the fundamental construct in some societies. In the Arab world, however, the nuclear family is often subordinate to the extended family (Hammad et al., 1999).

The traditional collectivist values emphasising the importance of familial ties date back to tribal pre-Islamic times (Nasir & Abdul-Haq, 2008). Islam, however, being the main religion in most Arab societies, extended the notion of the family to all Muslims considering them to be sisters and brothers in faith and humanity (Abudabbeh & Hays, 2006). Nevertheless, it does emphasise the independence of each family unit and the roles attributed to individual members of the family.

Multiple studies have been conducted to reflect the importance of the family in the Middle East (Ali et al., 1993; Kazarian, 2005; Starr, 1978), which is often considered a top priority, preceding that of commitment to self-development in some societies. This pattern is consistent across many Arab countries, emphasising the collectivist nature of values.

Given the extent of its impact, the family plays an important role in many facets of the individual members' lives. While emotional development and economic effects are commonly cited, the family also affects the mental and physical well-being and health of its members (Attum et al., 2020). It has the capacity to shape the understanding and meaning of health and illness, with a strong influence on decision-making (Attum et al., 2020; Nasir & Abdul-Haq, 2008). While traditional family structures remain prominent in many Arab countries, this is changing, particularly in urban areas. Present-day Arab family and marriage practices are showing more similarities to typical Western practices (Engelen & Puschmann, 2011). The change is attributed to economic hardships, growing costs of marriage ceremonies, prolonged education and the emancipation of women (Engelen & Puschmann, 2011).

This chapter will provide a discussion of family structures and functions in the Arab world. It will be followed by a discussion of the roles of constituent members and how they relate to health and healthcare. The discussion will include the challenges and possible interventions unique to the sociocultural features of the Arabian Gulf and the Middle East.

BACKGROUND

Family Structure and Function

The typical Arab family is defined as being extended, hierarchical and male-dominated (Faruqi, 1978; Hammad et al., 1999; Nasir & Abdul-Haq, 2008). The term 'extended' refers to intergenerational connections that are beyond immediate kinship. In a typical household, it includes grandparents, parents, children and grandchildren (Al-Thakeb, 1981, 1985; Farsoun, 1970; Fellous, 1981).

The second type of family structure is known as the clan or *hammula* (Hammad et al., 1999). This refers to all the joint families descending from the same paternal ancestor. An Arab village community usually consists of three to four such clans which may be called the *qabila*.

The status of the individual family member is reliant on the status of the family as a whole. Individual identity tends to be less important as compared with the affiliation to the family (Hammad et al., 1999). Besides the emotional interdependence, the extended family might share strong economic ties also (Nasir & Abdul-Haq, 2008). The 'traditional' structure of an Arab family, however, has been challenged by industrialisation and urbanisation forces (El-Haddad, 2003). The sociopolitical instability of the region has additionally affected the economic powers of family units, imposing increased patterns of global immigration on their individual members (El-Haddad, 2003). As such, it has been documented that traditionally defined families represent a minority in countries such as Bahrain, Kuwait, Jordan and Egypt (Al-Thakeb, 1981). Despite this, researchers have reported that emotional ties do still exist and surpass the absence of physical proximity.

The typical Arab family is also described as being hierarchical. The chain of command is vertical and male predominant. Authority and power of decision-making is determined by seniority and gender (Dhami & Sheikh, 2000; Kennan, 1998; Smadi, 2003). Fathers often uphold the highest capacity of decision-making on behalf of the family, especially in external affairs. Mothers in most cases are closer to the children and are responsible for arranging household matters (Haj-Yahia, 2000). This non-conjugal system is the norm in many societies and has been traditionally passed down through generations.

This structure existed well before Islam, paralleling tribal values, within the region, of power dominance of males (Nasir & Abdul-Haq, 2008). More recently, however, under the growing pressure of globalisation and expanding communication networks through social media (Al-Khraif et al., 2020; El-Haddad, 2003; Nasir & Abdul-Haq, 2008), typical gender roles have been challenged to include women in decision-making and involvement in external affairs.

Family and the Health/Illness Culture

Culture is defined as a collection of beliefs, customs, practices and social behaviour (Nasir & Abdul-Haq, 2008). It depicts the totality of norms and standards of practice in the majority of a society's building units, i.e., families. The culture shapes the understanding of disease process and health, treatment-seeking behaviour and compliance with medical treatment (Nasir & Abdul-Haq, 2008). For example, a study conducted by Ypinazar and Margolis (2006) revealed that the notion of illness is often used to describe 'organic' dysfunction with tangible disease manifestations in Arabian Gulf countries. In turn, 'good health' was defined as the absence of visible disease, with limited understanding of silent disease or role of preventative medicine (Ypinazar & Margolis, 2006). Such beliefs are often upheld by seniors within these countries, and this influences the decisions taken with regards to their health-seeking behaviours and that of their families.

Moreover, Arab families, especially Muslims, often perceive illness, suffering and pain as a test from God, by which their sins might be removed (Attum et al., 2020; Ezenkwele & Roodsari, 2013). This spirituality is often reflected in the care of the ill family member and is seen as a form of moral support and acceptance of the ill state. During these times, the family helps facilitate the worship practices of a patient, reminding them of the prayers to be recited during illness and helping them to withstand the effects of the disease (Ezenkwele & Roodsari, 2013).

These findings are supported by a study where participants viewed their health as having three main components; physical, spiritual and mental—that are greatly affected by the family (Ezenkwele & Roodsari, 2013; Ypinazar & Margolis, 2006). In addition to providing spiritual support, the roles of the family include providing physical care, emotional support and mediating interactions with the healthcare systems. The family has a great influence in supporting a sick family member in the hospital setting. Equally important, the family has been identified as an important player in mediating interactions with healthcare providers by discouraging or recommending particular treatments, based on their shared base of beliefs (Ezenkwele & Roodsari, 2013).

These beliefs extend to include multiple facets of healthcare like uptake of medications, utilisation of complementary medicine or use of traditional practices in Muslim teachings (Ezenkwele & Roodsari, 2013; Patterson et al., 2020). As such, inclusion of family in healthcare is of vital importance in delivering culturally competent care to patients.

The Western medical model emphasises the importance of individuality and autonomy with regards to health and health-related behaviours (Hamdy, 2006; Sorry et al., 2006). This emphasis does not always translate well in collectivist societies like Arab countries, which value group involvement in decision-making (Case Study 2.1). This affects the way information

---

CASE STUDY 2.1
BREAKING BAD NEWS

Abdulla is a 59-year-old man and has been diagnosed with glioblastoma. He has a poor prognosis. His children and his wife do not want the doctor to tell him his diagnosis and rather described his condition to him as a 'benign cyst' in the brain.

ANALYSIS

In the Western model of medical bioethics, the primary emphasis in clinical practice is the patient's autonomy and individuality in decision-making. However, in Arab societies and collectivist cultures, the preference is towards a family-centred approach to decision-making.

Families often conceal the truth from patients in an attempt to protect them from the negative consequences of losing hope. It also reflects the values ingrained in the culture of collective support and sacrifice.

This raises a question about the ethnocentricity of bioethics and the universal concept of society. There is evident plurality in perspectives regarding decision-making that is influenced by culture, religion, family relations and the collective memory of a society which should be understood by healthcare professionals.

---

is created, received and processed. It also determines the expectations of the role of a physician in providing treatment and medical advice. At a healthcare provider level, this creates a cognitive dissonance between the Western framework of medical education that medical schools adopt and the cultural manifestations in actual practice.

The effects of the family on health and healthcare will be explored further as the individual roles of the members are discussed below.

MARITAL PRACTICES
Traditional Marriages

Marriage is an important social institution and the basic foundation of every family (Nasir & Abdul-Haq, 2008). In the Arab culture, communal interests have played an important role in directing the decision to marriage and it is common for marriages to be arranged by the parents of the bride and groom. Arranged marriages may also be consanguineous.

Consanguineous Marriages

Close-kin marriage or consanguineous marriage is defined as the union between first-degree cousins (Modell & Darr, 2002). The rate in Arab countries is very high, reaching up to 70% in some countries (Hoodfar & Teebi, 1996; Teebi & El-Shanti, 2006). In the Arabian Gulf, it is estimated that rates are about 29% in Bahrain (Al-Arrayed, 1999), 30% in Kuwait (Al-Awadi et al., 1985) and 31% in Saudi Arabia (El-Hazmi et al., 1995). Contrary to popular belief, this form of marriage is not advocated by Islam and was practiced long before Islam came into being. It is also not restricted to Islamic Arab communities and is common in some Christian Arab communities like Lebanon (Nasir & Abdul-Haq, 2008).

The aims of this form of marriage are to consolidate familial ties, preserve economic power and lower matrimonial costs.

Several studies have reported a higher incidence of genetic diseases in Arab countries, related to consanguinity (Al-Gazali et al., 2006). Pregnancy outcomes are also more negative with a higher rate of neonatal mortality and congenital malformations (de Costa, 2002). Although there is widespread awareness of potential genetic consequences of close-kin marriage, as reported by multiple studies, the social imperative is significant and many partners proceed regardless of the anticipated outcomes (Al-Gazali, 2005; Raz & Star, 2004). Multiple Middle Eastern countries (Iran, Palestine, Jordan, KSA, UAE, Iraq and Bahrain) have implemented mandatory premarital screening and genetic counselling to identify carriers of recessively carried genes such as beta thalassaemia. Counselling is provided to at-risk couples to ensure that they understand the reproductive risk and available options. These programs were unsuccessful in discouraging at-risk marriages but successful in reducing the prevalence of affected births in countries providing prenatal detection and therapeutic abortion.

Polygynous Marriages

Polygynous marriage is defined as a marital relationship that involves more than one wife (Nasir & Abdul-Haq, 2008). The prevalence is variable in different regions, but it is trending down (Prothro & Diab, 1974). It is more common in Muslim societies that adhere closely to traditional lifestyles (Nasir & Abdul-Haq, 2008). It is permitted in Islamic law to marry up to four wives, provided that sufficient economic resources are available and all wives and families are treated equally. Polygynous marriages are associated with several health behaviours and conditions. For example, women in polygynous marriages are more likely to reject contraception due to 'fertility competition' between wives (Al-Krenawi & Lightman, 2000).

Other Marital Practices

White Marriage

White marriage refers to an informal physical and emotional relationship between two people. There is still inconclusive data regarding the scale of its practice, but it gained popularity as the financial requirements and social expectations of expensive wedding ceremonies have escalated in the Middle East. The concept remains controversial and faces immense opposition from scholars and religious authorities. It has also aroused much objection in the public sphere, being viewed as an immoral lifestyle. Discussion of the legal status is variable across the Middle Eastern sphere and is primarily influenced by the degree of secularism in individual countries. However, Muslim

doctrine considers any intimate relations between men and women that take place without marriage or outside of marriage to be haram (forbidden).

Temporary Marriage

This form of marriage is haram (forbidden) for a majority of Muslims and is not generally accepted by society. Added to this, there are many inter-sectarian differences and varying opinions regarding the concept of temporary marriage, making it a less acceptable option.

FERTILITY AND CHILDREARING

Fertility and childrearing are important factors in determining the acceptability of women within the family. It is a determining factor that influences the self-image of a female (Hammad et al., 1999; Nasir & Abdul-Haq, 2008). In traditional and self-enclosed Arab societies, motherhood is the only role permitted to women and is a gauge of her social, emotional and economic fulfilment (Hammad et al., 1999). As such, the social pressure to conceive is high and may result in closely spaced, frequent and multiple pregnancies until the 'correct' number and gender is attained (Gadalla et al., 1985; Khalaf & Callister, 1997). Women who delay marriage are often perceived as less socially favourable. Women who delay childbearing, however, can be seen as 'faulted' and pressured to prove their fecundity (Nasir & Abdul-Haq, 2008).

Given the above, the number of children in an Arab family is variable (2–7 children). This pattern is decreasing as Arab societies are opening up to other cultures. The values of educational attainment and extra-domestic roles of women are becoming more widespread and accepted, especially amongst individuals from high-socioeconomic status families. Patterns of high birth rate are declining with the introduction of programs of birth control and birth spacing. The support by Islamic scholars of the use of contraception methods, under specific circumstances, has contributed to positive perceptions regarding family planning (Roudi-Fahimi, 2004). Other factors determining effective use of family planning methods include involvement of the husband in decision-making, integration of contraception education in routine antenatal visits and postpartum contraception education.

Fertility and Emerging Challenges

Genetics and Physical Health

Understanding the demographic characteristics of the Arab population better explains the pattern of health indices related to children's health. These characteristics include high birth rates, childbearing at older maternal age and large family sizes. In addition, the extended structure of the Arab family displays unique distribution patterns for genetic diseases due to the vertical transmission of genetic mutations in the family given the high rates of consanguineous marriages.

The combination of these factors largely affects the prevalence and natural history of inherited diseases. Consanguinity, for example, has been linked to hearing loss, respiratory allergies, eczema, congenital heart defects and intellectual disability, among many other conditions (Modell & Darr, 2002). Most genetic diseases identified in Arab countries are related to single gene disorders. The prevalence of autosomal recessive diseases is 64% of the total diagnosed single gene disorders, followed by autosomal dominant (26%) and X-linked traits (6%) (Modell & Darr, 2002). These diseases pose a significant morbidity and mortality risk. For example, genetic diseases that are highly prevalent include all haemoglobin disorders (thalassaemia, sickle cell diseases and haemoglobin variants), which are cited as one of the common causes of death in some Arabian Gulf countries, including Saudi Arabia (Jastaniah, 2011). Saffi and Howard (2015) report that genetic counselling for beta thalassaemia has been implemented across eight Middle Eastern countries to reduce at-risk marriages and therefore reduce disease prevalence.

Children with genetic diseases often live with the manifestations of their underlying illness for a long time. In addition to physical limitations, the psychological effects of chronic diseases are equally significant. Children with chronic diseases have higher rates of anxiety, depression and general distress (Al-Gazali et al., 2006; Modell & Darr, 2002), and it also engenders an emotional reaction of guilt and grief over losing normal childhood and future. This, in turn, can affect the child's emotional development, which may be arrested.

The negative psychological effects of chronic illness can well extend to the psychological well-being of the parents. Caregivers, especially mothers, are reported to have a high prevalence of depression (Modell & Darr, 2002).

Adolescent Mothers

There is limited data on the prevalence of unwed pregnant adolescents, given that it is culturally and religiously unaccepted. Arab girls who become pregnant outside the wedding institution may encounter risk of violence and death (honour killings). According to the World Development Indicators in 2014, adolescent birth rates are variable in different Middle Eastern countries. For example, it is reported to be as high as 44.1 births per 1000 in Egypt and 10.5 births per 1000 in Saudi Arabia.

Given the potential risks faced by these young females, some governments in the Middle East, e.g. Jordan, offer an institutional model of congregate care. This model is the only out-of-home option currently available for adolescent mothers. However, institutionalising pregnant girls in a collectivist society where there is lack of family support and stable relationships may result in difficulties establishing healthy social networks, obtaining housing, finding employment or succeeding in marriage.

Parenting Style, Family Dynamics and Children's Health

The parenting style adopted in Arab families is described as authoritarian, especially amongst fathers (Checa & Abundis-Gutierrez, 2018; Nasir & Abdul-Haq, 2008). Mothers may have a higher tendency to adopt an authoritative parenting style than more liberal styles adopted by Western parents. Authoritarian parents provide an orderly environment, with close monitoring of their children's activities (Baumrind, 1991). The predominance of an authoritarian parenting style in Arab societies is consistent with the values of collectivist societies, as it emphasises giving priority to the welfare of the group over personal interests (Nasir & Abdul-Haq, 2008). Aref (2020) suggests that the predominant authoritarian parenting style in the Middle East and North Africa (MENA) region is less intense in urban areas compared with rural settings in the same country, whereas the authoritative style is mainly found in middle-class families with higher education backgrounds.

However, specific parenting practices have been associated with increased incidences of negative mental outcomes such as anxiety, depression, oppositional defiant disorders and personality disorders. A study in Saudi Arabia has shown that perceived parental cruelty, overprotection and neglect are associated with anxiety (Addelaim, 2003). Another example of a poor parental practice is triangulation which occurs when there is a propensity to focus attention on the child when there is a foreseen conflict between the parents. This disrupts the hierarchical structure and typical roles, which has been predicted to cause depression, anxiety and attention deficit and hyperactivity disorders in middle childhood (Nasir & Abdul-Haq, 2008). Yet, the level of adult awareness of children's vulnerability to psychological problems remains low in the Arabian Gulf (Nasir & Abdul-Haq, 2008).

Moreover, parenting styles are affected by family dynamics and structure. There is growing evidence supporting the association between family interactional patterns and children's physical, emotional and psychological development. In situations where there is excessive family conflict, early onset of disease during childhood and complex family structures (step-parents, divorced

parents, single parents, extended families), the patterns of familial interactions change.

THE EXTENDED FAMILY
Takaful

The extended family structure, unique to many Arab societies, is characterised by strong economic and emotional bonds, reinforced by physical proximity and shared living space. Although this arguably has changed under the influence of urbanisation, extended families continue to play an important role in provision of fiscal and moral support to individual members.

Family members' beliefs, experiences and perceptions are usually shared with each other, creating an influential reference point for individual members. In healthcare, for example, the extended family is often consulted in making an important decision regarding pursuit of a treatment, trust in healthcare and seeking alternative remedies (Attum et al., 2020). Their experiences are usually trusted and considered with high regard, as they are seen to be shared in the best interests of the individual member (Hammad et al., 1999) (Case Study 2.2).

However, the complexity of the structure of the extended family can affect the roles of individual members and impose restrictions on autonomy (Patterson et al., 2020). A study conducted in Jordan reported that a woman's structural position within the household is an indicator of individual autonomy in the context of the Arab Middle East (Doan & Bisharat, 1990). For example, a daughter-in-law has lower autonomy than the co-head of the house. Not only does this affect the parental ability to reinforce autonomous parental practices but it also has been shown to negatively correlate with health parameters like child nutrition. Extended families also play a mixed role in intimate partner violence; they can be perpetrators or protectors, depending on a range of factors, including supportive relatives, exposure and history of violence and whether the husband and wife reside with relatives (Clark et al., 2010).

Family Demographic Transitions

Globalisation coupled with economic and cultural pressures have led to evident changes in the

---

CASE STUDY 2.2
ROLE OF THE PHYSICIAN

Fatima is a 55-year-old female with left lower quadrant pain and positive rebound tenderness. A CT scan is requested to rule out acute diverticulitis. Her husband is refusing to proceed with imaging unless it is done by a female radiologist.

ANALYSIS

The healthcare provider is expected to understand the traditional gender roles within society and address these expectations. Although the female has the capacity to consent to the plan, she is unlikely to accept it, if it is met with opposition by her partner. Doing so might inflict conflict and disrupt the equilibrium of the relationship.

When faced with such a scenario, it is best approached by open communication and involvement of the partner in the decision-making process. The practitioner should attempt to understand the cause of objection and tackle it accordingly. Explaining that the boundaries of modesty and religious norms will be observed will most likely lead to acceptance of the plan. The cultural competency is mandated to prevent negative healthcare outcomes.

demographic structure of the Arab family. As Islamic countries undergo rapid modernisation, the family is undergoing radical transformation towards a nuclear structure. This is indicated by the increase in the mean age of first marriage, due to a notable increase in female education and integration into the workforce (Al-Khraif et al., 2020; Nasir & Abdul-Haq, 2008). Increased levels of education influence the duration of marriage, perceived ideal number of children, age of women at delivery of their last child, interval between consecutive pregnancies and history of abortions (Al-Khraif et al., 2020). With declining birth rates across the region, this has manifested in the form of smaller household sizes, delayed marriages, a rise in divorce and single parenthood, shifts in individual values and an increasing symmetry in gender roles and female autonomy.

In addition, movement from traditional or rural lifestyles to cities has also improved the social status and decision-making powers of women. This has created new opportunities for socialisation, cultural integration and intercultural marriages. This may result in changes in the composition of populations in some regions. Changes in the gender make-up of the workforce has many interconnected effects. Increased involvement of females leads to higher household incomes that may lead to improvement of health due to better healthcare, nutrition and living conditions (Nasir & Abdul-Haq, 2008). It is also postulated to improve the social status of a female. However, among some groups, fertility may be a woman's only acceptable option for social status and long-term security (NoFahim and Faris, 1992). Moreover, women are still expected to carry on with the traditionally mandated domestic responsibilities like childcare and household duties. This may create a double burden and increase mental health problems (Hattar-Pollara et al., 2000).

MALE HEALTH

A review of the literature on men's health in the Middle East highlights the following. First, there is a paucity of hard data and research in this area. Second, the Middle East is a collection of 18 countries (sources differ) with significantly varying socioeconomic statuses, so it can be challenging to speak on issues as if there is homogeneity. That said, there are areas of commonality, to varying degrees, regarding facets of Middle East culture and its impact on health and help seeking.

Background

Much has been written about Middle Eastern culture being traditional, collectivist, family-orientated and patriarchal. In addition, there is often the notion of masculinity as being the leader: strong, heroic, wise and protector of the family. Stigma and shame, particularly for men, can be associated with mental health issues, where a common belief is that the affected person has been possessed by Jinn spirits (Rassool, 2018) (Case study 2.3). Physical disability can be seen as a test from God, with some regarding it as a punishment, even though this does not form part of the belief of established religions, including Islam. Furthermore, sexual matters are often considered taboo for discussion, with sex outside marriage being frowned upon. All the preceding points add layers of complexity to the age-old problem, experienced in a number of cultures, of getting men to engage and discuss their health with healthcare providers, particularly with regard to mental and sexual health issues.

CASE STUDY 2.3
MEANING OF ILLNESS

Elias is a 23-year-old male with elated mood, grandiose delusions and hypersexuality. He was referred by his family physician to a psychiatrist to diagnose and manage suspected bipolar disorder. His family refused and report that he has been possessed by a spirit. They prefer to go to a religious 'healer' to have him cured.

ANALYSIS

Issues relating to mental health disorders are sensitive and should be handled with care. Many families refuse to acknowledge diagnosis of mental disorders out of fear of social stigma. 'Possession by a spirit' is more socially acceptable and is a better alternative for the family to explain the mental status of the ill person.

The provider might easily dismiss the family as being ignorant and fail to address the core issue. This requires deep understanding of family values, beliefs and support system to help tackle the stigma, reassuring the family that treatment of mental illness does not mean lack of faith. The family can be educated that religious and spiritual counsel can be sought in addition to medical treatment.

When the decision to access healthcare is made, timely access for men in the Middle East can be highly variable, both within and between countries. This can be due to significant variations in GDP between countries in the Middle East. In addition to a lack of financial resources, there can be a lack of suitably trained specialists. Further complicating the picture is the availability of different systems of healthcare including government-run schemes, private insurance and self-pay, often operating within the same country (Mukherji et al., 2020).

The current outlook for men's health in particular regions of the Middle East is concerning as there are profound socioeconomic changes occurring with rising GDP, swift urbanisation, sedentary lifestyles and an increase in consumption of a Western fast-food diet. The result is rising obesity and type 2 diabetes (Meo et al., 2019).

Rising Disease Incidence

The following is a brief exploration of three conditions that are on the rise for men in the Middle East region.

Prostate Cancer

Prostate cancer rates in the Middle East are currently lower than those in the rest of the world, but they are rising significantly. Various explanations have been offered to explain the current low figures, including the young age profile of the male population in Arab countries, genetic factors in mitigating prostate cancer risk and lower reported prostate-specific antigen levels in Arab men (Hilal et al., 2015). Unfortunately, reduced rates are likely to be also due to lack of patient awareness, deficiencies in regular screening and lack of robust population-based registries. As a result, a significant proportion of men present with locally advanced and metastatic prostate cancer at diagnosis (Mukherji et al., 2020).

A leading urologist at the Cleveland Clinic USA, Dr David Levy, rejects the theory of genetic protection for Arab men. He believes it is the Middle Eastern diet, rich in foods such as lentils, tomatoes and pomegranates that has helped keep prostate cancer rates low. Dr Levy highlighted that when Arab men adopt a Westernised lifestyle, their risk for prostate cancer rises to align with that of Westerners (Sanderson, 2018).

Type 2 Diabetes Mellitus

Another condition that has shown a dramatic rise in men in the Middle East is type 2 diabetes mellitus (T2DM). The *2021 International Diabetes Federation Atlas, 10th Edition*, estimates a world diabetes prevalence of 10.5% in adults of 20–79 years of age (IDF, 2021). However, a 2019 study, published in the *American Journal of Men's Health*, showed significantly elevated rates of T2DM in male populations of some Middle East countries. Examples include Bahrain (33.60%), Saudi Arabia (29.10%), UAE (25.83%) and Kuwait (25.40%) (Meo et al., 2019). These four countries comprise a majority of the six-member Gulf Cooperation Council (GCC) and have experienced profound societal changes that presage an ongoing increase in T2DM amongst the population. In addition to screening, there is an urgent need to devise informational healthcare campaigns to educate affected populations and reduce the incidence of T2DM. Both Yemen and Iran, Middle East countries with low GDPs compared with their GCC neighbours, showed a prevalence of T2DM in their male populations of under 10% (Meo et al., 2019). More specific information on T2DM and its impact on Middle East populations can be found in Chapter 4.

HIV Infection

The incidence of HIV infection is on the rise in the MENA region, making it one of only two regions in the world to see an increase in numbers (HIV statistics from reliable sources group the Middle East and North Africa as one region) (Mumtaz et al., 2022). Moreover, 2010–2021 saw an increase of 33% in new HIV infections. There is a lack of robust data on HIV in key populations who include sex workers, intravenous drug users (IDU), gay men, men who have sex with men (MSM) and prisoners (IN DANGER: UNAIDS Global AIDS Update, 2022). These are populations that often exist at the periphery of society, especially when there is stigma, supported by laws, related to them.

HIV testing resources are often misdirected at the low-risk general population, so reported incidence of HIV can be misleading. Acknowledging high-risk populations can be a sensitive issue for authorities. The result is that in over half of the countries in the region that have data, there is evidence of concentrated epidemics and sustained transmission in key populations such as MSM and IDU (Mumtaz et al., 2022). There are countries in the Middle East, such as Iran, that have adopted a multifaceted strategic approach, sometimes involving the input of culturally sensitive non-government organisations, to break the chain of transmission (Abu-Raddad et al., 2010).

SUMMARY AND TAKEAWAY POINTS

As a summary for this chapter, as it pertains to healthcare and the family, the following points are important to remember:

- Across the Middle East, men are often the decision-makers on women's healthcare needs. Though this is in decline, health practitioners should be sensitive to the fact that female members, particularly from more traditional family structures, may require the permission of a husband, father or brother for healthcare procedures to be performed.
- Inclusion of family in healthcare is vitally important in delivering culturally appropriate care to Arab patients.
- It is important for health practitioners to be aware that some patients may see illness as a test from God or in the case of mental illness, possession by Jinns. This can affect the treatment, ongoing follow-up or even the seeking of medical treatment in the first place by Arab patients.
- Consanguineous marriages across the region remain popular, resulting in increased rates of infant mortality and congenital malformations. However, an increase in premarital screening and genetic counselling has reduced the prevalence of certain genetic diseases.
- While HIV has been largely held in check across the developed world, there has been an increase across the MENA region. More investment in culturally sensitive strategic educational and support programs that target high-risk populations is required.
- Changing lifestyles and diet are resulting in increases in diseases such as prostate cancer and T2DM in a number of Middle Eastern countries.

REFERENCES

Abudabbeh, N., & Hays, P. (2006). Cognitive behavioral therapy with people of Arab heritage: *supervision* (pp. 141–159). Washington, DC: American Psychological Association.

Abu-Raddad, L.J., Akala, F.A., Semini, I., Riedner, G., Wilson, D., Tawil, O. (2010). Characterizing the HIV/AIDS Epidemic in the Middle East and North Africa: Time for Strategic Action. World Bank.

Addelaim, F. (2003). The relationship between anxiety and some parental treatment styles. *Arab Journal of Psychiatry*, 14(2), 116–126.

Al-Arrayed, S. S. (1999). Review of the spectrum of genetic diseases in Bahrain. *Eastern Mediterranean Health Journal*, 5(6), 435–440.

Al-Awadi, S. A., Moussa, M. A., Naguib, K. K., et al. (1985). Consanguinity among Kuwaiti population. *Clinical Genetics*, 27(5), 483–486.

Al-Gazali, L. I. (2005). Attitudes toward genetic counselling in the United Arab Emirates. *Community Genetics*, 8(1), 48–51.

Al-Gazali, L., Hamamy, H., & Al-Arrayad, S. (2006). Genetic disorders in the Arab World. *BMJ*, 333(7573), 831–834.

Ali, N. S., Khalil, H. Z., & Yousef, W. (1993). A comparison of American and Egyptian cancer patients' attitudes and unmet needs. *Cancer Nurse*, 16(3), 193–203.

Al-Khraif, R., Abdul Salam, A., & Abdul Rashid, M. F. (2020). Family demographic transition in Saudi Arabia: Emerging issues and concerns. *SAGE Open*, 10(1) 2158244020914556.

Al-Krenawi, A., & Lightman, E. S. (2000). Learning achievement, social adjustment, and family conflict among Bedouin-Arab children from polygamous and monogamous families. *The Journal of Social Psychology*, 140(3), 345–355.

Al-Thakeb, F. (1981). Size and composition of the Arab family: Census and survey data. *International Journal of Sociology of the Family*, 11(2), 171–178.

Al-Thakeb, F. (1985). The Arab family and modernity. Evidence from Kuwait. *Current Anthropology*, 26(5), 575–580.

Aref, A. (2020). United Nations Department of Economic and Social Affairs (UNDESA) Division for Inclusive Social Development Expert Group Meeting on "Families in development: Assessing progress, challenges and emerging issues. Focus on modalities for IYF+30 & parenting education" New York, 16–18. Available at https://www.un.org/development/desa/family/wp-content/uploads/sites/23/2020/06/Ahmed-Aref-Paper_Parenting-Styles-and-Programs-in-the-MENA-region_UNDESA-EGM-1.pdf. Accessed 11 August 2023.

Attum, B., Hafiz, S., Malik, A., et al. (2020). Cultural competence in the care of Muslim patients and their families. [Updated 2020 Jul 8]: *StatPearls [Internet]*. Treasure Island (FL): StatPearls Publishing. 2020 Jan-. Available at https://www.ncbi.nlm.nih.gov/books/NBK499933/. Accessed 31 July 2023.

Baumrind, D. (1991). The influence of parenting style on adolescent competence and substance use. *The Journal of Early Adolescence*, 11(1), 56–95.

Checa, P., & Abundis-Gutierrez, A. (2018). Parenting styles, academic achievement and the influence of culture. *Psychology and Psychotherapy: Research Study*, 1(4), 1–3.

Clark, C. J., Silverman, J. G., Shahrouri, M., Everson-Rose, S., & Groce, N. (2010). The role of the extended family in women's risk of intimate partner violence in Jordan. *Social Science & Medicine*, 70(1), 144–151.

De Costa, C. M. (2002). Consanguineous marriage and its relevance to obstetric practice. *Obstetrical & Gynecological Survey*, 57(8), 530–536. Aug 1.

Dhami, S., & Sheikh, A. (2000). The Muslim family: Predicament and promise. *The Western Journal of Medicine, 173*(5), 352–356.

Doan, R. M., & Bisharat, L. (1990). Female autonomy and child nutritional status: The extended-family residential unit in Amman, Jordan. *Social Science & Medicine, 31*(7), 783–789.

El-Haddad, Y. (2003). Major trends affecting families in the Gulf countries (pp. 1-24). na.

El-Hazmi, M. A., al-Swailem, A. R., Warsy, A. S., et al. (1995). Consanguinity among the Saudi Arabian population. *Journal of Medical Genetics, 32*(8), 623–626.

Engelen, T., & Puschmann, P. (2011). How unique is the Western European marriage pattern? A comparison of nuptiality in historical Europe and the contemporary Arab world. *The History of the Family, 16*(4), 387–400.

Ezenkwele, U. A., & Roodsari, G. S. (2013). Cultural competencies in emergency medicine: Caring for Muslim-American patients from the Middle East. *The Journal of Emergency Medicine, 45*(2), 168–174.

Farsoun, S. (1970). Family structure and society in modern Lebanon In L. E. Sweet American Museum of Natural History (Eds.), *Peoples and Cultures of the Middle East: an anthropological reader* (pp. 257–307). Garden City, NY: Published for the American Museum of Natural History [by] the Natural History Press 1970.

Faruqi, L. (1978). An extended family model from Islamic culture. *Journal of Comparative Family Studies, 9*(2), 243–256. Available at http://www.jstor.org/stable/41601050. Accessed 18 February 2021.

Fellous, M. (1981). Children for where? *Les Temps Modernes, 38*(424), 912–939.

Gadalla, S., McCarthy, J., & Campbell, O. (1985). How the number of living sons influences contraceptive use in Menoufia Governorate, Egypt. *Studies in Family Planning, 16*(3), 164–169.

Haj-Yahia, M. M. (2000). Wife abuse and battering in the sociocultural context of Arab society. *Family Process, 39*(2), 237–255.

Hamdy, S. (2006). *Our Bodies belong to God: Islam, medical science, and ethical reasoning in Egyptian life*. New York, NY: New York University.

Hammad, A., Kysia, R., Rabah, R., Hassoun, R., & Connelly, M. (1999). *Guide to Arab culture: Health care delivery to the Arab American community*. Dearborn, MI: Arab Community Center for Economic and Social Services (ACCESS).

Hattar-Pollara, M., Meleis, A. I., & Nagib, H. (2000). Multiple role stress and patterns of coping of Egyptian women in clerical jobs. *Health Care for Women International, 21*(4), 305–317.

Hilal, L., Shahait, M., Mukherji, D., Charafeddine, M., Farhat, Z., & Temraz, S. (2015). Prostate cancer in the Arab world: A view from the inside. *Clinical Genitourinary Cancer, 13*(6), 505–511. https://doi.org/10.1016/j.clgc.2015.05.010.

Hoodfar, E., & Teebi, A. S. (1996). Genetic referrals of Middle Eastern origin in a western city: inbreeding and disease profile. *Journal of Medical Genetics*, 212–215.

IDF DIABETES ATLAS. (2021). (10th ed.). International Diabetes Federation.

IN DANGER: UNAIDS Global AIDS (Update 2022). Geneva: Joint United Nations Programme on HIV/AIDS.

Kazarian, S. S. (2005). Family functioning, cultural orientation, and psychological well-being among university students in Lebanon. *The Journal of Social Psychology, 145*(2), 141–152.

Kennan, C. K., El-Haddad, A., & Balian, S. A. (1998). Factors associated with domestic violence in low-income Lebanese families. *Journal of Nursing Scholarship, 4*, 533–558.

Khalaf, I., & Callister, L. C. (1997). Cultural meanings of childbirth: Muslim women living in Jordan. *Journal of Holistic Nursing, 15*(4), 373–388.

Jastaniah, W. (2011). Epidemiology of sickle cell disease in Saudi Arabia. *Annals of Saudi Medicine, 31*(3), 289–293.

Meo, S. A., Sheikh, S. A., Sattar, K., Akram, A., Hassan, A., Meo, A. S., et al. (2019). Prevalence of type 2 diabetes mellitus among men in the Middle East: A retrospective study. *American Journal of Men's Health, 13*(3). https://doi.org/10.1177/1557988319848577.

Modell, B., & Darr, A. (2002). Genetic counselling and customary consanguineous marriage. *Nature Reviews. Genetics, 3*(3), 225–229. Mar.

Mukherji, D., Youssef, B., Dagher, C., El-Hajj, A., Nasr, R., Geara, F., et al. (2020). Management of patients with high-risk and advanced prostate cancer in the Middle East: Resource-stratified consensus recommendations. *World Journal of Urology, 38*(3), 681–693. https://doi.org/10.1007/s00345-019-02872-x.

Mumtaz, G. R., Chemaitelly, H., AlMukdad, S., Osman, A., Fahme, S., Rizk, N. A., et al. (2022). Status of the HIV epidemic in key populations in the Middle East and north Africa: Knowns and unknowns. *Lancet HIV, 9*(7), e506–e516. https://doi.org/10.1016/S2352-3018(22)00093-5.

Nasir, L. S., & Abdul-Haq, A. K. (2008). *Caring for Arab patients: A biopsychosocial approach*. Radcliffe Publishing.

NoFahim, H. I., & Faris, R. (1992). Child abuse as an inhibiting factor for family planning. *The Journal of the Egyptian Public Health Association, 67*(1-2), 1–11.

Patterson, J. E., Vakili, S., Richmond, E., & Abu-Hassan, H. H. (2020). Experiencing gender and culture differences in global healthcare settings: American students providing therapy in Jordan. *Journal of Feminist Family Therapy, 19*, 1–4. Apr.

Prothro, E. T., & Diab, L. N. (1974). *Changing Family Patterns in the Arab East*. Beirut: American University of Beirut.

Rassool, G. H. (2018). *Evil Eye, Jinn Possession, and Mental Health Issues: An Islamic Perspective* (1st ed.). Routledge. https://doi.org/10.4324/9781315623764.

Raz, A., & Star, M. (2004). Upright generations of the future: Traditions and medicalisation in community genetics. *Journal of Contemporary Ethnography, 33*(3), 296–322.

Roudi-Fahimi, F. (2004). *Islam and family planning*. Washington, DC: Population Reference Bureau. Jun 13.

Saffi, M., & Howard, N. (2015). Exploring the effectiveness of mandatory premarital screening and genetic counselling programmes for β-thalassaemia in the Middle East: A scoping review. *Public Health Genomics, 18*(4), 193–203.

Sanderson, D. (2018). Fast food putting Arab men at 'risk of prostate cancer'. *The National*. Available at https://www.thenationalnews.com/uae/health/fast-food-putting-arab-men-at-risk-of-prostate-cancer-1.783174. Accessed 6 August 2023.

Smadi, F. (2003). The Arabian Family in the light of Minuchin's systemic theory: An analytical approach. *Social Behavior and Personality*, *31*(5), 467–482.

Sorry, P., Schotsmans, P., & Dierickx, K. (2006). How international is bioethics? A quantitative retrospective study. *BMC Med Ethics*, *7*(1), E1.

Starr, P. (1978). Continuity and change in social distance: Studies from the Arab East - a research report. *Social Forces*, 1221–1227.

Teebi, A. S., & El-Shanti, H. I. (2006). Consanguinity: Implications for practice, research, and policy. *Lancet*, *367*(9515), 970–971.

Ypinazar, V. A., & Margolis, S. A. (2006). Delivering culturally sensitive care: The perceptions of older Arabian Gulf Arabs concerning religion, health, and disease. *Qualitative Health Research*, *16*(6), 773–787. Jul.

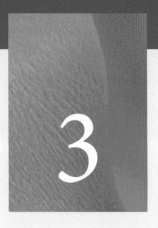

3 CONSUMER-DRIVEN HEALTHCARE

GARY E. DAY ■ AMINA AL MARZOUQI

CHAPTER OUTLINE

INTRODUCTION

Since the early 2000s, there has been a greater emphasis on the patient, or consumer, being central to decisions regarding not only their care and treatment options but also the cost of care. As more options for patient care become available, the increase in consumers' understanding of their own health needs through access to a greater number of information sources and the gradual increase in healthcare costs, means consumers are playing a larger part in healthcare decision-making. The concepts of patient- and consumer-centred healthcare start to become divergent when you consider that patient-centred care implies the patient is in the centre of care and being consulted on the decisions clinicians are making about their progress or treatment, whereas consumer-centred healthcare implies control over not only clinical decision-making but also financial decision-making.

While the Middle East is an ancient region of the world comprising many local and international cultures, the availability of high-quality, technological and data-driven healthcare is a more recent phenomenon. Additionally, the broader Middle East region is developing at different speeds, depending on national and international investment in health service provision and distribution. The fast pace of change in the development, funding, insuring and monitoring of primary, specialty and sub-specialty healthcare services in a culturally diverse region creates both opportunities and challenges for healthcare providers and consumers alike.

This chapter will explore the concept of consumer-driven healthcare (CDHC) and its understanding, uptake and application across the Greater Middle East.

BACKGROUND

Since the early 2000s, healthcare providers and insurers have been looking to shift some responsibility of health and healthcare to the individual. The initial concept of CDHC was initially conceived in the USA, primarily for the purpose of employers and insurers putting more choice in the hands of the employee through greater personal responsibility and at the same time reducing overall cost of health insurance premiums. Rook (2015) explains that CDHC is a name for the practice of setting up employee health plans with low premiums, high deductibles and savings accounts.

The primary goal of these healthcare insurance plans is to reduce costs for employers and encourage the individual to make more educated decisions about the care they seek, while at the same time increasing the number of individuals who have access to health insurance.

In systems where the employer or government are essentially the insurer, the concept of CDHC shifted the responsibility of the assessment of value-for-money and cost-effectiveness from the insurer to the individual. Robinson and Ginsburg (2009) argue that when in possession of adequate information and faced with appropriate incentives, consumers make better choices for their own health than does any third party. The philosophy of CDHC is promoted on the basis that it puts more power in the hands of the individual; however, this only works if the consumer has the necessary information to make informed decisions. 'The consumer-choice theory of cost containment assumes there is a free market in healthcare, that consumers are well informed about their choices, and that they will make more prudent choices if they are paying more of their costs' (Geyman, 2012, p. 574).

Consumers are faced with a plethora of options that enhance their healthcare choices and decisions including access to a range of modalities of care (in home, telemedicine), access to a wide array of personal healthcare data, availability of inexpensive wearable health devices and diagnostic apps, online shopping for medications and health products, direct access to medical specialists and a huge range of online medical resources. Consumers are able to tailor their healthcare, monitor their progress and consult with their physicians from the comfort and safety of their homes. Key to controlling costs, improving the quality of care and reducing iatrogenic incidents is to keep consumers out of hospital and doctors' offices (IBM Institute for Business Value, 2018). The globalisation and digitalisation of healthcare has created an environment where consumers have access to care and services from across the world.

The increase in health consumerism has grown in parallel with the ongoing evolution of health-related technology. The Middle East, particularly the United Arab Emirates (UAE), is not immune from the burgeoning growth and intrusion of technology that has driven much of the first-world healthcare systems. In the Gulf Cooperative Council (GCC) states, much of the growth over the last 50 years has been on the back of vast reserves of oil and gas. The rapid rise in sovereign and personal wealth as a result of these sought-after natural resources has also created a substantial burden of chronic disease such as coronary heart disease, obesity, hypertension (Taylor, 2009) and type 2 diabetes (Klautzer et al., 2014). This is particularly evident amongst the female population across the GCC countries (Alshaikh et. al., 2017).

Considerable numbers of the Greater Middle East population are caught in a conundrum of the trappings of affluence demonstrated by growing levels of chronic disease in the community while at the same time having greater ability to make healthcare choices supported by unparalleled access to technology and services. How the consumer makes personal health decisions with this two-edged sword of chronic disease management and data- and technology-driven healthcare will set the scene for how health services are developed, implemented and distributed across the Greater Middle East for decades to come.

Evidence-Base: Global/Regional

History of Consumer-Driven Healthcare

CDHC was derived in the United States over 20 years ago. The impetus for such an approach was driven by spiralling health costs and a growing awareness of the consumer to be more actively engaged in the process, either by self-determination or through more active approaches by health insurers and employers to engage the consumer in the decision-making process. The term CDHC refers to health plans in which individuals have a personal health account, such as a health savings account (HSA) or a health reimbursement arrangement (HRA), from which they pay medical expenses directly. The phrase is sometimes used more broadly to refer to defined contribution health plans, which allow employees to choose among various plans, often with a fixed dollar contribution from an employer (Herrick, 2005).

For more than 30 years, most USA health economists have accepted a conventional theory of health insurance based on the concept of moral hazard: an assumption is made that insured people overuse healthcare services because they have insurance. The trend towards CDHC in the early 2000s is advocated by its supporters based on this same premise, assuming that imprudent choices by patients can be avoided if they are held more financially responsible for their healthcare choices through larger co-payments and deductibles and other restrictions (Geyman, 2007). With more control over where to spend money on healthcare and armed with more information, it would not be unfair to think that there are endless possibilities for the health savvy consumer. Herzlinger (2002) points out however that when consumers apply pressure on an industry, whether it is retailing or banking, cars or computers, it invariably produces a surge of innovation that increases productivity, reduces prices, improves quality and expands choices. The essential problem with the healthcare industry is that it has been shielded from consumer control—by employers, insurers and the government. As a result, costs have exploded as choices have narrowed. While CHDC has had only moderate success in curbing costs and increasing choice in the USA, due primarily to the imbalance of power, information and moral hazard, CDHC in other countries with different approaches to health insurance has fared little better.

As healthcare has become more privatised in Europe, with a higher reliance on health insurance to stabilise healthcare expenditure, consumers have not benefitted from the global push to have the end user much more engaged in the healthcare decision-making process. Even in high-performing healthcare systems such as Switzerland and the Netherlands, the push for more efficient care through consumer choice has led to inequities in care due to high health insurance plan deductibles (Sandoval et al., 2020) as well as an inability for policy makers to realise reforms and gaps between the theoretical concepts of managed competition and the actual improvements in the health system (Okma & Crivelli, 2013).

With CDHC being devised by healthcare providers and insurers to curb spending while at the same time putting decision-making into the hands of the purchasers of healthcare, the last 20 years has shown that there may be more effective ways to increase consumer participation and control health expenditure. This notion is particularly critical in the Middle East as health insurance coverage varies greatly depending on employment type, the Emirate or country of residence and immigration status as well as nationality; and there

are multiple educational, social and cultural aspects that reduce informed decision-making and choice.

Creating Value in Healthcare

One of the key concepts of CDHC is creating value. Value can be viewed from whether the consumer (purchaser) felt they received a quality outcome for a fair price (the cost of any insurance and co-payment or deductible) or from the perspective of the insurance company/healthcare organisation (provider) believing they provided a service in an efficient manner. Value in healthcare must be thought of primarily from the consumer's perspective. As health insurance and the cost of care becomes more expensive, the end user needs to believe that there is a fair exchange between health outcomes and the ongoing cost of healthcare. The concept of value becomes more important as consumers spend more money to insure their health against a backdrop of an ageing population with an underlying burden of chronic disease. Putera (2017) posits that value is created from health outcomes which matter to patients relative to the cost of achieving those outcomes. The health outcomes should include all domains of health in a full cycle of care.

'Value' should always be defined around the customer, and in a well-functioning healthcare system, the creation of value for patients should determine the rewards for all other actors in the system. Since value depends on results, not inputs, value in healthcare is measured by the outcomes achieved, not the volume of services delivered, and shifting focus from volume to value is a central challenge (Porter, 2010, in Baumhauer & Bozic, 2016, p. 1375).

Value in healthcare, particularly in the Middle East, becomes difficult to determine when there is a lack of viable options for different aspects of care. With limited or scattered primary healthcare options and restricted private secondary and tertiary choices, consumers are often left with decisions that do not align with what could be considered value-based healthcare.

Health Insurance and Customer Choice

For a system where there is an expectation that the consumer becomes more active in their healthcare choices and can make informed decisions about care options and where they should spend their money, there needs to be substantial reform from the health providers and insurers. Herzlinger (2002) argues that CDHC requires that companies revamp their health benefits in six ways, namely: give employees incentives to shop intelligently; offer a real choice of insurance plans; charge employees prices that accurately reflect the company's costs; let providers set their own prices; adjust payments for each enrolee based on need; and provide relevant information. In many ways this may not serve large population groups across the Middle East, particularly lower paid expatriate workers and labourers, as they do not have equal access to information due to literacy and technology issues, to adequately inform customer choice.

Information Technology and Artificial Intelligence

One of the key enablers of a more engaged and knowledgeable health consumer over the last 20 years has been the rapid growth and penetration of information technology (IT), health applications and the outcomes of big data. It is also the case that while the consumer has been armed with more information about their condition, surgery and potential treatment options, hospitals, governments and insurers have gathered large amounts of patient- and population-level data to better understand the market. This data has been used in part to tailor health insurance plans, cost profiles and population health responses for patient groups. While the consumer has had access to their electronic health record and a wide array of online health information, they have not had access to the quality of health data that could help inform and support decision-making.

Beeuwkes et al. (2006) suggest that CDHC assumes that giving consumers greater financial responsibility for healthcare choices will lead them to demand accurate information about service costs and quality. Some insurance plans have launched programs to provide information on fees that they have negotiated for specific medical procedures and on prices for prescription drugs. Participants in CDHC plans appear to make greater use of this information. They are more likely to ask providers about costs and to pay attention to preventive services. Nevertheless, participants in consumer-directed plans generally reported that they lack sufficient information to support their decisions about costs or provider performance (Beeuwkes et al., 2006).

Accessible, high-speed internet and the availability of cheap, wearable devices has changed the landscape for consumers in the ways they interact with the healthcare system. Consumer wearables are providing patients with personalised health data, which could assist with self-diagnosis and behaviour change interventions, as well as provide real-time feeds via the internet to their physicians or nurses. While there has been an explosion in the acceptance, use and reliance of cost-effective wearable health devices over the last 10 years, there remains several concerns about the safety, reliability, confidentiality and security of using consumer wearables in healthcare (Piwek et al., 2016).

Despite the concerns, it cannot be ignored that it is now possible for the well-informed consumer to make individual choice and be an active participant in their own care, clinical decision-making and treatment. Herrick (2005) points to several direct health and decision-making benefits that integrated IT and the Internet have afforded the consumer, including:

■ Using the Internet to freely browse medical journals and libraries for information previously available only to professionals at a cost of thousands of dollars.
■ Obtaining a battery of more than 50 blood tests for as little as $90 by leaving a blood sample at a commercial testing centre.
■ E-mailing personal physicians to obtain a diagnosis rather than making an in-office visit.
■ Using the Internet to have test results evaluated or obtain a second opinion from a web-based physician.
■ Shopping online for lower-cost prescription drugs or over-the-counter equivalents, saving up to 90% off the cost of brand name prescriptions.

Regional

Technology plays a vital part in healthcare and will affect decision-making for consumers, regulators and healthcare providers. With the digitisation of data, regulators can plan for the future while providers can streamline processes and build on their research and analytics (Technology is Transforming Health Care in the UAE, 2017).

Healthcare industry planners and government health institution leaders are increasingly looking towards technology to provide this innovative, faster and more responsive approach. In line with UAE

Vision 2021, and to enable authentic, intelligent city living, the UAE wants its healthcare sector to be among the most innovative globally, sitting alongside key bright infrastructure elements to give its citizens and visitors the best possible healthcare outcomes.

The healthcare delivery system in the UAE is undergoing innovative transformation to meet the current and anticipated population growth needs with new state-of-the-art hospitals being designed and built. Insurance reforms shift the healthcare economic risk from a government-funded model to a more traditional managed care model. The UAE Health Authority has defined health data standards to ensure that providers and insurers are reporting data consistently; the health system in the UAE is leveraging this empirical data to drive population-based healthcare reforms and healthy lifestyle initiatives.

Hospitals are initiating and investing in new healthcare technologies, especially in the areas of software based, and therapeutic and diagnostic advanced technologies. The innovative initiatives are transforming and improving healthcare in the UAE (Hawkins, 2021).

SPECIFIC CHALLENGES/REGIONAL ASPECTS

Specific Challenges

There are number of challenges to the concept of a consumer-driven health plan (CDHP), whether it be globally or regionally specific. The first challenge is access to technology and being health literate. Although the availability of information upon which participants can make their healthcare decisions is critical to CDHPs, such information may be unavailable due to a lack of credible data and systematic, comprehensive methods of accumulating and disseminating such data. Even if credible data is available, it may not be equally accessible to all users. Furthermore, some may not be savvy enough to navigate the technology developed to disseminate information. This could result both in poor medical plan elections or personal decision-making made at the time of enrolment as well as poor ongoing treatment and healthcare provider choices made at the time of service. Another potential problem is that even if information is successfully gathered, individuals may not yet have the necessary skills to effectively evaluate

what they have gathered or been provided. Will personal healthcare and medical knowledge become more of a formal basic education requirement, or will it be left to those who wish to pursue such knowledge independently? (American Academy of Actuaries, 2004). Beeuwkes et al. (2006) lament the lack of health literacy by arguing that up to half of Americans find it difficult to understand health information, which likely hinders their ability to obtain high-quality care. Equally, research does not fully support the link between access to health data, consumer choice and health behaviour change. The small body of evidence available provides no consistent evidence that the public release of performance data changes consumer behaviour or improves care (Metcalfe et al., 2018).

Similarly, if the consumer has any number of chronic diseases or mental illness, full decision-making may not be possible. Consumers' lack of competence to participate was frequently perceived by mental health specialty providers to be a primary barrier to shared decision-making, while information provision on illness and treatment to consumers was cited by healthcare providers from all professions to be an important facilitator of shared decision-making (Chong et al., 2013).

Secondly, CDHC is affected by the cost of care. Consumers have a range of decision points about care including types of treatments or procedures, ease of access to healthcare, the cost and availability of suitable health insurance, the treating doctor and the cost of care. The United States has a dramatic 'cost of care' problem and is facing a significant trade-off between cost of care and access to care that is precipitated by the burgeoning numbers of uninsured in the United States. Likewise, Canada and the United Kingdom have a severe 'quality of care' problem and are facing a significant trade-off between quality of care and cost of care that is manifested by increasing healthcare tourism to the south (Brooke, 2000, Chinta & Chinta, 2013). Finally, Switzerland faces the trade-off between access to care and quality of care as market forces determine what to provide and what not to provide (Chinta & Chinta, 2013).

Although consumer choice is central to CDHC, it is easy to gloss over the fact that healthcare does not meet the conditions necessary for efficient consumer choice (Chinta & Chinta, 2013). Economic theory demonstrates that consumer choice enhances efficiency only if (1) individuals know with certainty the level of satisfaction they will obtain from a product or service, (2) they are rational, (3) they have sufficient information to make good choices (i.e., they know what choices are available and the opportunity costs of each choice) and (4) they are the best judges of their own welfare.

Consumer choice in many respects is limited by the country and the fundamental approach to insurance and the funding of health services. It could also be argued that those in the major metropolitan centres have far greater choice in relation to the variety and cost of healthcare services (due primarily to competition) than those in regional and remote locations (Case Study 3.1).

Finally, to ensure that consumers have access to the best quality healthcare, there needs to be a greater emphasis on understanding clinical outcomes, performance measures and the cost of care. Strategies must be developed to manage the evaluation of which outcomes relate to which performance. This is especially apparent in fragmented healthcare systems and for patients with long-term and multisetting care needs. Therefore, healthcare systems that strive to establish value-based care must collaborate beyond organisational boundaries to create clear patient trajectories (Elf et al., 2017). Thus, there are challenges that need to be addressed before value-based health services are likely to drive quality improvement and informed decision-making for people with complex long-term conditions (Elf et al., 2017).

Regional Aspects

Over the past few decades, Arab countries have witnessed marked improvements in the health status of their population, as evidenced by economic, social and health indicators. Unfortunately, this improvement has not been consistent across different socioeconomic groups. Sharp social inequalities and health inequities are found between rural and urban regions, income groups, gender and ethnic groups. It is striking to see that postnatal mortality may be five times more significant in children belonging to the poorest quintile in these countries than in children in the wealthiest quintile. Similarly, a child of an illiterate woman is three times more likely to die than a child of a woman with a secondary or higher level of education. Finally,

CASE STUDY 3.1
MEDICAL TOURISM IN THE MIDDLE EAST

One classic example of CDHC in the Greater Middle East is the rapid rise in medical tourism in the UAE (Bulatovic & Iankova, 2021). Medical tourism can be classified as either inbound (flying to the UAE) or outbound (flying elsewhere). Outbound medical tourism has largely been used where medical services are not available in the UAE (organ transplant or specialised cancer treatments) or where there has been a lack of suitably qualified specialists or there are long waiting periods.

Abu Dhabi and Dubai are identified in the top 10 worldwide destinations for medical tourism (Medical Tourism Association, 2020). As a part of its economic diversification strategy, the UAE has invested heavily in establishing world-class medical facilities, with high treatment standards for citizens as well as for people from outside, especially from the Middle East and Africa, who come to UAE on medical tourist visas (Ahmed et al., 2018). Inbound medical tourists have the ultimate choice in terms of CDHC as a majority of these consumers are self-funded (not covered by insurance) and have direct control over the costs of treatment.

Consumers identify the UAE as a medical tourism destination, particularly for cosmetic and aesthetic surgery, for a number of key reasons, namely: (1) the UAE is a major airline transport hub connecting the world, (2) a significant number of western trained Arabic surgeons work out of the UAE, (3) a significant level of choice across a range of specialties and price points, (4) there is significant investment in medical technology, (5) a high level of internationally accredited healthcare facilities and (6) due to the climate, political stability and availability of world-class hotels and accommodation, the UAE is seen as a perfect destination for a vacation and postoperative recuperation.

postnatal mortality is 2.5 times greater in rural areas than in cities. The World Health Organization (WHO), focusing on social determinants of health, highlighted the crucial importance of social determinants in their impact on access, utilisation and health status. There has been a total absence of sound and long-term social policies to combat poverty, deprivation, sex differences, social exclusion and unemployment in the social field. It has contributed to increased disparities within and between countries. Governments will need to address social policies to protect equity, promote solidarity and reduce inequalities (Kronfol, 2012). Equally, there needs to be a concerted effort to put more decision-making into the hands of consumers at the point of care. It should no longer be the case that healthcare is delivered to, or imposed on, consumers without their contribution to the decision-making process involving their own health.

Governments have an essential role in health development in the Arab region (Case Study 3.2). The efforts initiated by governments to build modern health systems must be continued and adapted to the new changes and challenges in the political, economic, social and cultural fields. Despite the pressures facing governments in managing the social sectors, Ministries of Health should continue to play their leadership role in health development. They should protect the social values of equity, solidarity and fairness. Health development should be coordinated between all concerned government ministries and agencies and all stakeholders by implementing and following the intersectoral cooperation approach, including academia, professional associations, the private sector and civil society organisations. Efforts should be made to promote the centrality of health in comprehensive socioeconomic development.

The private sector is assuming a growing role in both financing and delivery of healthcare. Intersectoral care must ensure that such actions are implemented under strong leadership and governance from governments. Government commitment is highly prevalent among healthcare providers across countries in the Middle East. Healthcare system strength is needed in a region that has endured years of ongoing conflict and is now into its third year of addressing the COVID-19 pandemic. An urgent reform to design and implement programs that tackle burnout among health professionals (Chemali et al., 2019) needs to be a priority to ensure that the local workforce do not undertake wholesale migration to more stable countries as well as making sure there is an active, patient-focused workforce in the country.

Equity is being fair in providing healthcare services according to the needs of different population groups. Healthcare services are essential to other social determinants such as education, employment, appropriate housing and other essential services (Hernández-Rincón et al., 2016). In 1978, the WHO initiated Primary Health Care (PHC) through the Al Mata Declaration (Somocurcio Vílchez, 1978). PHC is based

CASE STUDY 3.2
HEALTH INSURANCE REFORM IN THE UAE

The mass protests that swept the MENA region since December 2010 called for social justice and a dignified life and well-being for all citizens. Beyond the political and economic dimensions, these popular uprisings were also fuelled by a strong sense of discontent with struggling health systems that have not delivered on the promise for better, more affordable and equitable healthcare. Compared with other regions in the world, MENA countries have some of the lowest levels of public spending on health, which continue to translate into high levels of out-of-pocket expenses (Yabeck et al., 2017).

In the UAE, while health insurance is a mandatory requirement for all categories of citizens and residents and floor pricing for the premiums have already been fixed, with services such as pandemic coverage and the growing demand for mental healthcare to become an integral part of basic insurance covers, the health insurance industry as we knew it is set to turn on its head and become, in the process, more competitive and mature (Droesch, 2021). The Emirate of Abu Dhabi has taken concrete steps to reform health insurance by improving the access to health providers as well as freedom of choice. The growing cost of healthcare and the impact of the global financial crisis have meant that countries are no longer able to solely bear the cost (Hamidi et al., 2014).

The Abu Dhabi model has private sector involvement, but the government sets prices and benefits. The Abu Dhabi model adequately deals with the problem of adverse selection through making insurance coverage a mandatory requirement. There are issues with moral hazards, which are a combination of individual and medical practitioner behaviour that might affect the efficiency of the system (Hamidi et al., 2014). The current system works well, but with changing population trends (ageing population), demographics (mix of population), community health profile (chronic disease) and consumer demands (CDHC), the insurance system may come under financial pressure. According to Davidson (2015), when it comes to insurance failure, the reasons are often complex. There are those issues that now beset every modern health service: the influence of multinational corporations seeking to increase their profits by inflating the medical economy; newer/better imaging technologies that are so sensitive that they often demonstrate some minor 'abnormality', which then leads on to further investigations necessary only to reassure a now anxious patient; the all-pervasive influence of the pharmaceutical industry; and the impact of private medicine.

If these changes put more pressure on the healthcare insurance market in the UAE, the government may be forced to step in and put limits on its financial exposure.

on providing comprehensive and essential healthcare services accessible, affordable, acceptable and available to every individual. The PHC services were initiated to implement equity and reduce diversity among different groups of the population. Vulnerable groups within any country are the most suffering and deprived of essential healthcare services, especially promotive and preventive healthcare services. PHC implementation shows achievement and reduces inequity. Decentralisation of healthcare facilities is one of the essential principles of the PHC. The UAE and many other Arab countries implemented the decentralisation of the PHC services to implement equity and make needed healthcare services available to the population. The Sultanate of Oman achieved an outstanding target by reducing the under-five child mortality rate from more than 160 per 1000 in 1975 to less than 10 per 1000 in 2006 (De Maeseneer et al., 2008).

However, equity does not include accessibility or choice of the services, but the availability of the services needed by the population regardless of geographical areas. Disease and health problems are significant challenges facing humanity. Types of diseases have different trends based on many social factors. Across many Arab countries, there is an increasing number of lifestyle diseases caused primarily from smoking, diet and lifestyle habits. These lifestyle diseases have seen conditions such as diabetes and chronic renal failure amongst some of the highest rates in world (Islam et al., 2014).

CDHC is integrated within the PHC initiative by focusing on the health promotion and preventive services. Customer participation is considered to be the essential principle of PHC. Self-reliance focuses on the education and awareness level of individuals and communities. Healthcare systems need to encourage community participation to raise the awareness level and decrease the incidence of non-communicable diseases. Successful achievement of self-reliance are based on people-centred healthcare services (Sejin Ha, 2011). A PHC approach should define the population's needs and ensure the continuity of the services based on comprehensive preventive healthcare services. Despite the diversity of the healthcare delivery system in the UAE, more than 100 PHC centres provide a comprehensive care focussed on preventive services. Primary services are directed towards children and women within a systematic Women and Child Health Care Service, starting from premarital consultation to pre-natal, postnatal, a national immunisation programme and school healthcare (Bodolica & Spraggon, 2019).

SPECIFIC INTERVENTIONS

To improve CDHC in the Middle East, there needs to be a focus on refining and enhancing systems and structures that engage consumers in the care process. This is particularly important for those with chronic disease and mental health issues. A recent study suggests that changes may be necessary at several levels (i.e., consumer, provider and environment) to implement effective shared decision-making and interprofessional collaboration in mental healthcare (Chong et al., 2013).

One of the keys to greater consumer participation and therefore decision-making, particularly in chronic disease management, is to create the environment for behavioural change. Putting decision-making into the hands of consumers to make informed choices about their health status can be greatly enhanced by harnessing digital technology married to inexpensive wearable devices. Devices and programs using digital technology to foster or support behaviour change (digital interventions) are increasingly ubiquitous, being adopted for use in patient diagnosis and treatment, self-management of chronic diseases, and in primary prevention. They have been heralded as potentially revolutionising the ways in which individuals can monitor and improve their health behaviours and healthcare by improving outcomes, reducing costs and improving patient experience (Michie et al., 2017).

It is evident that as technology becomes much more affordable and almost 'disposable', wearable health devices are allowing consumers to be much more active in their decision-making about their healthcare options. Patients and practitioners regularly use digital technology (e.g., thermometers and glucose monitors) to identify and discuss symptoms. In addition, a third of general practitioners in the United Kingdom report that patients arrive with suggestions for treatment based on online search results, and in the United States, one in six (15%) consumers currently uses wearable technology, including smartwatches or fitness bands (Piwek et al., 2016).

The availability of predictive analytics and data to support CDHC is often seen as an important tool in allowing the consumer to make an informed healthcare choice. Predictive analytics, or the use of electronic algorithms to forecast future events in real time, makes it possible to harness the power of big data to improve the health of patients and lower the cost of healthcare. However, this opportunity raises policy, ethical and legal challenges (Cohen et al., 2014). If these challenges are addressed, consumers can have confidence in how the data is generated, stored and used.

Many Middle East countries have seen rapid growth in their populations and infrastructure over the last 50 years. This rapid growth, led initially by oil and gas discovery and production and more lately by financial and business hubs, has put both pressure and opportunity on the health and education sectors. In addition to state-funded and -operated healthcare services, private operators have provided much needed infrastructure to bring additional clinical specialisation and staff as the population and citizens needs and choice grows. For example, in Saudi Arabia, people are increasingly relying on private healthcare organisations to manage their healthcare needs. This trend will persist because of the essentials that drive demand, such as increased life expectancy, population growth and patients' need for treatment. Therefore, the private sector in Saudi Arabia offers attractive incentives to investors from commercial and social perspectives. While the government is the dominant force in the healthcare sector, the increasing population and health expenditures are forcing the government to enact considerable changes in the healthcare system (Yusuf, 2014). The increased focus on building infrastructure needs to also include integration of health records and information to allow for a more seamless health system, which creates greater opportunities for consumer choice irrespective of where it is accessed.

SUMMARY AND TAKEAWAY POINTS

To fully engage the community's participation in CDHC requires commitment to transparency, cost-effective clinical services, equitable access to primary, secondary and tertiary healthcare facilities, accessible and affordable health insurance and a commitment to putting in place supports for chronic disease prevention and management and ageing populations. Because

countries across the Middle East have different demographic profiles and organise their health systems and financing differently, no single approach will be successful, and regions need to find solutions that meet their local circumstances. Additionally, health policy, funding and systems need to be aligned to ensure consumers can be active and informed in decision-making about their own healthcare (Case Study 3.3).

CASE STUDY 3.3
HEALTHCARE QUALITY AND PATIENT EXPECTATIONS

Like developed healthcare systems across the globe, consumers in the Middle East look for the same level of service, quality and cost as those in first-world countries. Consumers expect more from health services irrespective of whether they are public or private services. In a recent study of UAE consumer perceptions of public and private hospitals, the perceived healthcare services in private hospitals and public hospitals do not significantly vary. Although patients were more satisfied with nursing care, the perceived satisfaction of patients with the quality of services provided by physicians and nurses as well as the quality of the hospital environment do not significantly vary in both public and private hospitals (Al-Neyadi et al., 2018).

In a recent 2014 report, Deloitte Consulting (2014) reports that outpatient satisfaction levels are trending downwards in the UAE. Consumers rated a visit to a healthcare provider as the second most dissatisfying consumer experience (17%) across a range of industry sectors (interaction with health insurers was rated worst at 18%). Consumers in the UAE have been spoilt for choice when it comes to shopping and retail. Consumers are starting to exert their power by making more demands on the healthcare provider–patient relationship and expecting to be treated in much the same way they are accustomed to being treated in their daily interactions with retailers. Deloitte Consulting (2014) points to three main themes that are shifting consumers expectation for better quality, service and outcomes. These include:

- Increased knowledge and awareness of choice
- Increasing expectation for value and cost transparency
- Increasing desire for a collaborative provider–patient relationship

Deloitte Consulting (2014) argues that if healthcare providers adopted these themes, as retailers have, consumers would get a much better quality of service.

In addition to the three themes, there is a fourth that can be considered that aligns with the retail experience, that being the ability to access high-quality online services. Much as retailers have moved to online shopping, particularly accelerated by COVID-19, healthcare consumers want ready access to online consultations, online health product purchasing as well as product, disease and lifestyle information.

Healthcare, as well as retail consumers are price sensitive, and this is a contributing factor to their perceptions of quality. Omna Health (2020) reported that despite having seen positive investments in infrastructure and services this year, the UAE unfortunately continues to grapple with issues around pricing, access and affordability, while regulation of medicines remains a challenge. Digitisation across the care pathway is aiding efficiencies and positively impacting patient care, while at the same time providing a quality patient experience.

Enhancing services for Middle East and North Africa (MENA) citizens requires forging a stronger social contract among public servants, citizens and service providers while empowering communities and local leaders to find 'best fit' solutions. Learning from the variations within countries, especially the outstanding local successes, can serve as a solid basis for new ideas and inspiration for improving service delivery (Brixi et al., 2015).

In summary, to improve and enhance CDHC, health services in the Greater Middle East requires:

- Provision of wider choice in the equitable access to health services.
- Continuing to develop, support and implement preventive health and primary health services that encourage greater consumer self-reliance and choice.
- Consumer access to health information that can assist in the decision-making process, through the use of 'wearables' and other information gathering approaches.
- Refining health insurance to make it more affordable, accessible and transparent, and provide incentives for consumers to maintain their health.
- Greater integration of the public and private healthcare sector as well as health records and information to allow greater consumer choice.
- Broadening approaches, education and usable information to enable consumers to be more health literate.

REFERENCES

Ahmed, G., Al Amiri, N., & Khan, W. (2018). Outward medical tourism: A case of UAE. *Theoretical Economics Letters*, *8*, 1368–1390.

Al-Neyadi, H. S., Abdallah, S., & Malik, M. (2018). Measuring patient's satisfaction of healthcare services in the UAE hospitals: Using SERVQUAL. *International Journal of Healthcare Management*, *11*(2), 96–105.

Alshaikh, M. K., Filippidis, F. T., Al-Omar, H. A., Rawaf, S., Majeed, A., & Salmasi, A. M. (2017). The ticking time bomb in lifestyle-related diseases among women in the Gulf Cooperation Council countries; Review of systematic reviews. *BMC Public Health*, *17*(1), 536.

American Academy of Actuaries, (2004). *The impact of consumer-driven health plans on health care costs: A closer look at plans with health reimbursement accounts*. Washington DC: Public Policy Monograph. January 2004.

Baumhauer, J. F., & Bozic, K. J. (2016). Value-based healthcare: Patient-reported outcomes in clinical decision making. *Clinical Orthopaedics and Related Research*, *474*, 1375–1378.

Beeuwkes, B. M., Damberg, C., Haviland, A., Kapur, K., Lurie, N., McDevitt, R., & Marquis, M. S. (2006). Consumer-Directed health care: Early evidence about effects on cost and quality. *Health Aff*, *25*(6), w516–w530.

Bodolica, V., & Spraggon, M. (2019). Toward patient-centered care and inclusive health-care governance: A review of patient empowerment in the UAE. *Public Health*, *169*, 114–124. https://doi.org/10.1016/j.puhe.2019.01.017.

Brixi, H., Lust, E., & Woolcock, M. (2015). *Trust, voice, and incentives: Learning from local success stories in service delivery in the Middle East and North Africa (English)*. Washington, D.C.: World Bank Group. Available at http://documents.worldbank.org/curated/en/381671468280164518/Trust-voice-and-incentives-learning-from-local-success-stories-in-service-delivery-in-the-MiddleEast-and-North-Africa.

Brooke, J. (2000). Full hospitals make Canadians wait and look south. *The New York Times*. Sect. 1, p. 3, col. 1, 16 January.

Bulatovic, I., & Iankova, K. (2021). Barriers to medical tourism development in the United Arab Emirates (UAE). *International Journal of Environmental Research and Public Health*, *18*, 1365.

Chemali, Z., Ezzeddine, F. L., Gelaye, B., Dossett, M. L., Salameh, J., Bizri, M., Dubale, B., & Fricchione, G. (2019). Burnout among healthcare providers in the complex environment of the Middle East: A systematic review. *BMC Public Health*, *19*(1). https://doi.org/10.1186/s12889-019-7713-1.

Chinta, D., & Chinta, R. (2013). Comparing health care systems in Canada/UK, USA and Switzerland to assess the direction of US health care reform. *GSTF Journal on Business Review (GBR)*, *2*(4), 171–176.

Chong, W. W., Aslani, P., & Chen, T. F. (2013). Shared decision-making and interprofessional collaboration in mental healthcare: A qualitative study exploring perceptions of barriers and facilitators. *Journal of Interprofessional Care*, *27*(5), 373–379.

Cohen, I. G., Amarasingham, R., Shah, A., Xie, B., & Lo, B. (2014). The legal and ethical concerns that arise from using complex predictive analytics in health care. *Health Aff*, 33(7). https://www.healthaffairs.org/doi/full/10.1377/hlthaff.2014.0048.

Davidson, R. (2015). Too much medicine in the Middle East? *British Journal of General Practice*, 65(637), 418. Available at https://bjgp.org/content/65/637/418.

Deloitte Consulting (2014). The Tail Wagging the Dog. How Retail is Changing Consumer Expectations of the Health Care Patient-Provider Relationship. Report available at https://www2.deloitte.com/tr/en/pages/life-sciences-and-healthcare/articles/how-retail-is-changing-consumer-expectations-of-the-health-care-patient-provider-relationship.html.

De Maeseneer, J., Moosa, S., Pongsupap, Y., & Kaufman, A. (2008). Primary health care in a changing world'. *British Journal of General Practice*, 58(556), 806–809. https://doi.org/10.3399/bjgp08X342697.

Droesch, J. (2021). What's next for health insurance in the Middle East post coronavirus? *Arabian Business* April, Available from https://www.arabianbusiness.com/comment/461603-whats-next-for-health-insurance-in-the-MiddleEast-post-coronavirus.

Elf, M., Flink, M., Nilsson, M., et al. (2017). The case of value-based healthcare for people living with complex long-term conditions. *BMC Health Services Research*, 17(24) Available at https://link.springer.com/article/10.1186/s12913-016-1957-6.

Geyman, J. P. (2007). Moral hazard and consumer-driven health care: A fundamentally flawed concept. *Journal of Law, Medicine & Ethics*, 37(2), 333–351.

Geyman, J. P. (2012). Cot-sharing under consumer-driven healthcare will not reform U.S. health care. *Journal of Law, Medicine & Ethics*, 40(3), 574–581.

Hamidi, S., Shaban, S., Mahate, A. A., & Younis, M. Z. (2014). Health insurance reform and the development of health insurance plans: The case of the Emirate of Abu Dhabi, UAE. *Journal of Health Care Finance*, 40(3), 47–66.

Hawkins, J.R., (2021). Healthcare IT in UAE: An innovative transformation. Asian Hospital & Health Care Management. Available at https://www.asianhhm.com/information-technology/healthcareit-uae.

Hernández-Rincón, E. H., Pimentel-González, J. P., Orozco-Beltrán, D., & Carratalá-Munuera, C. (2016). Inclusion of the equity focus and social determinants of health in health care education programmes in Colombia: A qualitative approach. *Family Practice*, 33(3), 268–273. https://doi.org/10.1093/fampra/cmw010.

Herrick, D.M., (2005). Consumer Driven Health Care: The Changing Role of the Patient. National Center for Policy Analysis. NCPA Policy Report No. 276, May 2005. Available at http://hrvirtualsolutions.com/st276.pdf.

Herzlinger, R. E. (2002). Let's put consumers in charge of health care. *Harvard Business Review*, 80(7), 44–50. Available at https://hbr.org/2002/07/lets-put-consumers-in-charge-of-health-care.

IBM Institute for Business Value (2018). Consumers at the Heart of Healthcare. Available at https://www.ibm.com/downloads/cas/5MWZ9BWQ.

Islam, S. M., Purnat, T. D., Phuong, N. T., Mwingira, U., Schacht, K., & Fröschl, G. (2014). Non-communicable diseases in developing countries: A symposium report. *Global Health*. https://doi.org/10.1057/9781137354785.

Klautzer, L., Becker, J., & Mattke, S. (2014). The curse of wealth-Middle Eastern Countries need to address the rapidly rising burden of diabetes. *International Journal of Health Policy and Management*, 2(3), 109–114.

Kronfol, N. M. (2012). Access and barriers to health care delivery in Arab countries: A review'. *Eastern Mediterranean Health Journal*. https://doi.org/10.26719/2012.18.12.1239.

Medical Tourism Association (2020). Medical Tourism Index. Available at https://www.medicaltourism.com/mti/home.

Michie, S., Yardley, L., West, R., Patrick, K., & Greaves, F. (2017). Developing and evaluating digital interventions to promote behavior change in health and health care: Recommendations resulting from an international workshop. *Journal of Medical Internet Research*, 19(6), e232. Available at https://www.jmir.org/2017/6/e232.

Metcalfe, D., Rios Diaz, A. J., Olufajo, O. A., Massa, M. S., Ketelaar, N., Flottorp, S. A., & Perry, D. C. (2018). Impact of public release of performance data on the behaviour of healthcare consumers and providers. *Cochrane Database of Systematic Reviews*, 9, Art. No. CD004538. https://doi.org/10.1002/14651858.CD004538.pub3.

Okma, K. G. H., & Crivelli, L. (2013). Swiss and Dutch "consumer-driven health care": Ideal model or reality? *Health Policy*, 109(2), 105–112. Available at https://www.sciencedirect.com/science/article/abs/pii/S0168851012002850.

Omna Health. (2020). Middle East Health Care Barometer. Available at https://insights.omnia-health.com/hospital-management/Middle-East-healthcare-barometer-2020.

Piwek, L., Ellis, D. A., Andrews, S., & Joinson, A. (2016). The rise of consumer health wearables: Promises and barriers. *PLoS Medicine*, 13(2), e1001953. Available at https://journals.plos.org/plosmedicine/article?id=10.1371/journal.pmed.1001953.

Porter, M. E. (2010). What is value in health care? *N Engl J Med.*, 363, 2477–2481.

Putera, I. (2017). Redefining health: Implication for value-based healthcare reform. *Cureus*, 9(3), e1067. Available at https://www.ncbi.nlm.nih.gov/pmc/articles/PMC5376155/.

Robinson, J. C., & Ginsburg, P. B. (2009). Consumer-driven health care: Promise and performance. *Health Aff*, 28(Supplement 2). Available at https://www.healthaffairs.org/doi/10.1377/hlthaff.28.2.w272.

Rook, D. (2015). *The Pros and Cons of Consumer-Driven Health Care*. JP Griffin Group. Available at https://www.griffinbenefits.com/blog/consumer-driven-healthcare-cdhc-cdhp.

Sandoval, J. L., Petrovic, D., Guessous, I., & Stringhini, S. (2020). Forgoing health care is associated with insurance deductibles in a consumer-driven health care system. *European Journal of Public Health*, 30(Supplement_5) Available at https://academic.oup.com/eurpub/article-abstract/30/Supplement_5/ckaa166.1381/5915661.

Sejin Ha, Y. J. L. (2011). Determinants of consumer-driven healthcare: Self-confidence in information search, health literacy, and trust in information sources. *International Journal of Pharmaceutical and Healthcare Marketing*. https://doi.org/10.1108/17506121111121550.

Somocurcio Vílchez, J. G. (1978). Primary health care: Report of the International Conference on Primary Health Care, Alma-Ata.

Revista Peruana de Medicina Experimental y Salud Pública, 171–172. https://doi.org/10.17843/rpmesp.2013.302.186.

Taylor, J. (2009). The changing health of the Middle East population through oil and automobiles. *European Heart Journal, 30*, 1291–1300.

Technology is Transforming Health Care in the UAE (2017). Hosting Data Fort. Available at https://www.ehdf.com/blog/technology-is-transforming-health-care-in-the-uae/.

Yabeck, A. S., Rabie, T. S., & Pande, A. (2017). Health sector reform in the Middle East and North Africa: Prospects and experiences. *Health Systems and Reform, Volume 3*. Available at https://www.tandfonline.com/doi/full/10.1080/23288604.2016.1272984.

Yusuf, N. (2014). Private and public healthcare in Saudi Arabia: Future challenges. *International Journal of Business & Economic Development, 2*(1), 114–118.

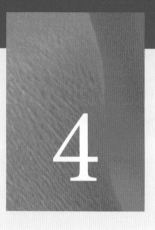

4

LIFESTYLE 1
Metabolic Syndromes—Type 2 Diabetes, Metabolic Syndrome and Polycystic Ovary Syndrome in the Arabian Gulf

ALEXANDRA E. BUTLER ■ STEPHEN L. ATKIN

INTRODUCTION

Recently there has been a shift in trends of both availability and consumption of food and dietary, physical activity and lifestyle behaviour patterns of people worldwide (Popkin, 2002, 2004). This has been better termed as a 'nutrition transition' (Popkin, 2002, 2004). There is increasing evidence that many middle- to high-income countries in the developing world are experiencing different stages of the nutrition transition. Populations with improving economic conditions, such as those in the Middle East and North Africa (MENA) region, are characterized by intake of high energy, high fat and carbohydrate diets; higher intake of processed foods; and a transition in technology that impacts both the workplace and leisure pursuits.

Of the five stages of nutrition transition presented at the Bellagio conference in 2002, this scenario equates to Pattern 4 in the nutrition transition (Popkin, 2002), resulting in high obesity, type 2 diabetes (T2D) and noncommunicable disease (NCD) prevalence in genetically predisposed populations.

BACKGROUND

The number of deaths from NCD, a category that includes cardiovascular disease (CVD) and chronic respiratory disease, cancer and diabetes, was projected to increase 15% worldwide according to the 2010 World Health Organization (WHO) survey to 2020 (Kelly et al., 2011). The WHO estimates that, by 2020, the number of deaths due to NCDs will reach approximately 44 million. The largest percentage increase, of over 20%, is expected to occur in Africa, South-east Asia and the Eastern Mediterranean regions (Kelly et al., 2011; Rahim et al., 2014), a geographical area centred around the MENA region.

Type 2 diabetes mellitus (T2DM) and obesity, in addition to CVD, are currently major health issues across the world, as the incidence and prevalence are increasing to alarming levels. The WHO reports that ~425 million people currently have diabetes globally and that, by 2045, this number will increase to ~629 million, equating to ~10% of the global adult population and making diabetes the seventh leading cause of death (2017). The majority of diabetes cases are T2DM, accounting for 90%–95%, and the increasing incidence of T2DM parallels that of obesity. Both of these conditions contribute to the development of CVD.

Weight gain is consequent upon the ingestion of calories exceeding the calories expended through physical activity (Institute of Medicine, 2004). The WHO has defined the overweight and obese condition as an 'abnormal or excessive fat accumulation that presents a risk to health' (World Health Organization, 2014). Body mass index (BMI), computed as weight (kg)/(height (m))^2, is used to classify individuals as overweight and obese: in adults, overweight being a BMI of $\geq$25 kg/m^2 and obese as a BMI of $\geq$30 kg/m^2 (World Health Organization, 2014).

According to the WHO, obesity prevalence globally has nearly doubled since 1980 (World Health Organization, 2014). In 2008 over 1.4 billion adults were classified as overweight with over 0.5 billion as obese (World Health Organization, 2013b). Obesity currently affects one in every four people across the globe. Figures from 2008 show that 35% of adults (defined as aged $\geq$20 years) were overweight and 11% obese (World Health Organization, 2014). Predictions about future obesity prevalence suggest that the condition will continue to rise rather than reduce, despite increased awareness surrounding the contributing factors to obesity. This has also resulted in an alarming rise in metabolic syndrome (MetS).

MetS is a common metabolic disorder with a cluster of risk factors for developing CVD (Isomaa et al., 2001; Lakka et al., 2002) and diabetes (Grundy, Hansen,

et al., 2004). There have been a number of definitions proposed for MetS, including those from the WHO (Alberti & Zimmet, 1998), National Cholesterol Education Program (NCEP) (Expert Panel on Detection, Evaluation, and Treatment of High Blood Cholesterol in Adults, 2001) and the International Diabetes Federation (2006). The risk factors common to all these definitions are dyslipidaemia, hypertension, dysglycaemia and abdominal obesity (Alberti et al., 2005). The most commonly used definition is that of the NCEP, defining MetS as having $\geq$3 of the following risk factors:

1. Elevated fasting plasma glucose (FPG) ($\geq$110 mg/dL). This threshold was lowered to an FPG of $\geq$100 mg/dL in 2004 (revised NCEP (rNCEP)), in order to be in alignment with the American Diabetes Association (ADA) criteria for impaired fasting glucose (IFG) (Grundy, Brewer, et al., 2004).
2. Central obesity, meaning waist circumference >102 cm for men and >88 cm for women. This threshold was also lowered from the more stringent 'greater than' to $\geq$102 cm for men and $\geq$88 cm for women.
3. Hypertension, defined as $\geq$130 mmHg systolic and $\geq$85 mmHg diastolic.
4. Diminished high-density lipoprotein (HDL) cholesterol, defined as <40 mg/dL for men and <50 mg/dL for women.
5. Elevated triglycerides, defined as $\geq$150 mg/dL for both men and women.

Worldwide, MetS prevalence is on the rise. This can be largely attributed to increasing levels of obesity and the nutrition transition, as noted earlier. The prevalence of MetS in adults >20 years in the United States was reported as 34% (Ervin, 2009). The risk of developing MetS was increased three-fold when comparing the age groups 20–39 years with those between 40 and 59 years (males: odds ratio (OR) = 2.70 (95% confidence interval (CI) = 1.96–3.73); females: OR = 3.20 (95% CI = 2.32–4.43)) (Ervin, 2009). Thirty percent of overweight males (BMI 25–29.9 kg/m^2) and 65% of obese males (BMI $\geq$ 30 kg/m^2) met the criteria for MetS (Ervin, 2009), illustrating the fact that MetS increases with increases in BMI.

COMPLICATIONS OF OBESITY, CARDIOVASCULAR DISEASE AND TYPE 2 DIABETES MELLITUS

Obesity has become one of the greatest challenges to sufferers as well as healthcare systems. Obesity significantly impacts health and well-being and is accompanied by various comorbidities including T2DM (Wilding, 2014), hypertension (Ho, 2001; Ledoux et al., 2010), dyslipidaemia (Howard et al., 2003), fatty liver (Patell et al., 2014), obstructive sleep apnoea (OSA) (Jordan et al., 2014), CVD (Chen et al., 2013; Ho, 2001), renal disease (Lin et al., 2014) and heightened risk of several cancers (Ashktorab et al., 2014; Renehan et al., 2008). Obesity negatively impacts mental health and well-being (Atlantis et al., 2009), leading to a reduced quality of life (Cameron et al., 2012; Jacobson et al., 1994). Further, obesity is associated with early mortality (World Health Organization, 2013a).

As mentioned above, obesity is classed as a risk factor for CVD. The development of CVD can occur as a result of several risk factors, some modifiable but others nonmodifiable (Gordon & Kannel, 1982; Kannel &

McGee, 1979b). Modifiable factors include smoking, a sedentary lifestyle, hypertension, dyslipidaemia and diabetes, as well as obesity (Kannel & McGee, 1979a). Diabetes, however, is undoubtedly the most significant indicator for development and severity of CVD.

Diabetes, unlike other chronic illnesses which usually do not affect multiple organ systems, is associated with serious microvascular and macrovascular complications. Classically, microvascular complications include nephropathy, retinopathy and neuropathy (Banerjee et al., 2013) while macrovascular complications include stroke, ischaemic heart disease (encompassing angina and infarction) (Goff et al., 2007) and peripheral vascular disease (predisposing to amputations) (Beach & Strandness, 1980; Melton et al., 1980). Diabetes is also associated with poor cognitive function (Palta et al., 2014) and dementia (Ninomiya, 2014) (underlying associations including multiple factors such as glucose levels, hypertension and vascular disease), depression (Goff et al., 2007), reduced quality of life (Rubin & Peyrot, 1999) and several major cancers (e.g. breast cancer) (Ashktorab et al., 2014; Renehan et al., 2008) as shown in Fig. 4.1. The high prevalence

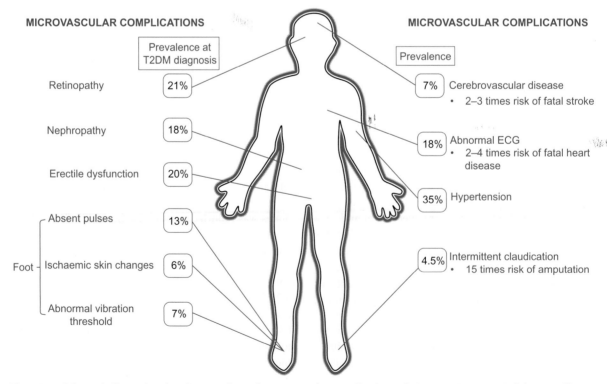

Fig. 4.1 ■ Schematic illustrating the microvascular and macrovascular complications of T2DM. *T2DM*, Type 2 diabetes mellitus.

of obesity and diabetes is a significant organizational and financial challenge to healthcare services and societies worldwide (World Health Organization, 2013a). It is beyond the scope of this chapter to detail the pharmaceutical treatment of T2DM which is outlined in Fig 4.2.

METABOLIC SYNDROME, CARDIOVASCULAR DISEASE, OBESITY AND TYPE 2 DIABETES MELLITUS IN THE MIDDLE EAST

It is projected that the levels of obesity, T2DM and CVD will continue to rise, particularly in the MENA region that encompasses the Gulf Cooperation Council (GCC) and is comprised of six Middle Eastern countries: Bahrain, Kuwait, Oman, Kingdom of Saudi Arabia (KSA), the United Arab Emirates (UAE) and Qatar. These countries share similarities in culture, background and geography.

Swift socioeconomic growth combined with dramatic lifestyle changes have impacted the health of the populations in the MENA region. MetS was found to affect ≥33% of the adult population in the GCC (Malik & Razig, 2008). Using the NCEP definition, prevalence of MetS was between 19.5% (Al-Lawati et al., 2003) and 37.2% (Al-Nozha et al., 2005) for men and 13.5% (Al-Qahtani et al., 2006) and 42.7% (Malik & Razig, 2008) for women.

The diabetes epidemic in the MENA region is considered to be a serious and increasing health problem. According to the International Diabetes Federation (2017), diabetes prevalence in the GCC countries is as follows: Qatar (23.3%), Kuwait (23.9%), KSA (23.4%), Bahrain (22.4%), UAE (18.9%) and Oman (10.2%). Over 90% of diabetes mellitus cases are T2DM. The high prevalence of diabetes will translate into serious vascular complications resulting in blindness (Lutty, 2013), end-stage renal disease (Nakagawa et al., 2011; Van Diepen et al., 2014) necessitating renal dialysis (Toppe et al., 2014) and transplantation, lower limb amputations (Lombardo et al., 2014), heart disease (Tuna et al., 2014) and stroke (Peters et al., 2014). Diabetes is thus associated with early mortality (Nakasone et al., 2009). The IDF estimates that healthcare expenditure to manage diabetes and prevent its complications in, for example,

Qatar is currently running at 2960 USD per person, which is about 18% of the total health expenditure. The IDF predicts that this percentage will double by 2030 (International Diabetes Federation, 2017).

Population Screening

The definition of population screening is 'the systematic application of a test or inquiry, to identify individuals at sufficient risk of a specific disorder to benefit from further investigation or direct preventive action, among persons who have not sought medical attention on account of symptoms of that disorder' (Wald, 2001).

Population screening has advantages, disadvantages and cost implications. Therefore there is an ethical obligation to maximize benefits and minimize harm. Wilson and Jungner, commissioned by the WHO in 1968, set the gold standard criteria for screening (Andermann et al., 2008). The criteria suggested, among other recommendations, that the condition/disease should be one that is an important health problem and that there needs to be a recognizable latent or early symptomatic phase. Both CVD and T2DM are important health issues that affect a large proportion of the population worldwide. These conditions also have a latent stage where they have either MetS or at least some of the MetS-associated risk factors. Screening can help identify people who have an undiagnosed/early disease, are at risk of developing the disease or are developing further complications of the disease. Screening can, therefore, decrease disease burden in the community, improve quality of life through early diagnosis of the disease and its complications and has a potential to save lives. It can also guide individuals to make informed choices regarding their health. However, it does not guarantee that a disease will not occur or that it can be cured if it does occur.

Prevalence of the Number of People at Risk for Development of Cardiovascular Disease Using the QRISK2 Calculator

The QRISK2 (Hippisley-Cox et al., 2008) is a risk calculator for CVD. It computes factors like age, blood pressure and cholesterol, utilizing an algorithm to give a 10-year risk of having a CVD-related event. The National Institute for Health and Care Excellence (NICE) in the UK recommendation is that lipid-lowering therapies should be initiated when a QRISK2

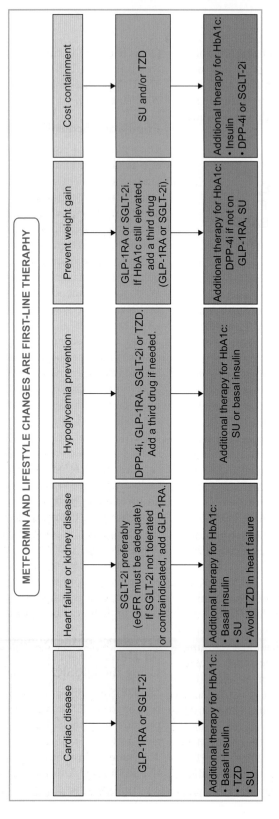

Fig. 4.2 ■ Recommended therapy for T2DM patients. First-line therapy is lifestyle intervention to manage weight and increase physical activity together with metformin. If HbA1c remains above target levels, then subsequent therapy is dependent upon whether there is established arteriosclerotic cardiovascular disease (ASCVD) or chronic kidney disease (CKD) or not. *DPP-4i*, Dipeptidyl peptidase-4 inhibitor; *eGFR*, estimated glomerular filtration rate; *GLP-1RA*, glucagon-like peptide-1 receptor antagonist; *HbA1c*, glycated haemoglobin A1c; *HF*, heart failure; *SGLT-2i*, sodium/glucose cotransporter 2 inhibitor; *SU*, sulfonylurea; *T2DM*, Type 2 diabetes mellitus; *TZD*, thiazolidinedione.

score is above 10 (National Clinical Guideline Centre, 2014). The QRISK2 is a simple tool that can be used in studies to evaluate the prevalence of individuals at risk for development of CVD. Accordingly, participants can take due action to help prevent CVD development (Case Studies 4.1 and 4.2).

Prevalence of Metabolic Syndrome

As discussed above, MetS is a metabolic disorder that increases the risk of CVD and diabetes. Screening for and identifying individuals with MetS risk factors will help identify early disease or those at risk of CVD and/or diabetes. It will help to develop strategies to help make the population in MENA more aware of health and lifestyle.

Point-of-care testing (POCT) is accomplished with portable devices that do not require dedicated space and can be used at different sites. This can be used to identify people who have MetS risk factors from blood samples that can include measurement of:

- HbA1c from a whole blood sample (1 μL) in 6 minutes
- Lipid profile from a blood sample (50 μL) in 3 minutes, which can include total cholesterol, low-density lipoprotein (LDL), HDL and triglyceride.

Diet

Diet and obesity contribute to the severity of CVD and T2DM (Apovian & Gokce, 2012). Research indicates that a large waist circumference is an accurate predictor that can be used to calculate the risk of development of diabetes and CVD (Czernichow et al., 2011;

CASE STUDY 4.1
THE USE OF TELEMEDICINE AND TELEMEDICINE DEVICES FOR NONCOMPLIANT DIABETIC PATIENTS DURING THE COVID-19 PANDEMIC

The COVID-19 pandemic restricted face to face medical consultations and encouraged the use of telemedicine to facilitate consultations. In the Middle East and North Africa (MENA) region the incidence of diabetes is high. A study was undertaken in 2021 to evaluate the impact of telemedicine consultations and telemedicine devices such as blood glucose monitors, vital signs monitoring (blood pressure, pulse oximetry, heart rates and automatic pill dispensers). These devices were provided to noncompliant diabetic patients to use in their homes and were linked to a dedicated mobile device in their home that automatically uploaded results to the diabetic clinic laptop and in turn to the clinical staff responsible for these patients. Patients were then contacted by the clinical staff about their results, to provide reminders and arrange for consultations.

The results demonstrated that the mean HbA1c decreased significantly from 10.3 to 7.4 after 3 months. Following the 3-month trial, 50% of patients achieved an HbA1c level of <7.

Addressing patient compliance is a struggle within the region. Telemedicine consultations and 'at home' devices may be the future focus.

Based on Farooqi, M. H., Abdelmannan, D. K., Albuflasa, M. M., Hamed, M. A., Xavier, M., Cadiz, T. J., & Nawaz, F. A. (2022). The impact of telemonitoring on improving glycemic and metabolic control in previously lost-to-follow-up patients with type 2 diabetes mellitus: a single center interventional study in the United Arab Emirates. *International Journal of Clinical Practice*, Art. No. 6286574.

CASE STUDY 4.2
DIABETES AND ARAB EMIGRANTS

While there has been a lot of focus on the rates of type 2 diabetes mellitus (T2DM) in the Middle East, there has been less consideration to those from the region who emigrate to other countries. In a recent cohort study of newly diagnosed diabetic patients, it was found that Middle Eastern emigrants represent a high-risk population for type 2 diabetes, with a severe insulin-deficient diabetes rate almost twice that of the local population.

While the increased risk of T2DM in the Middle East population can be partially attributed to obesity, family history, sedentary lifestyles and diet, the study found that ethnicity itself was a contributing factor.

The findings of this study raise important matters of health education, prevention and mitigation for health professionals and the population alike.

As a health professional:
- What education or health advice might you give Arabic families, in relation to diabetes, planning on moving to a western country?
- What diabetic screening, if any, would you consider for these types of patients?

Based on Bennet, L., Nilsson, C., Mansour-ALY, D., Christensson, A., Groop, L., & Ahlqvist, E. (2021). Adult-onset diabetes in Middle Eastern immigrants to Sweden: Novel subgroups and diabetic complications-The All New Diabetes in Scania cohort diabetic complications and ethnicity. *Diabetes Metabolism Research and Reviews*, 37(6), e3419.

Israni et al., 2012). Although there is broad variability in dietary patterns across the MENA region, there has been a shift towards a diet rich in fat and protein from animal sources with a decreasing consumption of whole grains, fruits and vegetables (Mehio Sibai et al., 2010). There is a need to identify specific areas of concern and implement strategies to educate the population about healthier dietary habits that fall within the cultural norms of the region.

Physical Activity

Physical activity definitively decreases risk factors for both CVD and T2DM (Lee et al., 2012; Luke et al., 2004). Data indicate that ~31% of the global population does not meet minimum guidelines for physical activity (Hallal et al., 2012). Research based on self-reported surveys indicates a higher inactivity rate in the MENA region compared with the global population; the variability from country to country ranges from overall 39% in Kuwait to 96.1% reported in the KSA (Mabry et al., 2010) and overall about 43% for the Eastern Mediterranean region (Hallal et al., 2012). There is, therefore, an urgent need to educate the population about how physical activity positively impacts their health and specifically how it reduces the risk for CVD and T2DM; however, there are specific challenges in the Middle East, particularly for women, to undertake physical activity in an Islamic society, such as childcare issues, family disapproval, family commitments, dress code and Ramadan/fasting/religious obligations.

Metabolic Syndrome Treatment and Management

The initial management of MetS involves lifestyle modifications, including changes in diet and exercise (DeBoer, 2019). The implementation of diet, exercise and potential pharmacologic interventions may inhibit the progression of MetS to diabetes mellitus (Tupper & Gopalakrishnan, 2007). Statins for dyslipidaemia, renin–angiotensin–aldosterone system inhibitors for arterial hypertension, metformin or sodium/glucose cotransporter 2 (SGLT-2) inhibitors or glucagon-like peptide 1 receptor agonists (GLP-1RAs) for glucose intolerance, and the GLP-1RA liraglutide for achieving body weight and waist circumference reduction have been recommended (Rask Larsen et al., 2018), but the

threshold for those interventions is less clear in young individuals and requires expert assessment.

OTHER METABOLIC CONDITIONS PARTICULARLY PREVALENT IN THE MIDDLE EAST AND NORTH AFRICA REGION: POLYCYSTIC OVARY SYNDROME

Polycystic ovary syndrome (PCOS), representing the commonest endocrine condition for women of reproductive age, has a wide array of distressing symptoms and signs, together with well-recognised biochemical abnormalities. These include irregular periods and infertility; increased androgen levels underlie the commonly noted hirsutism and acne (Ehrmann, 2005; Norman et al., 2007). Most women with PCOS are obese with increased incidence of impaired glucose tolerance (IGT) and T2DM. Women who suffer from PCOS have an elevated cardiovascular risk profile with hypertension, dyslipidaemia and insulin resistance (IR) (Moran & Teede, 2009; Sathyapalan & Atkin, 2011). IR is believed to be central to the underlying cause of PCOS, but the underlying pathophysiological mechanisms at the cellular level remain poorly understood. Insulin signalling is normal in PCOS and there are no abnormalities in insulin binding, insulin receptor expression or in second messenger intracellular signalling. However, tissue changes in the adipocyte function, such as glucose transport enhancement (Ciaraldi et al., 1992) and GLUT4 production (Rosenbaum et al., 1993), have been described (Biyasheva et al., 2009; Lord et al., 2006; Marsden et al., 2001). It is also recognised that women who have PCOS have increased risk for endometrial cancer due to amenorrhoea and oligomenorrhoea leading to relatively unopposed oestrogen (Norman et al., 2007). More recently, it has been recognised that they are also at higher risk for nonalcoholic fatty liver disease that may lead to hepatic inflammation and cirrhosis (Dawson et al., 2014).

The cause of PCOS remains unknown but it is thought that there is 78% heritability. Susceptibility gene mapping has been undertaken but many of the studies are small, fail to adjust for multiple testing and have been related to a number of small nucleotide polymorphisms (SNPs) based upon phenotypic association rather than those spanning the genome (Dunaif, 2016). Heredity-based association testing identified D19S884, a microsatellite marker mapping to intron 55 of the fibrillin-3 gene (Dunaif, 2016) but these studies have not provided the answer to the complex genetics of PCOS. Two genome-wide association studies (GWAS) in Chinese populations have identified 11 risk loci for PCOS that count for 17 SNPs that are related to the disease (Chen et al., 2011; Shi et al., 2012). These SNPs have been related to glucose and lipid metabolism as well as ovarian hormonal regulation and cell cycle regulation. These studies are supported by studies relating the genes to PCOS in non-Chinese populations (Eriksen et al., 2012; Simoni et al., 2008; Unsal et al., 2009; Welt et al., 2012). However, while studies have confirmed these markers to be associated with disease (Casarini & Brigante, 2014), the aetiology and relationship to the comorbidities remain lacking.

Known to be common in women of reproductive age (Kauffman et al., 2008), depending upon the guideline followed, the prevalence of PCOS has been determined to be between 6% (National Institute of Health (NIH) criteria) and 10% (Rotterdam and Androgen excess society guidelines) (Bozdag et al., 2016). Confusion over prevalence has resulted from the differing diagnostic criteria utilized causing, for example, a doubling of prevalence when employing the Rotterdam versus NIH criteria (March et al., 2010). Ethnic background also has influence upon the prevalence of PCOS; for example, South-east Asian women are frequently symptomatic at a younger age and with more severe phenotypic features and symptoms (Glintborg et al., 2010; Wijeyaratne et al., 2002). A recent analysis of a Biobank in the Middle East of 750 women between the ages of 10 and 40 found a prevalence of PCOS of 13.5% that would then likely reflect a prevalence of 21% if the Rotterdam criteria were used (Dargham et al., 2017). Thus the prevalence appears higher than other documented populations (Casarini & Brigante, 2014), and therefore with the greater potential for novel findings within the genotype or identified biomarkers.

The Rotterdam criteria suggest a wider definition for PCOS that requires two out of three criteria be present to make the diagnosis of PCOS and therefore leads to four potential phenotypes (Rotterdam ESHRE/ASRM-Sponsored PCOS Consensus Workshop Group, 2004). These four different phenotypes may have different metabolic profiles. For instance, it has been shown that those women with the non-hyperandrogenic phenotype show a milder phenotype with a milder metabolic profile compared to the other phenotypes (Zhang et al., 2009). The distribution of the different PCOS phenotypes in MENA women is unknown; however, from the PCOS women identified from the Qatar Biobank, 12% had IFG, 4% had diabetes and there was a marked metabolic phenotype with increased weight, systolic and diastolic blood pressure, IR and C-reactive protein (an indicator of inflammation) with a decreased HDL. This is in keeping with the prediction from GWAS with phenotype that a severe androgenic form is more common in the MENA countries (Casarini & Brigante, 2014).

Metabolic Consequences of Polycystic Ovary Syndrome

As noted earlier, women who have PCOS frequently demonstrate IGT and IR, and both are drivers of T2DM (Salley et al., 2007); this is especially true of women from the MENA region who have PCOS (Dargham et al., 2018). Approximately 50% of women with PCOS progress to frank MetS (Garruti et al., 2009). The prevalence of MetS in women with PCOS is remarkably high at ~40%–50% (Apridonidze et al., 2005). The evidence to date suggests that PCOS and its associated metabolic abnormalities differ between White and MENA subjects (Butler et al., 2020a). Additionally, the wide spectrum of associated complications in women who suffer from PCOS, examples being obesity, infertility, endometrial cancer and CVD, make PCOS a challenging and distressing health condition (Goodarzi et al., 2011; Mu et al., 2012).

THINKING GRID

A 21-year-old Bahraini woman who has been married for 6 months comes to you complaining that she cannot get pregnant. She reports her menarche at the age of 15 years but with irregular cycles, acne and hirsutism, and her BMI is 36 kg/m². The investigation and biochemistry profile confirm a diagnosis of polycystic ovary syndrome.

What types of discussions, advice and education would you have with this woman, particularly?

Therapeutic Approaches

The pharmaceutical treatment of PCOS should be tailored to the needs of the individual and are summarised in a recent review (Abdalla et al., 2020). Weight loss, though challenging, is central to PCOS management. Successful weight loss is effective in preventing CVD onset in PCOS (Wadden et al., 2005). Reduced caloric intake combined with increased physical activity is indicated although, disappointingly, rarely is body weight reduction of >10 kg achieved (Moran et al., 2011; Wadden et al., 2011). Drugs are primarily employed to treat associated conditions such as T2DM. Rather than a single approach, a combination of therapies (lifestyle intervention, metformin (Jensterle et al., 2020), GLP-1 receptor analogue therapy (Rasmussen & Lindenberg, 2014), SGLT-2 inhibitors (Javed et al., 2019b) and bariatric surgery (Eid et al., 2005; Escobar-Morreale et al., 2005)) seems to offer the greatest benefit. SGLT-2 inhibitors and GLP-1 RAs seem to offer advantages for improvement of metabolic parameters in women with PCOS and additional studies are required. Bariatric surgery is beneficial in certain women with PCOS to improve metabolic parameters and prevent T2DM.

CONTRIBUTORY FACTORS TO METABOLIC SYNDROME AND DIABETES: VITAMIN D DEFICIENCY

Vitamin D and Diabetes in Middle East and North Africa Region

Accumulating evidence suggests that vitamin D deficiency increases the risk of T2DM (Husemoen et al., 2012; Nakashima et al., 2016). Deficiency of vitamin D is associated with both IR and beta cell dysfunction (Chiu et al., 2004). As long ago as 1980, impaired insulin secretion was demonstrated in isolated perfused rat pancreas in the setting of vitamin D deficiency (Kadowaki & Norman, 1984). Later reports suggested that vitamin D deficiency could contribute to MetS and T2DM (Angellotti & Pittas, 2017; Berridge, 2017). Vitamin D appears to exert its antidiabetic effect through modulation of hepatic glucose and lipid metabolism via activation of calcium and the adenosine monophosphate-activated protein kinase (AMPK) pathway, and through promotion of beta cell function and survival (Leung, 2016).

A large prospective study of women, with 20 years of follow-up, reported an inverse relationship between vitamin D concentrations and the onset of diabetes (Pittas et al., 2006). Vitamin D deficiency in T2DM has also been correlated with microvascular complications of retinopathy, neuropathy and nephropathy (Bajaj et al., 2014; Wan et al., 2019), though there is still some debate.

Vitamin D_3 (cholecalciferol) is endogenously produced by UV-B irradiation of 7-dehydrocholesterol, while ergosterol is derived from the diet (primarily from mushrooms and fungi) and converted to previtamin D_2 (ergocalciferol) by UV-B light, though both are hydroxylated to $25(OH)D_3$ and $25(OH)D_2$, respectively, by multiple 25-hydroxylases in the liver (Bikle, 2014) (Fig. 4.3). 25(OH)D is transported to the kidney and converted to either the active $1,25(OH)_2D$ by 1 alpha hydroxylase, or to 24,25(OH)2D, that is also active, by the 24 alpha hydroxylase present in the renal tubular cells (Fig. 4.3) (Christakos et al., 2016). It has recently been reported that extrarenal tissues may also convert 25(OH)D to $1,25(OH)_2D$ although, notably, activation in renal and non-kidney tissues is regulated differently with macrophage production of $1,25(OH)_2D$ through the type 2 interferon response (Adams et al., 2014). $1,25(OH)_2D$ binds to the vitamin D receptor (VDR) but, to exert its effect (which may take several hours), it heterodimerizes with the retinoid X receptor (Christakos et al., 2016); however, reports suggest alternative, more rapid mechanisms of action through binding to membrane VDR or through the 1,25D-membrane-associated, rapid response steroid-binding protein receptor with activation of protein kinases A and C (Lösel & Wehling, 2003). Obesity can exacerbate vitamin D deficiency through decreased bioavailability due to deposition of vitamin D in the body fat compartments (Wortsman et al., 2000). In many countries, vitamin D_2 is available as a pharmaceutical and a supplement to counter vitamin D deficiency (Vieth, 1999).

While vitamin D deficiency is a global issue (Holick, 2006), cultural norms dictating full body coverage and high ambient temperatures precluding outdoor activity in the Middle East magnify the issue of vitamin D deficiency in these regions (Chakhtoura et al., 2018).

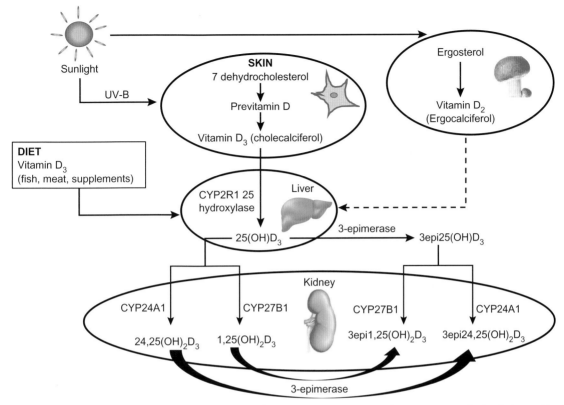

Fig. 4.3 ■ A simplified schematic representation of the synthesis and metabolism of vitamin D. 7-Dehydrocholesterol in the skin is converted to previtamin D_3 by UV-B and then is thermally isomerize to vitamin D_3. Transport of vitamin D_3 from the skin to the liver is mediated by vitamin D binding protein (DBP) where vitamin D_3 is hydroxylated at position 25 to 25(OH)D_3, DBP then transports 25(OH)D_3 to the kidney. 25(OH)D_3/DBP is filtered by the glomeruli and 25(OH)D_3 is taken up into the tubular cells, following DBP binding to megalin, a transmembrane protein. 25(OH)D_3 undergoes a second hydroxylation step by the 1 alpha hydroxylase Cyp27B1, converting to the active $1\alpha,25$ (OH)$_2D_3$, while 24 hydroxylase Cyp27A1 converts to 24,25(OH)$_2D_3$. Keratinocytes contribute to the 3-epimerase activity but the exact sites of activity remain unknown. 3epi25(OH)D_3 is converted by Cyp27A1 to 24,25(OH)D_3 and Cyp27B1 to 1,25(OH)D_3, in equal measure. Ergosterol (provitamin D_2) is plant based and is converted to ergocalciferol by UV-B light that then follows the same pathway as vitamin D_3 that is depicted with the *dotted arrow* to the liver to form 25(OH)D_2 and then transported to the kidney and epimerized to the D_2 metabolites.

Diagnosis is widely based upon measurement of total serum 25-hydroxyvitamin D (vitamin D_2 plus vitamin D_3), a value of <20 ng/mL (<48.4 nmol/L) being indicative of vitamin D insufficiency. Vitamin D replacement is commonplace usually with vitamin D_2 supplement, which is inexpensive, but there is evidence to suggest that the vitamin D_3 preparation is more effective. In addition, vitamin D testing is not covered routinely by insurance policies, and this also causes under-reporting. Certain ethnic groups appear to have low serum concentrations of 25(OH)D while maintaining healthy bone mineral density; Black Americans represent one such group, with typically low concentrations of 25(OH)D (Ginde et al., 2009; Mitchell et al., 2012; Mittelbrunn et al., 2011) and yet with a higher bone mineral density and a lower risk of osteoporosis and fractures than their White counterparts (Bischoff-Ferrari et al., 2004; Cauley et al., 2005, 2011; Zahiri et al., 2016).

Studies have previously shown that in patients from the MENA region, T2DM complications are associated with differing metabolites of vitamin D: diabetic retinopathy is associated with lower 25(OH)D_3 and

$1,25(OH)_2D_3$ concentrations, hypertension is associated with lower $1,25(OH)_2D_3$ and dyslipidaemia is associated with lower $25(OH)D_3$, $1,25(OH)_2D_3$ and $24,25(OH)_2D_3$ (Butler et al., 2020b), though whether this reflects ethnic differences is unclear.

Vitamin D and Polycystic Ovary Syndrome in the Middle East and North Africa Region

Vitamin D deficiency is very common in women with PCOS, with 67%–85% having serum concentrations of 25-hydroxyvitamin D (25(OH)D) <20 ng/mL, and levels have been reported to correlate with obesity and increased IR, as well as testosterone and dehydroepiandrosterone sulphate (DHEAS) levels (Hahn et al., 2006; Irani et al., 2015; Li et al., 2011; Muscogiuri et al., 2012). Studies have revealed that vitamin D replacement therapy (usually vitamin D_2 supplements) may have beneficial effects on IR and steroidogenesis of oestradiol and progesterone in obese women with PCOS (Lerchbaum & Obermayer-Pietsch, 2012; Selimoglu et al., 2010). Vitamin D has been associated with poorer glycaemic control and increased mortality (Osorio Landa et al., 2020). A recent small study in PCOS subjects alone in whom 50% were vitamin D insufficient suggested that vitamin D did not correlate with androgen levels, inflammation or IR (Mesinovic et al., 2020). Severe vitamin deficiency in this population is reported (Al-Dabhani et al., 2017) but severe vitamin D deficiency does not seem to correlate with, or exacerbate, the IR and cardiovascular risk parameters in PCOS. Vitamin D supplementation appears not to improve the metabolic parameters of PCOS in vitamin D deficient subjects (Javed et al., 2019a).

SUMMARY

Obesity is the major common factor in individuals in the MENA region that is multifactorial in its development and is reviewed in full in Chapter 5. This epidemic in obesity is reflected in the increase in MetS, the development of T2DM, the increase in the prevalence of PCOS and may be contributing to the development of vitamin D deficiency in this susceptible population. Lifestyle advice on diet and exercise remains critical and needs to be tailored to

the cultural norms and values of the MENA region for it to be impactful. However, with the development of metabolic-related conditions, pharmacological intervention may become warranted to help prevent long-term metabolic and disease-related sequelae.

REFERENCES

Abdalla, M. A., Deshmukh, H., Atkin, S., & Sathyapalan, T. (2020). A review of therapeutic options for managing the metabolic aspects of polycystic ovary syndrome. *Therapeutic Advances in Endocrinology and Metabolism*, 11 2042018820938305.

Adams, J. S., Rafison, B., Witzel, S., Reyes, R. E., Shieh, A., Chun, R., et al. (2014). Regulation of the extrarenal CYP27B1-hydroxylase. *The Journal of Steroid Biochemistry and Molecular Biology*, 144(Pt A), 22–27.

Al-Dabhani, K., Tsilidis, K. K., Murphy, N., Ward, H. A., Elliott, P., Riboli, E., et al. (2017). Prevalence of vitamin D deficiency and association with metabolic syndrome in a Qatari population. *Nutrition and Diabetes*, 7, e263.

Al-Lawati, J. A., Mohammed, A. J., Al-Hinai, H. Q., & Jousilahti, P. (2003). Prevalence of the metabolic syndrome among Omani adults. *Diabetes Care*, 26, 1781–1785.

Al-Nozha, M., Al-Khadra, A., Arafah, M. R., Al-Maatouq, M. A., Khalil, M. Z., Khan, N. B., et al. (2005). Metabolic syndrome in Saudi Arabia. *Saudi Medical Journal*, 26, 1918–1925.

Al-Qahtani, D. A., Imtiaz, M. L., Saad, O. S., & Hussein, N. M. (2006). A comparison of the prevalence of metabolic syndrome in Saudi adult females using two definitions. *Metabolic Syndrome and Related Disorders*, 4, 204–214.

Alberti, K., Zimmet, P., & Shaw, J. (2005). A new world-wide definition from the International Diabetes Federation Consensus. *Lancet*, 366, 1059–1062.

Alberti, K. G., & Zimmet, P. Z. (1998). Definition, diagnosis and classification of diabetes mellitus and its complications. Part 1: Diagnosis and classification of diabetes mellitus provisional report of a WHO consultation. *Diabetic Medicine*, 15, 539–553.

Andermann, A., Blancquaert, I., Beauchamp, S., & Dery, V. (2008). Revisiting Wilson and Jungner in the genomic age: A review of screening criteria over the past 40 years. *Bull World Health Organ*, 86, 317–319.

Angellotti, E., & Pittas, A. G. (2017). The role of vitamin D in the prevention of type 2 diabetes: To D or not to D? *Endocrinology*, 158, 2013–2021.

Apovian, C. M., & Gokce, N. (2012). Obesity and cardiovascular disease. *Circulation*, 125, 1178–1182.

Apridonidze, T., Essah, P. A., Iuorno, M. J., & Nestler, J. E. (2005). Prevalence and characteristics of the metabolic syndrome in women with polycystic ovary syndrome. *The Journal of Clinical Endocrinology and Metabolism*, 90, 1929–1935.

Ashktorab, H., Paydar, M., Yazdi, S., Namin, H. H., Sanderson, A., Begum, R., et al. (2014). BMI and the risk of colorectal adenoma in African-Americans. *Obesity (Silver Spring)*, 22, 1387–1391.

Atlantis, E., Goldney, R. D., & Wittert, G. A. (2009). Obesity and depression or anxiety. *BMJ*, 339, b3868.

Bajaj, S., Singh, R. P., Dwivedi, N. C., Singh, K., Gupta, A., & Mathur, M. (2014). Vitamin D levels and microvascular complications in type 2 diabetes. *Indian Journal of Endocrinology and Metabolism*, *18*, 537–541.

Banerjee, D., Leong, W. B., Arora, T., Nolen, M., Punamiya, V., Grunstein, R., et al. (2013). The potential association between obstructive sleep apnea and diabetic retinopathy in severe obesity-the role of hypoxemia. *PLoS One*, *8*, e79521.

Beach, K. W., & Strandness, D. E., Jr. (1980). Arteriosclerosis obliterans and associated risk factors in insulin-dependent and non-insulin-dependent diabetes. *Diabetes*, *29*, 882–888.

Berridge, M. J. (2017). Vitamin D deficiency and diabetes. *The Biochemical Journal*, *474*, 1321–1332.

Bikle, D. D. (2014). Vitamin D metabolism, mechanism of action, and clinical applications. *Chemistry & Biology*, *21*, 319–329.

Bischoff-Ferrari, H. A., Dietrich, T., Orav, E. J., & Dawson-Hughes, B. (2004). Positive association between 25-hydroxy vitamin D levels and bone mineral density: A population-based study of younger and older adults. *The American Journal of Medicine*, *116*, 634–639.

Biyasheva, A., Legro, R. S., Dunaif, A., & Urbanek, M. (2009). Evidence for association between polycystic ovary syndrome (PCOS) and TCF7L2 and glucose intolerance in women with PCOS and TCF7L2. *The Journal of Clinical Endocrinology and Metabolism*, *94*, 2617–2625.

Bozdag, G., Mumusoglu, S., Zengin, D., Karabulut, E., & Yildiz, B. O. (2016). The prevalence and phenotypic features of polycystic ovary syndrome: A systematic review and meta-analysis. *Human Reproduction*, *31*, 2841–2855.

Butler, A. E., Abouseif, A., Dargham, S. R., Sathyapalan, T., & Atkin, S. L. (2020a). Metabolic comparison of polycystic ovarian syndrome and control women in Middle Eastern and UK Caucasian populations. *Scientific Reports*, *10*, 18895.

Butler, A. E., Dargham, S. R., Latif, A., Mokhtar, H. R., Robay, A., Chidiac, O. M., et al. (2020b). Association of vitamin D(3) and its metabolites in patients with and without type 2 diabetes and their relationship to diabetes complications. *Therapeutic Advances in Chronic Disease*, *11* 2040622320924159.

Cameron, A. J., Magliano, D. J., Dunstan, D. W., Zimmet, P. Z., Hesketh, K., Peeters, A., et al. (2012). A bi-directional relationship between obesity and health-related quality of life: evidence from the longitudinal AusDiab study. *International Journal of Obesity (London)*, *36*, 295–303.

Casarini, L., & Brigante, G. (2014). The polycystic ovary syndrome evolutionary paradox: A genome-wide association studies-based, in silico, evolutionary explanation. *The Journal of Clinical Endocrinology & Metabolism*, *99*, E2412–E2420.

Cauley, J. A., Danielson, M. E., Boudreau, R., Barbour, K. E., Horwitz, M. J., Bauer, D. C., et al. (2011). Serum 25-hydroxyvitamin D and clinical fracture risk in a multiethnic cohort of women: the Women's Health Initiative (WHI). *Journal of Bone and Mineral Research*, *26*, 2378–2388.

Cauley, J. A., Lui, L. Y., Ensrud, K. E., Zmuda, J. M., Stone, K. L., Hochberg, M. C., et al. (2005). Bone mineral density and the risk of incident nonspinal fractures in black and white women. *Journal of the American Medical Association*, *293*, 2102–2108.

Chakhtoura, M., Rahme, M., Chamoun, N., & El-Hajj Fuleihan, G. (2018). Vitamin D in the Middle East and North Africa. *Bone Rep*, *8*, 135–146.

Chen, Y., Copeland, W. K., Vedanthan, R., Grant, E., Lee, J. E., Gu, D., et al. (2013). Association between body mass index and cardiovascular disease mortality in east Asians and south Asians: Pooled analysis of prospective data from the Asia Cohort Consortium. *BMJ*, *347*, f5446.

Chen, Z. J., Zhao, H., He, L., Shi, Y., Qin, Y., Shi, Y., et al. (2011). Genome-wide association study identifies susceptibility loci for polycystic ovary syndrome on chromosome 2p16.3, 2p21 and 9q33.3. *Nature Genetics*, *43*, 55–59.

Chiu, K. C., Chu, A., Go, V. L., & Saad, M. F. (2004). Hypovitaminosis D is associated with insulin resistance and beta cell dysfunction. *The American Journal of Clinical Nutrition*, *79*, 820–825.

Christakos, S., Dhawan, P., Verstuyf, A., Verlinden, L., & Carmeliet, G. (2016). Vitamin D: Metabolism, molecular mechanism of action, and pleiotropic effects. *Physiological Reviews*, *96*, 365–408.

Ciaraldi, T. P., El-Roeiy, A., Madar, Z., Reichart, D., Olefsky, J. M., & Yen, S. S. (1992). Cellular mechanisms of insulin resistance in polycystic ovarian syndrome. *The Journal of Clinical Endocrinology and Metabolism*, *75*, 577–583.

Czernichow, S., Kengne, A. P., Huxley, R. R., Batty, G. D., De Galan, B., Grobbee, D., et al. (2011). Comparison of waist-to-hip ratio and other obesity indices as predictors of cardiovascular disease risk in people with type-2 diabetes: A prospective cohort study from ADVANCE. *European Journal of Cardiovascular Prevention and Rehabilitation*, *18*, 312–319.

Dargham, S. R., Ahmed, L., Kilpatrick, E. S., & Atkin, S. L. (2017). The prevalence and metabolic characteristics of polycystic ovary syndrome in the Qatari population. *PLoS One*, *12*, e0181467.

Dargham, S. R., Shewehy, A. E., Dakroury, Y., Kilpatrick, E. S., & Atkin, S. L. (2018). Prediabetes and diabetes in a cohort of Qatari women screened for polycystic ovary syndrome. *Sci Rep*, *8*, 3619.

Dawson, A. J., Sathyapalan, T., Smithson, J. A., Vince, R. V., Coady, A. M., Ajjan, R., et al. (2014). A comparison of cardiovascular risk indices in patients with polycystic ovary syndrome with and without coexisting nonalcoholic fatty liver disease. *Clinical Endocrinology (Oxford)*, *80*, 843–849.

Deboer, M. D. (2019). Assessing and managing the metabolic syndrome in children and adolescents. *Nutrients*, *11*, 1788.

Dunaif, A. (2016). Perspectives in polycystic ovary syndrome: From hair to eternity. *The Journal of Clinical Endocrinology and Metabolism*, *101*, 759–768.

Ehrmann, D. A. (2005). Polycystic ovary syndrome. *The New England Journal of Medicine*, *352*, 1223–1236.

Eid, G. M., Cottam, D. R., Velcu, L. M., Mattar, S. G., Korytkowski, M. T., Gosman, G., et al. (2005). Effective treatment of polycystic ovarian syndrome with Roux-en-Y gastric bypass. *Surgery for Obesity and Related Diseases*, *1*, 77–80.

Eriksen, M. B., Brusgaard, K., Andersen, M., Tan, Q., Altinok, M. L., Gaster, M., & Glintborg, D. (2012). Association of polycystic ovary syndrome susceptibility single nucleotide polymorphism rs2479106 and PCOS in Caucasian patients with PCOS or hirsutism as referral diagnosis. *European Journal of Obstetrics, Gynecology, and Reproductive Biology*, *163*, 39–42.

Ervin, R. B. (2009). Prevalence of metabolic syndrome among adults 20 years of age and over, by sex, age, race and ethnicity, and body mass index: United States, 2003-2006. *National Health Statistics Reports, 13*, 1–7.

Escobar-Morreale, H. F., Botella-Carretero, J. I., Alvarez-Blasco, F., Sancho, J., & San Millán, J. L. (2005). The polycystic ovary syndrome associated with morbid obesity may resolve after weight loss induced by bariatric surgery. *The Journal of Clinical Endocrinology and Metabolism, 90*, 6364–6369.

Expert Panel on Detection, Evaluation, and Treatment of High Blood Cholesterol in Adults. (2001). Executive Summary of The Third Report of The National Cholesterol Education Program (NCEP) Expert Panel on Detection, Evaluation, and Treatment of High Blood Cholesterol in Adults (Adult Treatment Panel III). *Journal of the American Medical Association, 285*, 2486–2497.

Garruti, G., Depalo, R., Vita, M. G., Lorusso, F., Giampetruzzi, F., Damato, A. B., & Giorgino, F. (2009). Adipose tissue, metabolic syndrome and polycystic ovary syndrome: From pathophysiology to treatment. *Reprod Biomed Online, 19*, 552–563.

Ginde, A. A., Liu, M. C., & Camargo, C. A., Jr (2009). Demographic differences and trends of vitamin D insufficiency in the US population, 1988-2004. *Archives of Internal Medicine, 169*, 626–632.

Glintborg, D., Mumm, H., Hougaard, D., Ravn, P., & Andersen, M. (2010). Ethnic differences in Rotterdam criteria and metabolic risk factors in a multiethnic group of women with PCOS studied in Denmark. *Clinical Endocrinology (Oxford), 73*, 732–738.

Goff, D. C., Jr, et al., Gerstein, H. C., Ginsberg, H. N., Cushman, W. C., Margolis, K. L., Byington, R. P., et al. (2007). Prevention of cardiovascular disease in persons with type 2 diabetes mellitus: Current knowledge and rationale for the Action to Control Cardiovascular Risk in Diabetes (ACCORD) trial. *The American Journal of Cardiology, 99*, 4i–20i.

Goodarzi, M. O., Dumesic, D. A., Chazenbalk, G., & Azziz, R. (2011). Polycystic ovary syndrome: Etiology, pathogenesis and diagnosis. *Nature Reviews Endocrinology, 7*, 219–231.

Gordon, T., & Kannel, W. B. (1982). Multiple risk functions for predicting coronary heart disease: The concept, accuracy, and application. *American Heart Journal, 103*, 1031–1039.

Grundy, S. M., Hansen, B., Smith, S. C., Jr, Cleeman, J. I., Kahn, R. A., & American Heart Association; National Heart, Lung, and Blood Institute, (2004). Clinical management of metabolic syndrome: Report of the American Heart Association/National Heart, Lung, and Blood Institute/American Diabetes Association conference on scientific issues related to management. *Circulation, 109*, 551–556.

Grundy, S. M., Brewer, H. B., Jr, Cleeman, J. I., Smith, S. C., Jr, Lenfant, C., & American Heart Association; National Heart, Lung, and Blood Institute, (2004). Definition of metabolic syndrome: Report of the National Heart, Lung, and Blood Institute/American Heart Association conference on scientific issues related to definition. *Circulation, 109*, 433–438.

Hahn, S., Haselhorst, U., Tan, S., Quadbeck, B., Schmidt, M., Roesler, S., et al. (2006). Low serum 25-hydroxyvitamin D concentrations are associated with insulin resistance and obesity in women with polycystic ovary syndrome. *Experimental And Clinical Endocrinology & Diabetes, 114*, 577–583.

Hallal, P. C., Andersen, L. B., Bull, F. C., Guthold, R., Haskell, W., Ekelund, U., & Lancet Physical Activity Series Working Group, (2012). Global physical activity levels: Surveillance progress, pitfalls, and prospects. *Lancet, 380*, 247–257.

Hippisley-Cox, J., Coupland, C., Vinogradova, Y., Robson, J., Minhas, R., Sheikh, A., et al. (2008). Predicting cardiovascular risk in England and Wales: Prospective derivation and validation of QRISK2. *BMJ, 336*, 1475–1482.

Ho, S. C. C., Chen, Y. M., Woo, J. L., Leung, S. S., Lam, T. H., & Janus, E. D. (2001). Association between simple anthropometric indices and cardiovascular risk factors. *International Journal of Obesity and Related Metabolic Disorders, 25*, 1689–1697.

Holick, M. F. (2006). High prevalence of vitamin D inadequacy and implications for health. *Mayo Clinic Proceedings, 81*, 353–373.

Howard, B. V., Ruotolo, G., & Robbins, D. C. (2003). Obesity and dyslipidemia. *Endocrinology and Metabolism Clinics of North America, 32*, 855–867.

Husemoen, L. L., Thuesen, B. H., Fenger, M., Jørgensen, T., Glümer, C., Svensson, J., et al. (2012). Serum 25(OH)D and type 2 diabetes association in a general population: A prospective study. *Diabetes Care, 35*, 1695–1700.

Institute of Medicine. (2004). *Preventing childhood obesity: Health in the balance.* Washington DC: The National Academies Press.

International Diabetes Federation. (2006). The IDF consensus worldwide definition of the metabolic syndrome. Brussels, Belgium.

International Diabetes Federation. (2017). *IDF diabetes atlas [Online].* Belgium: International Diabetes Federation. Available at http://www.diabetesatlas.org.

Irani, M., Seifer, D. B., Grazi, R. V., Julka, N., Bhatt, D., Kalgi, B., et al. (2015). Vitamin D Supplementation decreases TGF-beta1 bioavailability in PCOS: A randomized placebo-controlled trial. *The Journal of Clinical Endocrinology and Metabolism, 100*, 4307–4314.

Isomaa, B., Almgren, P., Tuomi, T., Forsén, B., Lahti, K., Nissén, M., et al. (2001). Cardiovascular morbidity and mortality associated with the metabolic syndrome. *Diabetes Care, 24*, 683–689.

Israni, A. K., Snyder, J. J., Skeans, M. A., Kasiske, B. L., & PORT Investigators, (2012). Clinical diagnosis of metabolic syndrome: Predicting new-onset diabetes, coronary heart disease, and allograft failure late after kidney transplant. *Transplant International, 25*, 748–757.

Jacobson, A. M., De Groot, M., & Samson, J. A. (1994). The evaluation of two measures of quality of life in patients with type I and type II diabetes. *Diabetes Care, 17*, 267–274.

Javed, Z., Papageorgiou, M., Deshmukh, H., Kilpatrick, E. S., Mann, V., Corless, L., et al. (2019a). A randomized, controlled trial of vitamin D supplementation on cardiovascular risk factors, hormones, and liver markers in women with polycystic ovary syndrome. *Nutrients, 11*, 188.

Javed, Z., Papageorgiou, M., Deshmukh, H., Rigby, A. S., Qamar, U., Abbas, J., et al. (2019b). Effects of empagliflozin on metabolic parameters in polycystic ovary syndrome: A randomized controlled study. *Clinical Endocrinology (Oxford), 90*, 805–813.

Jensterle, M., Kravos, N. A., Ferjan, S., Goricar, K., Dolzan, V., & Janez, A. (2020). Long-term efficacy of metformin in overweight-obese PCOS: Longitudinal follow-up of retrospective cohort. *Endocr Connect, 9*, 44–54.

Jordan, A. S., Mcsharry, D. G., & Malhotra, A. (2014). Adult obstructive sleep apnoea. *Lancet*, *383*, 736–747.

Kadowaki, S., & Norman, A. W. (1984). Dietary vitamin D is essential for normal insulin secretion from the perfused rat pancreas. *The Journal of Clinical Investigation*, *73*, 759–766.

Kannel, W. B., & Mcgee, D. L. (1979a). Diabetes and cardiovascular disease. The Framingham study. *Journal of the American Medical Association*, *241*, 2035–2038.

Kannel, W. B., & Mcgee, D. L. (1979b). Diabetes and cardiovascular risk factors: The Framingham study. *Circulation*, *59*, 8–13.

Kauffman, R. P., Baker, T. E., Baker, V. M., DiMarino, P., & Castracane, V. D. (2008). Endocrine and metabolic differences among phenotypic expressions of polycystic ovary syndrome according to the 2003 Rotterdam consensus criteria. *American Journal of Obstetrics and Gynecology*, *198*, 670. e1-7; discussion 670 e7-10.

Kelly, C., Kent, B., Nolan, G., & McNicholas, W.T. (2011). The relationship of obstructive sleep apnoea syndrome with renal function. *Irish journal of medical science*, Conference: UCD School of Medicine and Medical Science, SMMS, Summer Student Research Awards 2011, SSRA Dublin Ireland. Conference Start: 20111005 Conference End: 20111005. Conference Publication:, S521-S522.

Lakka, H. M., Laaksonen, D. E., Lakka, T. A., Niskanen, L. K., Kumpusalo, E., Tuomilehto, J., et al. (2002). The metabolic syndrome and total and cardiovascular disease mortality in middle-aged men. *Journal of the American Medical Association*, *288*, 2709–2716.

Ledoux, S., Coupaye, M., Essig, M., Msika, S., Roy, C., Queguiner, I., et al. (2010). Traditional anthropometric parameters still predict metabolic disorders in women with severe obesity. *Obesity (Silver Spring)*, *18*, 1026–1032.

Lee, I. M., Shiroma, E. J., Lobelo, F., Puska, P., Blair, S. N., Katzmarzyk, P. T., & Lancet Physical Activity Series Working Group, (2012). Effect of physical inactivity on major non-communicable diseases worldwide: An analysis of burden of disease and life expectancy. *Lancet*, *380*, 219–229.

Lerchbaum, E., & Obermayer-Pietsch, B. (2012). Vitamin D and fertility: A systematic review. *European Journal of Endocrinology*, *166*, 765–778.

Leung, P. S. (2016). The potential protective action of vitamin D in hepatic insulin resistance and pancreatic islet dysfunction in type 2 diabetes mellitus. *Nutrients*, *8*, 147.

Li, H. W., Brereton, R. E., Anderson, R. A., Wallace, A. M., & Ho, C. K. (2011). Vitamin D deficiency is common and associated with metabolic risk factors in patients with polycystic ovary syndrome. *Metabolism*, *60*, 1475–1481.

Lin, B., Shao, L., Luo, Q., Ou-Yang, L., Zhou, F., Du, B., et al. (2014). Prevalence of chronic kidney disease and its association with metabolic diseases: A cross-sectional survey in Zhejiang province, Eastern China. *BMC Nephrology*, *15*, 36.

Lombardo, F. L., Maggini, M., De Bellis, A., Seghieri, G., & Anichini, R. (2014). Lower extremity amputations in persons with and without diabetes in Italy: 2001-2010. *PLoS One*, *9*, e86405.

Lord, J., Thomas, R., Fox, B., Acharya, U., & Wilkin, T. (2006). The effect of metformin on fat distribution and the metabolic syndrome in women with polycystic ovary syndrome--a randomised, double-blind, placebo-controlled trial. *BJOG*, *113*, 817–824.

Lösel, R., & Wehling, M. (2003). Nongenomic actions of steroid hormones. *Nature Reviews. Molecular Cell Biology*, *4*, 46–56.

Luke, A., Philpott, J., Brett, K., Cruz, L., Lun, V., Prasad, N., Zetaruk, M., & CASM AdHoc Committee on Children's Fitness, (2004). Physical inactivity in children and adolescents: CASM AdHoc Committee on Children's Fitness. *Clinical Journal of Sport Medicine*, *14*, 261–266. discussion 260.

Lutty, G. A. (2013). Effects of diabetes on the eye. *Invest Ophthalmol Vis Sci*, *54* ORSF81-7.

Mabry, R. M., Reeves, M. M., Eakin, E. G., & Owen, N. (2010). Gender differences in prevalence of the metabolic syndrome in Gulf Cooperation Council Countries: A systematic review. *Diabetic Medicine*, *27*, 593–597.

Malik, M., & Razig, S. A. (2008). The prevalence of the metabolic syndrome among the multiethnic population of the United Arab Emirates: A report of a national survey. *Metabolic Syndrome and Related Disorders*, *6*, 177–186.

March, W. A., Moore, V. M., Willson, K. J., Phillips, D. I., Norman, R. J., & Davies, M. J. (2010). The prevalence of polycystic ovary syndrome in a community sample assessed under contrasting diagnostic criteria. *Human Reproduction*, *25*, 544–551.

Marsden, P. J., Murdoch, A. P., & Taylor, R. (2001). Tissue insulin sensitivity and body weight in polycystic ovary syndrome. *Clinical Endocrinology (Oxford)*, *55*, 191–199.

Mehio Sibai, A., Nasreddine, L., Mokdad, A. H., Adra, N., Tabet, M., & Hwalla, N. (2010). Nutrition transition and cardiovascular disease risk factors in Middle East and North Africa countries: Reviewing the evidence. *Annals of Nutrition & Metabolism*, *57*, 193–203.

Melton, L. J., 3rd, Macken, K. M., Palumbo, P. J., & Elveback, L. R. (1980). Incidence and prevalence of clinical peripheral vascular disease in a population-based cohort of diabetic patients. *Diabetes Care*, *3*, 650–654.

Mesinovic, J., Teede, H. J., Shorakae, S., Lambert, G. W., Lambert, E. A., Naderpoor, N., et al. (2020). The relationship between vitamin D metabolites and androgens in women with polycystic ovary syndrome. *Nutrients*, *12*, 1219.

Mitchell, D. M., Henao, M. P., Finkelstein, J. S., & Burnett-Bowie, S. A. (2012). Prevalence and predictors of vitamin D deficiency in healthy adults. *Endocrine Practice*, *18*, 914–923.

Mittelbrunn, M., Gutiérrez-Vázquez, C., Villarroya-Beltri, C., González, S., Sánchez-Cabo, F., González, M. Á., et al. (2011). Unidirectional transfer of microRNA-loaded exosomes from T cells to antigen-presenting cells. *Nature Communications*, *2*, 282.

Moran, L., & Teede, H. (2009). Metabolic features of the reproductive phenotypes of polycystic ovary syndrome. *Hum Reprod Update*, *15*, 477–488.

Moran, L. J., Hutchison, S. K., Norman, R. J., & Teede, H. J. (2011). Lifestyle changes in women with polycystic ovary syndrome. *Cochrane Database of Systematic Reviews*, CD007506.

Mu, N., Zhu, Y., Wang, Y., Zhang, H., & Xue, F. (2012). Insulin resistance: A significant risk factor of endometrial cancer. *Gynecologic Oncology*, *125*, 751–757.

Muscogiuri, G., Policola, C., Prioletta, A., Sorice, G., Mezza, T., Lassandro, A., et al. (2012). Low levels of 25(OH)D and insulin-resistance: 2 unrelated features or a cause-effect in PCOS? *Clinical Nutrition*, *31*, 476–480.

Nakagawa, T., Tanabe, K., Croker, B. P., Johnson, R. J., Grant, M. B., Kosugi, T., et al. (2011). Endothelial dysfunction as a potential contributor in diabetic nephropathy. *Nature Reviews Nephrology*, 7, 36–44.

Nakashima, A., Yokoyama, K., Yokoo, T., & Urashima, M. (2016). Role of vitamin D in diabetes mellitus and chronic kidney disease. *World Journal of Diabetes*, 7, 89–100.

Nakasone, H., Kako, S., Endo, H., Ito, A., Sato, M., Terasako, K., et al. (2009). Diabetes mellitus is associated with high early-mortality and poor prognosis in patients with autoimmune hemolytic anemia. *Hematology*, 14, 361–365.

National Clinical Guideline Centre (UK). (2014). *Lipid modification: cardiovascular risk assessment and the modification of blood lipids for the primary and secondary prevention of cardiovascular disease.* London: National Institute for Health and Care Excellence (UK).

Ninomiya, T. (2014). Diabetes mellitus and dementia. *Current Diabetes Reports*, 14, 487.

Norman, R. J., Dewailly, D., Legro, R. S., & Hickey, T. E. (2007). Polycystic ovary syndrome. *Lancet*, 370, 685–697.

Osorio Landa, H. K., Pérez Díaz, I., Laguna Bárcenas, S. D. C., López Navarro, J. M., Abella Roa, M. F., Corral Orozco, M., et al. (2020). Association of serum vitamin D levels with chronic disease and mortality. *Nutricion Hospitalaria*, 37, 335–342.

Palta, P., Schneider, A. L., Biessels, G. J., Touradji, P., & Hill-Briggs, F. (2014). Magnitude of cognitive dysfunction in adults with type 2 diabetes: A meta-analysis of six cognitive domains and the most frequently reported neuropsychological tests within domains. *Journal of the International Neuropsychological Society*, 20, 278–291.

Patell, R., Dosi, R., Joshi, H., Sheth, S., Shah, P., & Jasdanwala, S. (2014). Non-alcoholic fatty liver disease (NAFLD) in obesity. *Journal of Clinical and Diagnostic Research*, 8, 62–66.

Peters, S. A., Huxley, R. R., & Woodward, M. (2014). Diabetes as a risk factor for stroke in women compared with men: A systematic review and meta-analysis of 64 cohorts, including 775 385 individuals and 12 539 strokes. *Lancet*, 383, 1973–1980.

Pittas, A. G., Dawson-Hughes, B., Li, T., Van Dam, R. M., Willett, W. C., Manson, J. E., et al. (2006). Vitamin D and calcium intake in relation to type 2 diabetes in women. *Diabetes Care*, 29, 650–656.

Popkin, B. (2002). An overview on the nutrition transition and its health implications: The Bellagio meeting. *Public Health Nutrition*, 5, 93–103.

Popkin, B. (2004). The nutrition transition: An overview of world patterns of change. *Nutrition Reviews*, 62, S140–S143.

Rahim, H. F., Sibai, A., Khader, Y., Hwalla, N., Fadhil, I., Alsiyabi, H., et al. (2014). Non-communicable diseases in the Arab world. *Lancet*, 383, 356–367.

Rask Larsen, J., Dima, L., Correll, C. U., & Manu, P. (2018). The pharmacological management of metabolic syndrome. *Expert Review of Clinical Pharmacology*, 11, 397–410.

Rasmussen, C. B., & Lindenberg, S. (2014). The effect of liraglutide on weight loss in women with polycystic ovary syndrome: An observational study. *Frontiers in Endocrinology (Lausanne)*, 5, 140.

Renehan, A. G., Tyson, M., Egger, M., Heller, R. F., & Zwahlen, M. (2008). Body-mass index and incidence of cancer: A systematic review and meta-analysis of prospective observational studies. *Lancet*, 371, 569–578.

Rosenbaum, D., Haber, R. S., & Dunaif, A. (1993). Insulin resistance in polycystic ovary syndrome: Decreased expression of GLUT-4 glucose transporters in adipocytes. *The American Journal of Physiology*, 264, E197–E202.

Rotterdam ESHRE/ASRM-Sponsored PCOS Consensus Workshop Group, (2004). Revised 2003 consensus on diagnostic criteria and long-term health risks related to polycystic ovary syndrome (PCOS). *Hum Reprod*, Jan., 19(1), 4–17. doi: 10.1093/humrep/deh098. PMID: 14688154.

Rubin, R. R., & Peyrot, M. (1999). Quality of life and diabetes. *Diabetes Metabolism Research and Reviews*, 15, 205–218.

Salley, K. E., Wickham, E. P., Cheang, K. I., Essah, P. A., Karjane, N. W., & Nestler, J. E. (2007). Glucose intolerance in polycystic ovary syndrome--a position statement of the Androgen Excess Society. *The Journal of Clinical Endocrinology and Metabolism*, 92, 4546–4556.

Sathyapalan, T., & Atkin, S. (2011). Review topic on mechanisms in endocrinology recent advances in the cardiovascular aspects of polycystic ovary syndrome. *European Journal of Endocrinology*, 166, 575–583.

Selimoglu, H., Duran, C., Kiyici, S., Ersoy, C., Guclu, M., Ozkaya, G., et al. (2010). The effect of vitamin D replacement therapy on insulin resistance and androgen levels in women with polycystic ovary syndrome. *Journal of Endocrinological Investigation*, 33, 234–238.

Shi, Y., Zhao, H., Shi, Y., Cao, Y., Yang, D., Li, Z., et al. (2012). Genome-wide association study identifies eight new risk loci for polycystic ovary syndrome. *Nature Genetics*, 44, 1020–1025.

Simoni, M., Tempfer, C. B., Destenaves, B., & Fauser, B. C. (2008). Functional genetic polymorphisms and female reproductive disorders: Part I: Polycystic ovary syndrome and ovarian response. *Human Reproduction Update*, 14, 459–484.

Toppe, C., Möllsten, A., Schön, S., Jönsson, A., & Dahlquist, G. (2014). Renal replacement therapy due to type 1 diabetes; time trends during 1995-2010 - A Swedish population based register study. *Journal of Diabetes and its Complications*, 28, 152–155.

Tuna, M., Manuel, D. G., Bennett, C., Lawrence, N., van Walraven, C., Keely, E., et al. (2014). One- and five-year risk of death and cardiovascular complications for hospitalized patients with hyperglycemia without diagnosed diabetes: An observational study. *Journal of Hospital Medicine.*

Tupper, T., & Gopalakrishnan, G. (2007). Prevention of diabetes development in those with the metabolic syndrome. *The Medical Clinics of North America*, 91, 1091–1105. viii-ix.

Unsal, T., Konac, E., Yesilkaya, E., Yilmaz, A., Bideci, A., Ilke Onen, H., et al. (2009). Genetic polymorphisms of FSHR, CYP17, CYP1A1, CAPN10, INSR, SERPINE1 genes in adolescent girls with polycystic ovary syndrome. *Journal of Assisted Reproduction and Genetics*, 26, 205–216.

Van Diepen, M., Schroijen, M. A., Dekkers, O. M., Rotmans, J. I., Krediet, R. T., Boeschoten, E. W., et al. (2014). Predicting mortality in patients with diabetes starting dialysis. *PLoS One*, 9, e89744.

Vieth, R. (1999). Vitamin D supplementation, 25-hydroxyvitamin D concentrations, and safety. *The American Journal of Clinical Nutrition*, 69, 842–856.

Wadden, T. A., Berkowitz, R. I., Womble, L. G., Sarwer, D. B., Phelan, S., Cato, R. K., et al. (2005). Randomized trial of lifestyle modification and pharmacotherapy for obesity. *The New England Journal of Medicine, 353,* 2111–2120.

Wadden, T. A., Volger, S., Sarwer, D. B., Vetter, M. L., Tsai, A. G., Berkowitz, R. I., et al. (2011). A two-year randomized trial of obesity treatment in primary care practice. *The New England Journal of Medicine, 365,* 1969–1979.

Wald, N. J. (2001). Guidance on terminology. *Journal of Medical Screening, 8,* 56.

Wan, H., Wang, Y., Zhang, K., Chen, Y., Fang, S., Zhang, W., et al. (2019). Associations between vitamin D and microvascular complications in middle-aged and elderly diabetic patients. *Endocrine Practice, 25,* 809–816.

Welt, C. K., Styrkarsdottir, U., Ehrmann, D. A., Thorleifsson, G., Arason, G., Gudmundsson, J. A., et al. (2012). Variants in DENND1A are associated with polycystic ovary syndrome in women of European ancestry. *The Journal of Clinical Endocrinology and Metabolism, 97,* E1342–E1347.

Wijeyaratne, C. N., Balen, A. H., Barth, J. H., & Belchetz, P. E. (2002). Clinical manifestations and insulin resistance (IR) in polycystic ovary syndrome (PCOS) among South Asians and Caucasians: Is there a difference? *Clinical Endocrinology (Oxford), 57,* 343–350.

Wilding, J. P. (2014). The importance of weight management in type 2 diabetes mellitus. *Int J Clin Pract.*

World Health Organization. (2013a). *Diabetes.* World Health Organization.

World Health Organization. (2013b). *Obesity and overweight.* World Health Organization.

World Health Organization. (2014). *Obesity and overweight.* World Health Organization.

Wortsman, J., Matsuoka, L. Y., Chen, T. C., Lu, Z., & Holick, M. F. (2000). Decreased bioavailability of vitamin D in obesity. *The American Journal of Clinical Nutrition, 72,* 690–693.

Zahiri, Z., Sharami, S. H., Milani, F., Mohammadi, F., Kazemnejad, E., Ebrahimi, H., et al. (2016). Metabolic syndrome in patients with polycystic ovary syndrome in Iran. *International Journal of Fertility & Sterility, 9,* 490–496.

Zhang, H. Y., Zhu, F. F., Xiong, J., Shi, X. B., & Fu, S. X. (2009). Characteristics of different phenotypes of polycystic ovary syndrome based on the Rotterdam criteria in a large-scale Chinese population. *BJOG, 116,* 1633–1639.

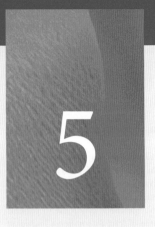

5

LIFESTYLE 2
Obesity, Body Image and Nutrition

EMAN TAWASH

CHAPTER OUTLINE

INTRODUCTION

Obesity is a complex, 'modern' condition and increasing global health concern (Isakova et al., 2018), somewhat ironically replacing the late 20th century's focus on undernutrition, with 70% of the adult population now considered to be overweight or obese (WHO (World Health Organization), 2016).

Obesity affects both sexes, all age groups and all socioeconomic levels (Azzeh et al., 2017) and can negatively impact an individual's physical and mental health and quality of life as well as contribute to a decline in life expectancy. Millions of people with obesity suffer premature disability and serious noncommunicable diseases such as cardiovascular disease, stroke, type 2 diabetes and several types of cancer (Blüher, 2019). People with obesity may even encounter social discrimination; avoid public places; live with depression, shame, guilt and social isolation; and are also less likely to be less successful in their working lives (Sarwer & Polonsky, 2016).

The impact of globalisation and concomitant socioeconomic changes has had a considerable impact on people's lifestyles and nutritional habits. Moreover, it is also important to recognise distinct regional differences in obesity prevalence and trends that might help identify societal causes of obesity including political, socioeconomic, cultural and physical factors which promote obesogenic environments. Having a better understanding of these factors can help provide guidance on the most promising intervention strategies as obesity and its related diseases are largely preventable. Further, prompt and proactive global interventions are needed, as the longer a person is overweight, the more difficult it may be to reverse the process, as the body's ability to burn fat may become somewhat compromised (Whittle et al., 2015).

BACKGROUND

Obesity: Definition and Classification

Overweight and obesity are defined as abnormal or excessive accumulations of fat that present a risk to an individual's health (Fitzpatrick et al., 2018). Overweight and obesity usually result from an energy imbalance between calorie intake and expenditure, especially with decreased levels of physical activity with these excess calories stored in the body as fat (Alharbi et al., 2017). Obesity can occur at any age, even in young children. For adults, a body mass index (BMI) equal to or over 25 is considered overweight, and a BMI equal to or over 30 is obese. Severe obesity is defined when a BMI is greater than 40. The Centres for Disease Control and Prevention (CDC, 2020) subdivide obesity into three categories:

- Class 1: BMI of 30 to <35
- Class 2: BMI of 35 to <40
- Class 3: BMI of 40 or higher

Class 3 obesity is sometimes categorised as 'extreme' obesity carrying the greatest risk of other health problems.

Numerous studies have confirmed obesity as a multifactorial disorder (Lin et al., 2018) including genetics (Karra et al., 2013); stress; medications such as steroids, anticonvulsants and mood stabilisers (Domecq et al., 2015); and environmental factors (Kit et al., 2014). Sleep deprivation has also been identified as a contributing factor to obesity due to its negative metabolic consequences (Agrawal, 2016).

EPIDEMIOLOGY OF OBESITY

Obesity was once considered a problem only in high-income countries; however, it is steadily affecting many low- and middle-income countries, especially in urban areas (WHO, 2021). Since 1980, WHO has reported significant increases in every region with the epidemiology differing according to the age of the obesity epidemic. In developing countries, it is estimated that over 115 million people suffer from obesity-related problems. Children in low- and middle-income countries are also more vulnerable to obesity because of poor diet and limited opportunities for physical activity (Mirmiran et al., 2010). From an early age, these children are exposed to high-fat, high-sugar, high-salt, energy-dense and micronutrient-poor foods, which tend to be lower in cost but are also lower in nutrient quality (WHO, 2021).

In the Middle East, obesity has reached alarming levels, thereby increasing the incidence of noncommunicable diseases with the latter accounting for 50% of the total causes of death (Musaiger, 2011a). According to WHO (2017), nine Arab countries have ranked highest in obesity statistics among adults: Kuwait (37.9%), Jordan (35.5%), Saudi Arabia (35.4%), Qatar (35.1%), Libya (32.5%), Egypt and Lebanon (32%), United Arab Emirates (UAE, 31.7%) and Iraq (30.4%). Accordingly, related diseases such as diabetes have increased exponentially, for example, diabetes rates are projected to increase by 96.2% by 2035, creating significant pressures on healthcare systems.

The six Arabian Gulf countries have a very high prevalence of obesity and being overweight. Around 30% or more of the population in these countries are obese, and more than 60% have a weight range of $25\,kg/m^2$ higher than normal (Samara et al., 2019). According to the United Nations, Kuwait has been ranked the highest when it comes to the obesity index in the Gulf (42% of adults obese)—the world's 10th most obese population per capita—closely followed by Saudi Arabia (35%) and Qatar (33%) (Al Busaidi et al., 2019).

LIFESPAN AND SEX

A global estimation of obesity from 1980 to 2013 found that the peak age of obesity in developing countries was about 45 years for men and 55 years for women (Ng et al., 2014). In the Arabian Gulf countries, obesity has increased continuously over time (Azzeh et al., 2017). For example, the prevalence of obesity in men ranged from 16% (Oman) to 39% (Kuwait) with women 22% (Oman) to 53% (Kuwait) (Musaiger, 2011a). Most recent statistics showed that the highest global prevalence of obesity in women is reported in Saudi Arabia (Alharbi et al., 2017). Notably, women may have higher rates of obesity, but men have higher rates of being overweight (WHO, 2021).

In the Eastern Mediterranean Region (EMR), the prevalence of obesity among preschool children has increased significantly during the past three decades and it was estimated that about 23.5 million school children were overweight or obese during 1992–2001 with this proportion almost doubling to 41.7 million in 2010 (Musaiger, 2011a). Being overweight in the Arabian Gulf countries among preschool children

CASE STUDY 5.1
MARYAM AND OBESITY

Maryam is a 40-year-old female, married with five children. She was working as a school administrator until she had her first baby. She lives in a small house in Manama-Bahrain with her family and a housemaid who helps her with domestic work and cooking. Maryam was recently diagnosed with type 2 diabetes and based on her height and weight, she had a body mass index (BMI) of 40 kg/m^2. During her follow-up visits to the diabetes clinic, the nurse found that Maryam's blood glucose was always high. The nurse discussed with Maryam that she needs to reduce her weight to improve her diabetes.
1. What factors contributed to Maryam's diabetes?
2. Considering the above factors, what strategies should be considered to help Maryam reduce her weight?

ranged from 1.9% (Oman) to 13.2% (Bahrain), while obesity prevalence in children and adolescents was 5%–14% (Alharbi et al., 2020). In school-age children specifically, the prevalence of obesity ranged from 7.1% (Qatar) to 24.8% (Kuwait).

The prevalence of overweight and obesity by sex in this age group does not exhibit the same trend. In countries such as Bahrain, Kuwait and Qatar, the prevalence of being overweight was higher among girls than among boys. In the UAE, the prevalence of overweight and obesity was higher in boys than in girls (Musaiger, 2011a), while in Saudi Arabia the prevalence of obesity among school boys aged 6–14 years has increased seven times—from 3.4% in 1988 to 24.5% in 2005 (Al-Hazzaa, 2007). Generally, the prevalence of overweight and obesity in the Middle East is greater among boys than among girls from Saudi Arabia, the Islamic Republic of Iran, Lebanon, Kuwait and Pakistan. Such differences may reflect different cultural habits and attitudes towards nutrition and physical activity (Bellizzi et al, 2002).

THE IMPACT OF OBESITY

Obesity is the sixth most important risk factor for worldwide disease burden and is strongly associated with diabetes, cerebral and cardiovascular diseases, various cancers, sleep apnoea and musculoskeletal disorders (Badran & Laher, 2011). Adults, children and adolescents all suffer from short-term and long-term health consequences (Villarosa et al., 2018).

People with obesity are more likely to have high blood pressure and high cholesterol levels, which are risk factors for cardiovascular disease and stroke, with hypertension likely to cause about 12.8% of the total of all global deaths (Ahmed et al., 2014). Furthermore, elevated blood pressure is reported to be more prevalent in children with obesity (Yi et al., 2015) and also affects the ability of insulin to control blood sugar levels in the body which, in turn, raises the risk of insulin resistance (Bays et al., 2007).

Obesity may increase the risk of cancer in different body organs including the kidney, prostate, uterus, breast, colon, rectum, liver and pancreas, with those with a BMI of more than 40 compared to those with normal weight, having death rates from cancer that were 52% higher for men and 62% higher for women (Calle et al., 2003). Obesity may also cause infertility in men and women (Al-Othman et al., 2015) due to hormonal abnormalities and ovulation dysfunction (Bosdou et al., 2016).

More recently, obesity increases the risk of developing severe symptoms related to bacterial and viral infections including coronavirus disease 2019 (COVID-19). People who have had severe cases of COVID-19 may require treatment in intensive care units or even mechanical assistance to breathe (Albashir, 2020). Furthermore, obesity increases the risk for mental illnesses such as clinical depression, anxiety and other mental disorders (Rajan & Menon, 2017) with a meta-analysis also confirming that obesity increases the risk of depression (Luppino et al., 2010).

Obesity is also associated with social disadvantages, unemployment and reduced socioeconomic efficiency, thus progressively creating an economic burden (Blüher, 2019) with weight discrimination also becoming a manifestation of such social inequity (Alberga et al., 2016). This weight bias contributes to a violation of human rights where children and adults living with obesity are treated unequally at educational institutions, at work and within healthcare facilities simply because of their body size (O'Hara, 2013) (Case Study 5.1).

FACTORS CONTRIBUTING TO OBESITY IN THE ARABIAN GULF

The discovery of oil in the 1930s resulted in significant growth in incomes in the Arabian Gulf, resulting in rapid urbanisation and much improved living conditions. This increase in wealth led to dramatic changes in the socioeconomic structure of the Gulf communities (Alharbi et al., 2020) bringing with it significant prosperity and easier lifestyles in terms of working environment, types of work, transport, access to cheap migrant labour, more sedentarism and the adoption of Westernised style fast food (Badran & Laher, 2011). Fifty years ago, obesity was not familiar to the people of the Gulf; however, these changes created an 'obesogenic environment' and were unsurprisingly, followed by the emergence of metabolic conditions or other noncommunicable diseases (Amin et al., 2014).

Obesity is known to result from environmental factors including a lack of physical activity, changes in dietary patterns and technological advances, combined with a lack of supportive policies in sectors such as health, agriculture, transport, urban planning, environment, food processing, distribution, marketing, promotion and pricing, as well as education (WHO, 2021). The structure of people's diet has shifted towards caloric dense foods with more fat, salt and added sugar and a decline in the intake of fruits and vegetables (Amin et al., 2014). For example, data have shown an increase in fat supply in the Middle East countries exceeding 40% in Kuwait and United Arab Emirates (Musaiger, 2011b). Although there is a perception that the shift from traditional foods to more Westernised foods has contributed to obesity, it is important to note that many indigenous fast foods contain a considerable amount of fat and energy (Alzaman & Ali, 2016) with a study from Bahrain demonstrating many local fast foods have higher a proportion of fat, salt and calories than Western fast foods (Musaiger & D'Souza, 2007).

There are a number of other factors that have contributed to the increase in obesity in the greater Middle East including but not limited to:

- Accessible and readily available fast food that is high in fats, sugar and carbohydrates (Badran & Laher, 2011).
- Increasing food portion sizes including 'up size' options and 'all-you-can-eat' buffets (Benton, 2015).
- More women are now involved in the Gulf Cooperation Council (GCC) countries' workforce, and thus have less time for food preparation, with the frequency of eating food prepared outside the home increasing (Alzaman & Ali, 2016).
- Food tends to be a family-focused endeavour in the Gulf with restaurants being very busy during weekends and holidays (Musaiger & D'Souza, 2007).
- Many neighbourhoods have little or no access to fresh, healthy foods and a lot of fresh food tends to be very expensive with fruit and vegetables largely imported (Musaiger et al., 2012). Local food production is clearly challenging due to the hot climate and lack of fresh water but local initiatives such as farmers' markets and aquaponic farms, for example, Bahrain Line Aquaponic Centre, are encouraging and offer hope going forward.
- Television commercials and images promote unhealthy foods which may influence the viewers' food choices (Madanat et al., 2007) with television food advertisements mostly related to fast foods, chocolate and sweets (Musaiger, 2011a).
- Eating breakfast reduces the risk of becoming overweight or obese (Szajewska & Ruszczyn, 2010). However, skipping or intake of a poor nutritional value breakfast has become something of a habit in the region.
- WHO (2009) reported a high prevalence of inactivity among most countries of the EMR contributing to the high rates of obesity. The shift from occupations requiring physical activity and heavy manual work such as farming, diving, carpentry and animal husbandry to the service sector and high technology work that requires little energy expenditure has led to a more sedentary lifestyle in the Gulf (Bener, 2010). Likewise, people living in isolated rural areas in the UAE and Oman have lower obesity rates because they still maintain a Bedouin lifestyle and eat traditional foods (Badran & Laher, 2011).
- With the availability of extensive road networks, most people in the Gulf use their own cars for transportation (Alzaman & Ali, 2016), while more people are less likely to walk or cycle, not least due to the extremes of temperature. The extreme outdoor temperatures force people to remain indoors and resort to using cars to travel even relatively short distances. There is also a lack of sidewalks and safe bike trails, and many

neighbourhoods do not have safe areas to walk or exercise. The lack of public transportation and appropriate bus stations that accommodate the weather is another factor that discourages people from walking even a small distance to take the bus.

- Nonactive, indoor activities are also highly associated with weight gain, for example, mobile phones, computers, etc. (AlNohair, 2014), with one study claiming that 57% of obese adolescents consumed their main meals while watching television—a habit that tends to lead to overeating (Musaiger, 2011a).

- More recently, smoking cigarettes and shisha has become increasingly popular in the Gulf with Moradi-Lakeh et al. (2016) reporting a higher prevalence of overweight and obesity in heavy smokers and daily users of shisha.

- Obesity increases in illiterate people due to the lack of appreciation of the health risks associated with obesity (Badran & Laher, 2011) and not being exposed to information about proper nutrition and healthy food choices (Al Slamah et al., 2017).

- In general, married couples are more likely to be overweight or obese, which could be due to decreased activity and an increase in food intake which is reinforced by eating together (AlNohair, 2014). Obesity is also found to be common among the inherited diseases resulting from parents' consanguinity, which is very common in the GCC. Alharbi et al. (2020) suggested that participants in Saudi Arabia were more prone to develop obesity if they had first-cousin consanguineous parents.

- Multiparity is very common in the GCC and has led to more obesity among women. Women are likely to gain 4.55 kg or more 1 year postpartum due to gestational weight gain, decreased physical activity and increased food intake (Badran & Laher, 2011).

- Wearing the traditional long and wide dress either for men or women (abaya) in the Gulf countries may indirectly contribute to obesity as it hides weight gain and may reduce motivation to lose weight (Musaiger & Qashqari, 2005) with Al-Tawil et al. (2007) noting that the prevalence

> ## CASE STUDY 5.2
> ### WHAT CAUSED SALMAN'S OBESITY?
>
> Salman is a 2-year-old boy from Kuwait. When he was born, his weight was 4 kg and his length was 50.5 cm. All his family members commented on how beautiful and healthy he looked, and his mother expressed pride in hearing this. During Salman's visit to the child welfare clinic, he maintained a height in the 74th percentile and a weight in the 95th percentile on the growth charts. 'He likes to play and eats very well. He loves eating potato chips, and pizza' his mother said. Although Salman is developing well, the nurse feels it is important to caution his mother to be attentive to his caloric intake and to ensure that he remains active.
> 1. Comparing Salman's data with the WHO child growth standard, how would you evaluate Salman's weight?
> 2. Why do you think the nurse is concerned about Salman's weight?

of obesity was greater among women who wore gowns or the abaya, than those who wore trousers outside the home.

- Women in the GCC may face more cultural impediments to undertaking exercise and sports compared to men due to childcare and home commitments as well as negative attitudes by family members (Musaiger, 2011a). Further, exercise facilities may be limited (Samara et al., 2015) and the sedentary lifestyle may also be aggravated by a high dependency on migrant labour for domestic chores (Badran & Laher, 2011) (Case Study 5.2).

RAMADAN AND FASTING

Specific cultural practices related to diet are also identified to increase the prevalence of obesity in the Middle East. For example, sharing plates with family members is common and may encourage overeating via a lack of portion control (Al-Tawil et al., 2007). Food plays a large part in socialisation, hospitality and families in the GCC with most traditional meals consisting of rice (high carbohydrates) and red meat (high fat). During the Holy month of Ramadan, when Muslims fast between the hours of daylight, large high-calorie meals (mostly lamb stewed with wheat berries) are prepared for iftar (breaking fasting) every night. Traditional dishes, particularly rich desserts, are considered the most important aspect of the meal. Social gatherings, usually buffet style, are frequent at iftar and suhur (predawn meal) and are associated with heavy eating. Fasting has many health benefits (Rouhani & Azadbakht, 2014); however, the unhealthy eating habits that people associate with Ramadan have led to more obesity. Furthermore, during Ramadan, people invert the normal day–night routine that alters their sleep patterns, and sleep deprivation is noted to have metabolic effects that predispose individuals to weight gain (Cooper et al., 2018).

OBESITY AND BODY IMAGE

The influence of men in determining women's attitudes towards body size is another important issue in some countries in the Middle East. For example, 43% of Qatari women reportedly believed that men preferred overweight women (Musaiger et al., 2012). Culturally, there is also a perception among some parents in the Gulf that being overweight is a sign of high social status, fertility and prosperity (Badran & Laher, 2011).

More recently, it has been suggested that perceived 'Western' standards of beauty have contributed to Arab females' apparent preoccupation with thinness and body image dissatisfaction and may also be evidence of growing conflict between Western values and Arabic traditions. For example, 66% of UAE adolescents, especially girls, displayed body image dissatisfaction while expressing the desire to be thin (Eapen et al., 2006). Similarly in Bahrain, Al-Sendi et al. (2004) demonstrated that adolescents' weight-related beliefs and attitudes exist at two ends of the spectrum: a tolerance of obesity at one end and exaggerated concern for its occurrence at the other, while in Saudi Arabia, 36.8% of overweight women perceived themselves as normal weight (Musaiger, 2011a).

The current trend of being weight-centric, in which weight is viewed worldwide as a proxy for health and beauty, has arguably contributed to individuals who are overweight or obese experiencing weight discrimination (Alberga et al., 2016). People with obesity are often blamed for their weight status by society, due to the belief that obesity is wholly controlled by individuals. Furthermore, there is a lot of focus through media portrayals, public health programmes and campaigns on glamorising thinness and demonising fatness to reflect the health consequences of obesity (Puhl et al.,

2013). Participants who viewed negative, stereotypical photographs of obese people expressed more negative attitudes towards them (Fortner, 2017) with obese people thought to be lazy, unmotivated, unintelligent, less competent, noncompliant and lacking self-discipline. These stereotypes are predominant and are rarely challenged, especially in Western society, leaving obese persons vulnerable to social prejudice, unfair treatment and an impaired quality of life (Puhl & Heuer, 2012).

A lack of understanding can lead to negative attitudes and stigma towards people of all ages who suffer from obesity. Children and adolescents with obesity are exposed to many forms of weight stigma, including verbal teasing, social exclusion and physical bullying by peers. Moreover, this weight stigma creates different expectations from adults including coaches, teachers, healthcare providers and even parents. Accordingly, obese children are more likely to have low self-esteem, depression, anxiety and a poor body image. Rankin et al. (2016) found that children suffering from obesity face negative attitudes from peers and have higher rates of suicidal thoughts and behaviours while adolescents who were unfairly treated due to their physical appearance had higher blood pressure (Matthews et al., 2005). All areas of children's lives are affected by weight discrimination which correspondingly greatly reduces their quality of life (Sahoo et al., 2015).

OBESITY INTERVENTIONS

Long-term weight management is extremely challenging due to interactions between individuals' biology, behaviour and the obesogenic environment they may live in (Hall & Kahan, 2018). Substantial weight loss is possible across a range of interventional modalities; however, sustaining a long-term weight loss is very challenging and weight regain is typical (Loveman et al., 2011). The goal of obesity interventions is to reach and stay at a healthy weight. Maintaining a healthy weight through dietary changes (80%) and increased physical activity (20%) is one way to prevent or reduce obesity. People with obesity need 150–300 minutes a week of moderate-intensity physical activity to maintain a modest loss of weight and prevent further weight gain (Swift et al., 2014). Changing eating and physical activity habits can be very hard; however, they are key when managing obesity. Even modest weight loss, as small as 5%–10%, can reduce the risk of developing complications related to obesity (Ryan & Yockey, 2017).

Many nonclinical weight management programs are available and can be self-managed, ranging from books and websites to chain weight-loss programmes and support groups. However, very often people with obesity find it more helpful to work with health professionals to help them make changes in their eating and activity habits and guide them with resources and support. These may include obesity specialists, nurses, dietitians and behavioural counsellors. Antiobesity medications such as phentermine and topiramate enhance adherence to a low-calorie diet by stopping the hunger and lack of fullness signals that appear when trying to lose weight (Roberts et al., 2017). Increasing evidence has shown that antiobesity medications can result in greater weight loss; however, they have a high cost, may cause adverse outcomes including cancer and people regain weight when they stop taking them (Tak & Lee, 2020).

It has been reported that 579,517 bariatric metabolic operations and 14,725 endoluminal procedures are performed annually worldwide (Angrisani et al., 2017). In the Middle East and North African (MENA) region, bariatric procedures are recommended for people with a BMI of 40 or 35 kg/m² with obesity-related comorbidities (Inocian et al., 2021). Endoscopic bariatric procedures significantly reduce patients' stomach volume or alter other parts of the digestive tract to treat obesity and related comorbidities (Castro & Guerron, 2020). Currently, bariatric procedures are considered the only effective, safe and durable therapeutic option for most patients with obesity (Reges et al., 2018) with the expected weight loss varying from 5% to 20% of total body weight loss (Wolfe et al., 2016).

The Middle East has seen a considerable increase in the provision of a highly profitable cosmetic surgery market. The growing numbers of bariatric surgeries, including sleeve gastrectomy, gastric bypass and the placement of gastric bands, are becoming much more commonplace among the indigenous populations who view it as a quick fix, with GCC countries undertaking the highest percentage of bariatric procedures in the world (Alyouhah et al., 2020). Unfortunately, bariatric surgery has arguably become something of a fashion for those who view regime, exercise and a healthy lifestyle

---

CASE STUDY 5.3
FATIMA AND BARIATRIC SURGERY

Fatima is a 35-year-old mother of three who has suffered from obesity problems since childhood. After failing several nonsurgical attempts to lose weight, she decided to undergo bariatric surgery. Before the surgery, her BMI was 42 kg/m². Nine months after the surgery, Fatima visited the outpatient clinic and was happy that she reached her weight loss goal. The nurse still advised Fatima to continue following up with her nutritionist and primary care provider.
1. Discuss the selection criteria for bariatric surgery.
2. Why is it important for Fatima to follow the nurse's advice?

---

as a challenging and cumbersome process and there is much work still to be done to fully address the problem of obesity in the Middle East. There is also a pressing need to incorporate culture-specific care for patients undergoing bariatric surgery to ensure improved outcomes (Inocian et al., 2021) (Case Study 5.3).

SUMMARY AND TAKEAWAY POINTS

Obesity is a complicated global health concern associated with many serious comorbidities, including diabetes and cardiovascular disease, and premature mortality:

- Although the prevalence of obesity has increased in almost every country in the world, regional differences exist in both obesity prevalence and trends. Understanding the drivers of these regional differences might help provide guidance for the most promising intervention strategies.
- The obesity pandemic is attributed to many factors including genetics, changes in the global food system and increased sedentary behaviours.
- Economic development, urbanisation and improved living conditions in the GCC and other Arab countries accompanied by cultural barriers and a lack of public awareness of healthy eating habits and increased sedentary lifestyle have led to greater consumption of unhealthy foods and decreased physical activity, with all of these factors increasing the prevalence of obesity across the last five decades.
- A major challenge for the GCC and other Arab countries is to translate knowledge of the main

causes of increased obesity prevalence in their countries into effective policies and actions in order to facilitate healthier individual choices.

■ Government policymakers must acknowledge that the increased prevalence of obesity is not a failure of an individual's drive to resist unhealthy foods and physical activity and should design preventive strategies accordingly.

■ Obesity-related issues and preventative strategies should incorporate culture-specific information to enhance relevance and improve outcomes.

REFERENCES

Agrawal, S. (2016). *Obesity, bariatric and metabolic surgery: A practical guide.* Switzerland: Springer International Publishing. https://doi.org/10.1007/978-3-319-04343-2.

Ahmed, H. G., Ginawi, I. A., & Al-hazimi, A. M. (2014). Prevalence of hypertension in Hail region, KSA: In a comprehensive survey. *International Journal of Sciences: Basic and Applied Research* (IJSBAR), 17(2), 288–296. Available at https://www.gssrr.org/index.php/JournalOfBasicAndApplied/article/view/2539. Accessed 23 August 2023.

Albashir, A. (2020). The potential impacts of obesity on COVID-19. *Clinical Medicine*, 20(4), e109–e113. https://doi.org/10.7861/clinmed.2020-0239.

Alberga, A. S., Russell-Mayhew, S., Ranson, K. M., & McLaren, L. (2016). Weight bias: A call to action. *Journal of Eating Disorders*, 4, 34. https://doi.org/10.1186/s40337-016-0112-4.

Al Busaidi, N., Shanmugam, P., & Manoharan, D. (2019). Diabetes in the Middle East: Government health care policies and strategies that address the growing diabetes prevalence in the Middle East. *Current Diabetes Reports*, 19(2), 8. https://doi.org/10.1007/s11892-019-1125-6.

Alharbi, K. K., Al-Sheikh, Y. A., Alsaadi, M. M., Mani, B., Udayaraja, G. K., Kohailan, M., et al. (2020). Screening for obesity in the offspring of first-cousin consanguineous couples: A phase-I study in Saudi Arabia. *Saudi Journal of Biological Sciences*, 27, 242–246. https://doi.org/10.1016/j.sjbs.2019.09.001.

Alharbi, K. K., Syed, R., Alharbi, F. K., & Khan, I. A. (2017). Association of apolipoprotein epolymorphism with impact on overweight university pupils. *Genetic Testing Molecular Biomarkers*, 21(1), 53–57. https://doi.org/10.1089/gtmb.2016.0190.

Al-Hazzaa, H. M. (2007). Prevalence and trends in obesity among schoolboys in Central Saudi Arabia between 1988 and 2005. *Saudi Medical Journal*, 28(10), 1569–1574.

AlNohair, S. (2014). Obesity in Gulf countries. *International Journal of Health Science*, 8(1), 79–83. https://doi.org/10.12816/0006074.

Al-Othman, S., Haoudi, A., Alhomoud, S., Alkhenizan, A., Khoja, T., & Al-Zahrani, A. (2015). Tackling cancer control in the Gulf Cooperation Council countries. *The Lancet Oncology*, 16(5), e246–e257. https://doi.org/10.1016/S1470-2045(15)70034-3.

Al-Sendi, A. M., Shetty, P., & Musaiger, A. O. (2004). Body weight perception among Bahraini adolescents. *Child: Care, Health and Development*, 30(4), 369–376. https://doi.org/10.1111/j.1365-2214.2004.00425.x.

Al Slamah, T., Nicholl, B. I., Alslail, F. Y., & Melville, C. A. (2017). Self-management of type 2 diabetes in Gulf Cooperation Council countries: A systematic review. *PloS One*, 12(12). https://doi.org/10.1371/journal.pone.0189160.

Al-Tawil, N. G., Abdulla, M. M., & Abdul Ameer, A. J. (2007). Prevalence of and factors associated with overweight and obesity among a group of Iraqi women. *Eastern Mediterranean Health Journal*, 13(2), 420–429. https://apps.who.int/iris/handle/10665/117263.

Alyouhah, N., Chen, W., & Kamel, D. (2020). Tackling obesity in the GCC: Increasing popularity of bariatric surgery to replace a healthy lifestyle, better understanding for policies and regulations. Proceedings of the Industrial Revolution & Business Management: 11th Annual PWRDS. https://doi.org/10.2139/ssrn.3659136

Alzaman, N., & Ali, A. (2016). Obesity and diabetes mellitus in the Arab world. *Journal of Taibah University Medical Sciences*, 11(4), 301–309. https://doi.org/10.1016/j.jtumed.2016.03.009.

Amin, T. T., Al-Hammam, A. M., Almulhim, N. A., Al-Hayan, M. I., Al-Mulhim, M. M., et al. (2014). Physical activity and cancer prevention: Awareness and meeting the recommendations among adult Saudis. *Asian Pacific Journal of Cancer Prevention*, 15, 2597–2606. https://doi.org/10.22034/APJCP.2017.18.1.135.

Angrisani, L., Santonicola, A., Iovino, P., et al. (2017). Bariatric surgery and endoluminal procedures: IFSO Worldwide Survey 2014. *Obesity Surgery*, 27, 2279–2289. https://doi.org/10.1007/s11695-017-2666-x.

Azzeh, F. S., Bukhari, H. M., Header, E.A., Ghabashi, M. A., Al-Mashi, S. S. & Noorwali, N. M. (2017). Trends in overweight or obesity and other anthropometric indices in adults aged 18–60 years in western Saudi Arabia. *Annals in Saudi Medicine*, 37(2): https://doi.org/10.5144/0256-4947.2017.106.

Badran, M., & Laher, I. (2011). Obesity in Arabic-speaking countries. *Journal of Obesity*, 686430. https://doi.org/10.1155/2011/686430.

Bays, H. E., Chapman, R. H., & Grandy, S. (2007). The relationship of body mass index to diabetes mellitus, hypertension and dyslipidaemia: Comparison of data from two national surveys. *International Journal of Clinical Practice*, 61(5), 737–747. https://doi.org/10.1111/j.1742-1241.2007.01336.x.

Bellizzi, M. C., et al. (2002). Prevalence of childhood and adolescent overweight and obesity in Asian and European countries. In C. ChenW. H. (2002). Dietz (Eds.), *Obesity in childhood and adolescence (Nestle Nutrition Workshop Series. Pediatric Program* (Vol. 49, pp. 23–35). Philadelphia: Lippincott Williams and Wilkins.

Bener, A. (2010). Colon cancer in rapidly developing countries: Review of the lifestyle, dietary, consanguinity and hereditary risk factors. *Oncology Reviews*, 5(1), 1–11. https://doi.org/10.1007/s12156-010-0061-0.

Benton, D. (2015). Portion size: What we know and what we need to know. *Critical Reviews in Food Science and Nutrition*, 55(7), 988–1004. https://doi.org/10.1080/10408398.2012.679980.

Blüher, M. (2019). Obesity: Global epidemiology and pathogenesis. *Nature Reviews Endocrinology*, 15, 288–298. https://doi.org/10.1038/s41574-019-0176-8.

Bosdou, J. K., Kolibianakis, E. M., Tarlatzis, B. C., & Fatemi, H. M. (2016). Sociocultural influences on fertility in the Middle East: The role of parental consanguinity, obesity and vitamin D deficiency. *Fertility Sterility*, 106(2), 259–260. https://doi.org/10.1016/j.fertnstert.2016.04.010.

Calle, E. E., Rodriguez, C., Walker-Thurmond, K., & Thun, M. J. (2003). Overweight, obesity, and mortality from cancer in a prospectively studied cohort of U.S. adults. *The New England Journal of Medicine*, 348(17), 1625–1638. https://doi.org/10.1056/NEJMoa021423.

Castro, M., & Guerron, A. D. (2020). Bariatric endoscopy: Current primary therapies and endoscopic management of complications and other related conditions. *Mini-invasive Surgery*, 4(47). https://doi.org/10.20517/2574-1225.2020.14.

Centres for Disease Control and Prevention (CDC) (2020). *Physical activity*. Available at https://www.cdc.gov/physicalactivity/basics/adults/index.htm.

Cooper, C. B., Neufeld, E. V., Dolezal, B. A., & Martin, J. L. (2018). Sleep deprivation and obesity in adults: A brief narrative review. *BMJ Open Sport & Exercise Medicine*, 4(1). https://doi.org/10.1136/bmjsem-2018-000392.

Domecq, J. P., Prutsky, G., Leppin, A., Sonbol, M. B., Altayar, (2015). Drugs commonly associated with weight change: A systematic review and meta-analysis. *Journal of Clinical Endocrinology and Metabolism*, 100(2), 363–370. https://doi.org/10.1210/jc.2014-3421.

Eapen, V., Mabrouk, A. A., & Bin-Othman, S. (2006). Disordered eating attitudes and symptomatology among adolescent girls in the United Arab Emirates. *Eating Behaviors*, 7(1), 53–60. https://doi.org/10.1016/j.eatbeh.2005.07.001.

Fitzpatrick, K. M., Shi, X., Willis, D., & Niemeier, J. (2018). Obesity and place: Chronic disease in the 500 largest US cities. *Obesity Research & Clinical Practice*, 12(5), 421–425. https://doi.org/10.1016/j.orcp.2018.02.005.

Fortner, S. A. (2017). *Effect of exposure to body-based imagery on weight bias and body image satisfaction in college students. Thesis*. Oregon State University.

Hall, K. D., & Kahan, K. (2018). Maintenance of lost weight and long-term management of obesity. *Medical Clinics of North America.*, 102(1), 183–197. https://doi.org/10.1016/j.mcna.2017.08.012.

Inocian, E. P., Nolfi, D. A., Felicilda-Reynaldo, R. F., Bodrick, M., et al. (2021). Bariatric surgery in the Middle East and North Africa: Narrative review with focus on culture-specific considerations: Review Article. *Surgery for Obesity and Related Diseases*, 17(2021), 1933–1941. https://doi.org/10.1016/j.soard.2021.06.015.

Isakova, J., Talaibekova, E., Vinnikov, D., Aldasheva, N., Mirrakhimov, E., & Aldashev, A. (2018). The association of Val109Asp polymorphic marker of intelectin 1 gene with abdominal obesity in Kyrgyz population. *BMC Endocrine Disorders*, 18(1), 15. https://doi.org/10.1186/s12902-018-0242-6.

Karra, E., O'Daly, O. G., Choudhury, A. I., Yousseif, A., Millership, S., et al. (2013). A link between FTO, ghrelin, and impaired brain food-cue responsivity. *The Journal of Clinical Investigation*, 123(8), 3539–3551. https://doi.org/10.1172/JCI44403.

Kit, B. K., Ogden, C. L., & Flegal, K. M. (2014). Epidemiology of obesity In W. Ahrens & I. Pigeot (Eds.), *Handbook of epidemiology*. New York: Springer. https://doi.org/10.1007/978-0-387-09834-0-55.

Lin, B. Y., Genden, K., Shen, W., Wu, P. -S., Yang, W. -C., Hung, H. -F., et al. (2018). The prevalence of obesity and metabolic syndrome in Tibetan immigrants living in high altitude areas in Ladakh, India. *Obesity Research & Clinical Practice*, 12(4), 365–371. https://doi.org/10.1016/j.orcp.2017.03.002.

Loveman, E., Frampton, G. K., Shepherd, J., et al. (2011). The clinical effectiveness and cost-effectiveness of long-term weight management schemes for adults: A systematic review. *Health Technology Assessment*, 15(2), 1–182. https://doi.org/10.3310/hta15020.

Luppino, F. S., de Wit, L. M., Bouvy, P. F., Stijnen, T., Cuijpers, P., Penninx, B., & Zitman, F. G. (2010). Overweight, obesity, and depression a systematic review and meta-analysis of longitudinal studies. *Arch Gen Psychiatry*, 67(3), 220–229. https://doi.org/10.1001/archgenpsychiatry.2010.2.

Madanat, H. N., Brown, R. B., & Hawks, S. R. (2007). The impact of body mass index and Western advertising and media on eating style, body image and nutrition transition among Jordanian women. *Public Health Nutrition*, 10(10), 1039–1046. https://doi.org/10.1017/S1368980007666713.

Matthews, K. A., Salomon, K., Kenyon, K., & Zhou, F. (2005). Unfair treatment, discrimination, and ambulatory blood pressure in Black and White adolescents. *Health Psychology*, 24(3), 258–265. https://doi.org/10.1037/0278-6133.24.3.258.

Mirmiran, P., Sherafat-Kazemzadeh, R., Jalali-Farahani, S., & Azizi, F. (2010). Childhood obesity in the Middle East: A review. *Eastern Mediterranean Health Journal*, 16(9), 1009–1017.

Moradi-Lakeh, M., El-Bcheraoui, C., Tuffaha, M., Daoud, F., Al Saeedi, M., Basulaiman, M., et al. (2016). The health of Saudi youths: Current challenges and future opportunities. *BMC Fam Pract*, 17, 26. https://doi.org/10.1186/s12875-016-0425-z.

Musaiger, A. O. (2011a). Overweight and obesity in Eastern Mediterranean region: Prevalence and possible causes. *Journal of Obesity*, 2011, 407237. https://doi.org/10.1155/2011/407237.

Musaiger, A. O. (2011b). Food Consumption Patterns in the Eastern Mediterranean Region. Arab Center for Nutrition Manama-Bahrain. Available at file:///C:/Users/eahmed/Downloads/Food_Consumption_Patterns_in_the__Eastern_Mediterranean_Region5%20(1).pdf.

Musaiger, A. O., & D'Souza, R. (2007). Nutritional profile of local and western fast foods consumed in Bahrain. *Ecology of Food and Nutrition*, 46(2), 143–161. https://doi.org/10.1080/03670240701328150.

Musaiger, A. O., & Qashqari, K. (2005). The relation between dressing and obesity among women in Saudi Arabia. *Arab Journal of Food and Nutrition*, 6, 292–302.

Musaiger, A. O., Takruri, H. R., Hassan, A. S., & Abu-Tarboush, H. (2012). Food-based dietary guidelines for the Arab Gulf countries. *Journal of Nutrition & Metabolism*, 2012, 905303. https://doi.org/10.1155/2012/905303.

Ng, M., Fleming, T., Robinson, M., Thomson, B., Graetz, N., Margono, C., et al. (2014). Global, regional, and national prevalence of overweight and obesity in children and adults during 1980–2013: A systematic analysis for the Global Burden of Disease Study 2013. *Lancet*, 384, 766–781. https://doi.org/10.1016/S0140-6736(14)60460-8.

O'Hara, L. G. J. (2013). Human rights casualties from the "War on Obesity": Why focusing on body weight is inconsistent with a human rights approach to health. *Fat Stud*, *1*, 32–46.

Puhl, R. M., & Heuer, C. A. (2012). The stigma of obesity: A review and update. *Obesity*, *17*, 941–964. https://doi.org/10.1038/oby.2008.636.

Puhl, R., Luedicke, J., & Peterson, J. L. (2013). Public reactions to obesity-related health campaigns: A randomized controlled trial. *American Journal of Preventive Medicine.*, *45*(1), 36–48. https://doi.org/10.1016/j.amepre.2013.02.010.

Rajan, T. M., & Menon, V. (2017). Psychiatric disorders and obesity: A review of association studies. *Journal of Postgraduate Medicine*, *63*(3), 182–190. https://doi.org/10.4103/jpgm.JPGM_712_16.

Rankin, J., Matthews, L., Cobley, S., Han, A., Sanders, R., Wiltshire, H. D., & Baker, J. S. (2016). Psychological consequences of childhood obesity: Psychiatric comorbidity and prevention. *Adolescent Health, Medicine and Therapeutics*, *7*, 125–146. https://doi.org/10.2147/AHMT.S101631.

Reges, O., Greenland, P., Dicker, D., et al. (2018). Association of bariatric surgery using laparoscopic banding, Roux-en-Y gastric bypass, or laparoscopic sleeve gastrectomy vs usual care obesity management with all-cause mortality. *JAMA*, *319*(3), 279–290. https://doi.org/10.1001/jama.2017.20513.

Roberts, C. A., Christiansen, P., & Halford, J. C. G. (2017). Tailoring pharmacotherapy to specific eating behaviours in obesity: Can recommendations for personalised therapy be made from the current data. *Acta Diabetol*, *54*, 715–725. https://doi.org/10.1007/s00592-017-0994-x.

Rouhani, M. H., & Azadbakht, L. (2014). Is Ramadan fasting related to health outcomes? A review on the related evidence. *Journal of Research in Medical Science: The Official Journal of Isfahan University of Medical Sciences*, *19*(10), 987–992.

Ryan, D. H., & Yockey, S. R. (2017). Weight loss and improvement in comorbidity: Differences at 5%, 10%, 15%, and Over. *Current Obesity Reports.*, *6*(2), 187–194. https://doi.org/10.1007/s13679-017-0262-y.

Sahoo, K., Sahoo, B., Choudhury, A. K., Sofi, N. Y., Kumar, R., & Bhadoria, A. S. (2015). Childhood obesity: Causes and consequences. *Journal of Family Medicine and Primary Care*, *4*(2), 187–192. https://doi.org/10.4103/2249-4863.154628.

Samara, A., Andersen, P. T., & Aro, A. R. (2019). Health promotion and obesity in the Arab Gulf states: Challenges and good practices. *Journal of Obesity*, article ID 4756260. https://doi.org/10.1155/2019/4756260.

Samara, A., Aro, A. R., Alrammah, T., & Nistrup, A. (2015). Lack of facilities rather than sociocultural factors as the primary barrier to physical activity among female Saudi university students. *International Journal of Women's Health*, *7*, 279–286. https://doi.org/10.2147/IJWH.S80680.

Sarwer, D. B., & Polonsky, H. M. (2016). The psychosocial burden of obesity. *Endocrinology and Metabolism Clinics of North America.*, *45*(3), 677–688. https://doi.org/10.1016/j.ecl.2016.04.016.

Swift, D., Johannsen, N., Lavie, C., Earnest, C., & Church, T. (2014). The role of exercise and physical activity in weight loss and maintenance. *Progress in Cardiovascular Diseases*, *56*, 441–447. https://doi.org/10.1016/j.pcad.2013.09.012.

Szajewska, H., & Ruszczynski, M. (2010). Systematic review demonstrating that breakfast consumption influences body weight outcomes in children and adolescents in Europe. *Critical Reviews in Food Science and Nutrition*, *50*(2), 113–119. https://doi.org/10.1080/10408390903467514.

Tak, J. Y., & Lee, S. Y. (2020). Anti-obesity drugs: Long-term efficacy and safety: An updated review. *World J Mens Health*, *39*, 208–221. https://doi.org/10.5534/wjmh.200010.

Villarosa, A. R., George, D., Ramjan, L. M., Srinivas, R., & George, A. (2018). The role of dental practitioners in addressing overweight and obesity among children: A scoping review of current interventions and strategies. *Obesity Research & Clinical Practice*, *12*(5), 405–415. https://doi.org/10.1016/j.orcp.2018.07.002.

Whittle, A. J., Jiang, M., Peirce, V., Relat, J., Virtue, S., et al. (2015). Soluble LR11/SorLA represses thermogenesis in adipose tissue and correlates with BMI in humans. *Nature Communications*, *6*, 8951. https://doi.org/10.1038/ncomms9951.

Wolfe, B. M., Kvach, E., & Eckel, R. H. (2016). Treatment of obesity: Weight loss and bariatric surgery. *Circulation Research.*, *118*(11), 1844–1855. https://doi.org/10.1161/CIRCRESAHA.116.307591.

WHO (World Health Organization) (2009). Regional data on non-communicable diseases. Available at http://www.emro.who.int/ncd/. Accessed 31 January 2021.

WHO (2016). Obesity and diabetes: The slow-motion disaster. Keynote address at the 47th meeting of the National Academy of Medicine. Available at https://www.who.int/director-general/speeches/. Accessed 31 January 2021.

WHO (2017). World health statistics: Monitoring health for the SDGs. Geneva. Available at https://www.who.int/gho/publications/world_health_statistics/2017/EN_WHS2017_TOC.pdf.

WHO (2021). Obesity. Available at https://www.who.int/health-topics/obesity#tab=tab_1. Accessed 15 January 2021.

Yi, Z., Rong, L. W., Chong, S., Qian, F., & Ming, S. X. (2015). Prevalence and correlates of elevated blood pressure in Chinese children aged 6-13 years: A nationwide school-based survey. *Biomedical and Environmental Sciences*, *28*(6), 401–409. https://doi.org/10.3967/bes2015.057.

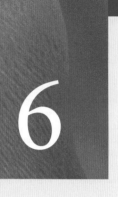

6

WOMEN'S HEALTH IN THE ARABIAN GULF AND GREATER MIDDLE EAST
Achievements and Challenges

GHUFRAN JASSIM

INTRODUCTION

Improvements in women's health are closely linked to changing social and political norms that have set the foundation for the current Arabian Gulf women's health movement.

This chapter discusses the achievements as well as challenges in healthcare delivery to women and girls in the Gulf Corporation Countries (GCC). Further, it puts emphasis on women's health by introducing the perspective of cultural frameworks that relate to holistic approaches to women's health and healthcare. At the end of this chapter, you will realise how cultural identities intersect to influence health.

In this chapter, challenges and gaps in providing holistic healthcare to women are discussed as well as potential solutions and suggestions for healthcare providers and policy makers in the GCC to optimise healthcare delivery to women.

Lastly, information about culturally sensitive healthcare practices and health literacy will be introduced to improve the communication between women and healthcare providers during healthcare encounters.

For centuries women's health has been largely interchangeable with that of women's reproductive health. Although vital, reproductive health is not the only component of women's health. There is an increasing amount of evidence that the definition of women's health should be more inclusive to more accurately reflect the sex and gender differences in all areas of health and disease (Regitz-Zagrosek, 2012). The term 'women's health' refers to all health conditions for which there is evidence in women, compared to men, of differing risks, presentations and/or responses to treatment, as well as those reproductive issues exclusive to women (American Medical Women's Association, 2016). Although the notion of women's health took decades to be brought to fruition in the West, it is just starting to emerge in the Middle East and GCC states. It is fundamental to separate the two geographical areas when it comes to women's health because the challenges, achievements and gaps are hugely different. GCC states constitute a case study of a Middle Eastern context.

This chapter will shed light on the ways in which Arabian Gulf states targeted women's health and well-being, including its gaps and challenges. It will also explore the sociocultural attitudes and perceptions of women's well-being, as well as the ways in which this is linked to other sociodemographic factors related to women.

The GCC states are known for their massive capital flows and resources as well as ambitious economic reforms strategies. In terms of foreign trade in 2013, the GCC economy was rated fifth in the world. The GCC (i.e., Bahrain, Kuwait, Oman, Qatar, the Kingdom of Saudi Arabia (KSA) and the United Arab Emirates (UAE)) aligned their national development plans with the eight millennium development goals (MDGs) proposed by the United Nation (UN) and the 17 sustainable development goals (SDGs) with commitment to fulfilling these goals (Daher-Nashif & Bawadi, 2020).

The World Health Organization's (WHO, 2016) 2015 report on the MDGs indicates that all GCC countries reduced measles, mumps and rubella (MMR) by roughly half between 1999 and 2015 (Daher-Nashif & Bawadi, 2020; UNICEF, 2018). This was attributed to improvements in healthcare services, prevention and public awareness. However, it is also likely to be the result of an improvement in human development index (HDI) components, such as life expectancy, education and income.

MATERNAL AND CHILD HEALTH

The maternal and child health services in the GCC are well developed but largely limited to preventive services such as immunisations, antenatal, postnatal and premarital check-ups. Immunisation rates in the GCC states are among the highest in the world, reaching up to 99% immunisation (UNICEF, 2018). Couples are routinely offered premarital testing for common genetic blood disorders (e.g. sickle cell anaemia, thalassaemia, sickle cell anaemia) and infectious diseases (e.g. hepatitis B, hepatitis C and HIV/AIDS). Such testing has become compulsory and is a legal requirement of marriage in all states in the Arabian Gulf with the exception of Oman (Al-Balushi & Al-Hinai, 2018; el-Hazmi et al., 1995). The aim of these check-ups is to alert couples to any potential health risks of hereditary blood disorders in their future offspring. As discussed in more detail later in this chapter, this is extremely important in the GCC because the area has one of the highest rates of consanguinity in the world (el-Hazmi et al., 1995). About half of all marriages across Gulf nations are between cousins, and their frequency is increasing with first-cousin marriage being the most frequently encountered pattern (el-Hazmi et al., 1995).

Postnatal check-ups are provided to women at 6 weeks postnatal and encompass numerous interventions. These services include but are not limited to cervical cancer screening, breastfeeding and contraception counselling. Reports from the GCC have shown that the uptake of these interventions is less than 30%, with no reminder system in place to alert mothers to the postnatal check-up due date (Jassim et al., 2018; So et al., 2018). Unfortunately, cervical screening tends to be only offered on an opportunistic rather than planned basis. Furthermore, these services are offered to married women who gave birth recently which means that unmarried women, divorced, widowed and married women with no children might miss out on the opportunity for cervical cancer screening due to the propensity to focus services on married women and families, given the cultural context (Stein et al., 2005).

It is imperative that healthcare policy makers in the Arabian Gulf review these fundamental issues and provide clear guidelines for the utility and scope of cervical cancer screening. Such policies and guidelines patently need to attend to the needs of the indigenous and expatriate populations that make up the majority of the workforce in the Arabian Gulf, thereby appropriately accounting for globalisation and multiculturalism.

There is arguably a degree of hesitancy in introducing the human papilloma virus (HPV) vaccine in the Arabian Gulf states and this may be, in part, due to the apparent perception of parents that the HPV vaccine may 'encourage' premarital sexual behaviour (Trim et al., 2012). Conversely, all attitude studies regarding HPV vaccine in the region have demonstrated very positive public attitudes (Husain et al., 2019; Hussain et al., 2016; Ortashi et al., 2013). Further, the HPV vaccine was introduced in the UAE, with whom we (Bahrainis) share the same norms, values, religion and culture.

Therefore, healthcare policy makers should consider acting immediately upon the available evidence and introduce HPV vaccine without any further delay or hesitancy to the target population in the GCC states that have not enlisted the vaccine among their immunisation schedule yet.

THINKING GRID

- What would be the best strategy for introducing HPV vaccine in the national immunisation schedule?
- How could we increase the uptake for cervical cancer screening?

Despite the advancement of healthcare parameters related to women's health in the GCC, maternal mortality rates, child vaccination rates and postnatal uptake rates are not the only indicators of women's health and wellbeing. There are various cultural practices in the region impacting upon women's health which may be ignored or understated due to a societal reluctance to address these issues, as well as cultural and religious sensitivities. These practices constitute an integral part of the culture and norms in the Arabian Gulf states and are embedded within the community. No lights have been shed on these practices despite the significant impact they are likely to have on women's health. For example, nonattendance for screening appointments is very high and often women are known to refuse the medical examination of genitals and breasts due to their sensitive nature. This is more evident when the healthcare provider is a male or when the patient is covered (wearing hijab or face veil) (Alqufly et al., 2019; Attum, 2022). The cultural mores and sensibilities around intimacy, embarrassment and remaining covered, especially to male genders, are undoubtedly likely to contribute to late presentation in 'women's cancers' resulting in more advanced disease.

In addition to the issues outlined above, there are other challenges and gaps facing women's health in the GCC where actions and plans need to be considered, such as urinary and faecal incontinence which is the focus of the next chapter.

CONTRACEPTION USE

The rate of contraceptive use in Arabian Gulf states is still low (United Nation, 2019). According to the UN report on contraceptive use in 2019, the percentage of women of reproductive age (15–49 years) using any birth spacing was 19.6% in Oman, 18.6% in Saudi Arabia, 32.2% in Bahrain, 33.4% in UAE, 35.5% in Kuwait and 29% in Qatar (United Nations, 2019). In general, reversible contraceptive methods are acceptable in Islam, the main religion in the Arabian Gulf, but irreversible permanent methods, intrauterine device as well as the morning after pills are considered more controversial (Atighetchi, 1994; Shaikh et al., 2013). Further, the ruling on employing the loop (or intrauterine contraceptive device (IUCD): small plastic devices that are wrapped in copper or contains female sex hormones) and the morning after pill is somewhat different to the general ruling on other reversible contraception (Atighetchi, 1994; Shaikh et al., 2013). Notably, 'any method that may prevent a fertilised egg from implanting itself into the womb will not be allowed except in certain medical conditions, for which one should consult a reliable scholar of knowledge and piety' (Shaikh et al., 2013). Despite this, while the loop (or IUCD) is available and widely practiced, emergency contraception (EC) is not.

The estimated prevalence of the IUCD (known as the loop) use among women of reproductive age (15–49 years) was 7.7% in Qatar, 3.2% in Saudi Arabia, 2% in Oman (United Nations, 2019). No data were available for Bahrain, UAE and Kuwait (United Nations, 2019). The data on utilisation, practices and attitudes of EC among women in the Arabian Gulf states are sparse (Karim et al., 2015). EC can play a vital role in preventing unintended pregnancies. Hence, a better understanding of the culturally specific factors affecting the use of EC needs to be addressed. Further, the legislations for its use and availability need to be updated.

THINKING GRID

- What are the barriers for using contraception among women?
- Do schools have the capacity and are equipped to discuss contraception? To both girls and boys? In a culturally sensitive way?

The limited number of published reports from the region shows low knowledge prevalence of the variety of contraceptive techniques despite a greater acceptance of their usage (Al-Musa et al., 2019; Al Kindi & Al Sumri, 2019; Alhusain et al., 2018; Arbab et al., 2011; Ghazal-Aswad et al., 2001) and prevailing misconceptions regarding its use (Al-Kindi et al., 2019; Al-Musa et al., 2019; Alhusain et al., 2018; Farzaneh, 2012). For example, some women believe that they are unlikely to become pregnant because they are breast-feeding, approaching menopause or having infrequent intercourse (Farzaneh, 2012). Also, some women lack knowledge about the pros and cons of each contraceptive method. Others are ambivalent about whether to use contraception which could be explained by fatalistic attitudes common in the Arab region and also by women's subordinate position in the family and in society (Farzaneh, 2012).

Access to more information and education is needed and should ideally commence as early as school years. Healthcare practitioners can play a pivotal role in providing culturally appropriate contraceptive advice which could lead to an improvement in women's knowledge base and in contraceptive utilisation. Efforts are recommended to raise awareness regarding newer forms of contraceptives including EC methods. Community outreach awareness campaigns on the availability and proper use of contraceptives is highly recommended but would need to attend to local cultural contexts and sensitives.

Further studies focusing on perceptions and beliefs among men and women (including unmarried individuals) regarding contraception are needed to better understand the cultural barriers and beliefs. Family planning programmes should also reach out to broader audiences, such as religious and community leaders, and use the media to advocate for the health and well-being benefits of family planning and of responsible parenthood.

SEXUAL HEALTH SERVICES

In this region, children tend to be the fulcrum around which women's health is screened and managed. For example, maternal and child health services are well established in the GCC and are dominated by pre- and postnatal check-ups, children's vaccination schedules and the routine assessment of developmental milestones in stark contrast to the limited provision of sexual health services. Issues related to sexual health may arise at any point in a women's life: before marriage, early at marriage, during birth spacing and the decline in sexual desire following menopause or life-threatening diagnoses such as breast cancer—yet none

of these addressed in a transparent and structured way (Alomair et al., 2020). As indicated previously, such issues may be neglected because of the embarrassment and stigma associated with intimacy and gender preference (Alomair et al., 2020, 2021). Further, unmarried women face greater difficulties in accessing or obtaining contraception as the labelling of 'sexual' or 'reproductive' health services makes it uncomfortable for them to access those services as unmarried women. This is because in Islam premarital sex (fornication) and sex outside marriage (adultery) is absolutely forbidden (Quran 24:2).

There are very few sexual health clinics in the region per se and those which exist are mainly referred to as sexually transmitted infections (STI) clinics, focussing on the treatment of STIs such as HIV, syphilis and gonorrhoea.

Safer sex, such as the use of male or female condoms, can prevent STIs as well as unwanted or unintended pregnancy. However, the current approaches to sex education among the youth of the region focusses on sexual abstinence only, given the strict prohibition of premarital sex. However, focussing on abstinence-only sexual health awareness without contraceptive sex education is unlikely to wholly prevent teenage pregnancies (Smerecnik et al., 2010).

Such abstinence-only approaches were commonplace in the Western world for some considerable time in the late 20th century, often at the behest of religious bodies such as the Roman Catholic church. However, gradually religious bodies slowly reduced their vocal opposition to nonabstinence approaches as they began to recognise the health and well-being benefits of proactive sexual healthcare from preadolescence (Ott & Santelli, 2007). However, it is important to state that it is vital to engage with religious leaders to agree upon a culturally appropriate way to address this very sensitive issue.

Through a better understanding of the cultural context and its prevailing impact upon sexual health including polygamy, nonabstinence programmes and the provision of structured prevention and follow-up programmes is key to attending to the implicit and explicit sensitivities and religious objections. Sexual health is undoubtedly one of the areas that requires considerable transformation and restructuring. Numerous steps could be taken to reduce the stigma associated with sexual health such as providing integrated services; reinforcing STI care as a component of holistic health; reframing sexual health in campaigns; educating the public; providing wider options to aid disclosure and partner notification practices; promoting sexual health as both a preventive and counselling service; employing highly confidential medical records accessed by clinic providers only and the rolling out self-testing services whenever possible. The involvement of religious and community leaders to advocate safer sex practices and raise awareness of risky sexual behaviours is also key—with all of those initiatives being critical to achieving a more equitable and improved sexual health services that can exist productively and transparently within the existing cultural context (Smerecnik et al., 2010).

In short, women's health is largely overlooked throughout the lifespan from adolescence to post menopause. The challenges of addressing these issues and women's natural concerns regarding intimacy, privacy, embarrassment and body image are multiplied 10-fold in a predominantly conservative society.

THINKING GRID

- How could sexual health clinics be launched without stigmatising attendees?
- How could safe sex be discussed without crossing the red lines of culture, religion, norms and values?

ABORTION

Abortion is an essential component of women's healthcare—a safe and critically important part of healthcare that needs to be addressed—yet it remains an uncomfortable topic and one that may be shrouded in some unspoken thoughts, beliefs and stigma, specific to the region.

Many factors influence a woman's decision to have an abortion. They include, but are not limited to, contraceptive failure, barriers to contraceptive use and access, rape, foetal anomalies, illness during pregnancy and exposure to teratogenic medications (American College of Obstetricians and Gynecologists, 2014).

While the debate continues even in Western societies, the Muslim-majority Middle East and North Africa (MENA) region shows remarkable variation

in abortion legislation, and religious scholars diverge notably in their theological reasoning (Maffi & Tønnessen, 2019). In most Arabian Gulf states, abortion is legal only in cases where there is a threat to a woman's and/or foetus' life. The impact of abortion bans on women's health in the MENA region is understudied, and reliable data on unsafe abortion in countries where access to safe abortion is difficult or nonexistent are lacking with states where abortion is illegal and not routinely collecting data on that topic (or at least do not make them public) (Maffi & Tønnessen, 2019).

Very few publications exist on abortion in MENA countries, and these tend to either give a broad overview of the legislation of different states or evaluate Islam's position on abortion (Maffi & Tønnessen, 2019). Detailed fieldwork-based studies on actual medical practices, political debates, local legal implementation, moral and social norms, and the trajectories of individual women in MENA countries are very rare (Maffi & Tønnessen, 2019). Therefore, there is a need to fill this gap by offering new insights into national and local practices present in the MENA region.

Based on most studies from MENA region and South-east Asian countries, religion was identified as one of the key determinants of people's attitudes towards abortion and plays a crucial role in people's readiness to accept or refute this practice (Rehnström Loi et al., 2015; Saadeh et al., 2021). The overall attitude towards abortion was negative and conservative, except if the pregnancy was a threat to the mother's life. Induced abortion due to unplanned/unwanted pregnancy was not seen as a justification, especially after the ensoulment or the breathing of the soul into the foetus which occurs after 120 days according to most religious scholars (Lenfest, 2018; Rehnström Loi et al., 2015; Saadeh et al., 2021). The right to abortion dilemma is not exclusive to the Middle East and MENA region. In June 2022, The US Supreme Court overturned Roe v. Wade—the decision that had guaranteed a constitutional right to an abortion for nearly 50 years (BBC, 2022)

Doctors who treat women suffering such problems are arguably forced to manoeuvre between their commitment to medical ethics and their compliance with strict government laws and policies. The legalisation of abortion is not a magic bullet but it is nonetheless important for the advancement of women's sexual and reproductive rights in the Arabian Gulf and MENA region (Livni, 2019; Maffi & Tønnessen, 2019).

THINKING GRID

- In view of the rapidly changing legislations for abortion, what are the implications anticipated on women's health?
- What are the possibilities and challenges for developing a regional culturally appropriate consensus on abortion?

WELL WOMEN CLINIC

The notion of the well women clinics, which focuses on regular health check-ups, health screening services (e.g. breast cancer, cervical cancer and bone density screening), diagnosing and managing ongoing normal physiological problems such as menopause, women specific evaluation and treatment, are not yet well developed in the GCC. With the exception of UAE, there is a limited number of well women clinics providing these services utilising a holistic approach under one roof. Women presenting with these problems are often referred to gynaecologists, surgeons, internal medicine or all of them. The Saudi Arabia healthcare sector will launch in November 2022 a women's well-being smartphone application resulting in tailored and personalised healthcare according to patient's need (News, 2022). It is forecasted that future demand in healthcare in the GCC will be evolving around setting up a comprehensive women's service that addresses the healthcare needs of women of all ages and provides new services for women beyond the traditional maternity care.

DO MUSLIM WOMEN NEED SAVING?

American anthropologist Lila Abu-Lughod made the strident case in her 2013 text that Muslim women—many of them Arab—do not need to be liberated by the West. Gender inequality is not just about religion or culture but rather it emanates from a compelling mix of circumstances that are not only found in the Arab world. Arab women are unique. They are not homogenous. They come from a mix of demography,

understandings, attitudes, cultures and religion. They have agency and an identity and that is important within the context of this chapter—Muslim women are not victims or oppressed, but there is a notable gender gap and gender inequality affects many aspects including the utilisation of, and access to, healthcare. While women and men may encounter similar health problems, the fact remains that such problems are likely to impact women differently (Abu-Lughod, 2015).

For example, women are more likely to die following a heart attack than men, have UTI problems, STIs are more serious in women than in men, women are more likely to have mental health problems, specifically depression and anxiety, and are also privy to a range of specific reproductive health concerns such as polycystic ovarian syndrome (PCOS), endometriosis and uterine fibroids. They are more likely to prioritise the health of their husbands and family than that of their own, not least delaying accessing healthcare for a myocardial infarction (MI). Whilst unique and compassionate, they are also vulnerable, with the Arab world host to a large refugee population, half of whom are women and who are at a higher risk of rape, illness and sex trafficking.

Arab women do not need to be 'saved' or portrayed as victims, but they do need to be better understood, appreciated and included and most of all have *all* their healthcare needs addressed appropriately.

SUMMARY

The younger population in the Arabian Gulf are more career-oriented and more highly educated and thus, more likely to be receptive to health education, knowledge-sharing and informed decision-making. GCC states also have the potential for regional cooperation and economic integration, which would allow them to speak with a shared voice and shared legislations in view of their shared norms, values and social determinants of health. That said, it would be misleading to generalise the findings and discussion to all women in the Middle East or Arab region due to the vast variation in political, economic and social determinants of health.

Much of the work on maternal and child health in the region was clear and well-developed, in sharp contrast to the opportunity for (all) women to be able to freely access sexual and reproductive healthcare services. Sociocultural values, attitudes, perceptions and the over-riding cultural context of the region under-standably predominate, and the tensions between the focus on 'reproductive' health versus 'sexual' health (for all) impacts the health and well-being of a significant proportion of the population, who may, *or may not*, be a wife, child-bearer, mother or sister. The lack of a collective vision for well-being for all needs to be fully addressed—the GCC states should seize the opportunity and act instantly to exult in their prosperity and demonstrate their ability to be magnanimous and caring in all aspects of health and well-being.

REFERENCES

Abu-Lughod, L. (2015). Do Muslim Women Need Saving? Ethnicities, 15(5), 759–777. https://doi.org/10.1177/1468796814561357.

Al-Balushi, A. A., & Al-Hinai, B. (2018). Should premarital screening for blood disorders be an obligatory measure in Oman? *Sultan Qaboos University Medical Journal*, 18(1), e24–e29. https://doi.org/10.18295/squmj.2018.18.01.004.

Al-Kindi, R. M., Kannekanti, S., Natarajan, J., Shakman, L., Al-Azri, Z., & Al-Kalbani, N. I. (2019). Awareness and attitude towards the premarital screening programme among high school students in Muscat, Oman. *Sultan Qaboos University Medical Journal*, 19(3), e217–e224. https://doi.org/10.18295/squmj.2019.19.03.007.

Al-Musa, H. M., Alsaleem, M. A., Alfaifi, W. H., Alshumrani, Z., Alzuheri, N. S., Aslouf, A. S., et al. (2019). Knowledge, attitude, and practice among Saudi primary health care attendees about family planning in Abha, Kingdom of Saudi Arabia. *Journal of Family Medicine and Primary Care*, 8(2), 576–582. https://doi.org/10.4103/jfmpc.jfmpc_363_18.

Al Kindi, R. M., & Al Sumri, H. H. (2019). Prevalence and sociodemographic determinants of contraceptive use among women in Oman. *Eastern Mediterranean Health Journal*, 25(7), 495–502. https://doi.org/10.26719/emhj.18.064.

Alhusain, F., Alkaabba, F., Alhassan, N., Alotaibi, S., Breakeit, S., Musaudi, E., et al. (2018). Patterns and knowledge of contraceptive methods use among women living in Jeddah, Saudi Arabia. *Saudi Journal for Health Sciences*, 7(2), 121–126. https://doi.org/10.4103/sjhs.sjhs_8_18.

Alomair, N., Alageel, S., Davies, N., & Bailey, J. V. (2020). Factors influencing sexual and reproductive health of Muslim women: A systematic review. *Reproductive Health*, 17(1), 33. https://doi.org/10.1186/s12978-020-0888-1.

Alomair, N., Alageel, S., Davies, N., & Bailey, J. V. (2021). Barriers to sexual and reproductive wellbeing among Saudi women: A qualitative study. *Sexuality Research and Social Policy*, 19, 860–869. https://doi.org/10.1007/s13178-021-00616-4.

Alqufly, A. E., Alharbi, B. M., Alhatlany, K. K., & Alhajjaj, F. S. (2019). Muslim female gender preference in delaying the medical care at emergency department in Qassim Region, Saudi Arabia. *Journal of Family Medicine and Primary Care*, 8(5), 1658–1663. https://doi.org/10.4103/jfmpc.jfmpc_141_19.

Arbab, A. A., Bener, A., & Abdulmalik, M. (2011). Prevalence, awareness and determinants of contraceptive use in Qatari women. *Eastern Mediterranean Health Journal*, 17(1), 11–18.

American Medical Women's Association. (2016). An Expanded Definition of Women's Health H-525.976. *Council on Science and Public Health*. Available at https://policysearch.ama-assn.org/policyfinder/detail/An%20Expanded%20Definition%20of%20Women's%20Health%20H-525.976?uri=%2FAMADoc%2FHOD-525.976.xml.

Atighetchi, D. (1994). The position of Islamic tradition on contraception. *Med Law*, 13(7-8), 717–725.

Attum, B., Hafiz, S., Malik, A., & Shamoon, Z. (2022). Cultural competence in the care of Muslim patients and their families: *StatPearls [Internet]*. Treasure Island (FL): StatPearls Publishing. Available at https://www.ncbi.nlm.nih.gov/books/NBK499933/.

BBC. (2022). Roe v Wade: US Supreme Court ends constitutional right to abortion [Press release]. Available at https://www.bbc.com/news/world-us-canada-61928898.

Daher-Nashif, S., & Bawadi, H. (2020). Women's health and well-being in the United Nations sustainable development goals: A narrative review of achievements and gaps in the Gulf states. *International Journal of Environmental Research and Public Health*, 17(3), 1059. https://doi.org/10.3390/ijerph17031059.

el-Hazmi, M. A., al-Swailem, A. R., Warsy, A. S., al-Swailem, A. M., Sulaimani, R., & al-Meshari, A. A. (1995). Consanguinity among the Saudi Arabian population. *Journal of Medical Genetics*, 32(8), 623–626. https://doi.org/10.1136/jmg.32.8.623.

Farzaneh, R.-F. A., Abdul Monem; Lori, Ashford; Maha, El-Adawy. (2012). Women's need for family planning in Arab countries. Available at https://www.who.int/evidence/resources/policy_briefs/UNFPAPBunmentneed2012.pdf.

Ghazal-Aswad, S., Rizk, D. E., Al-Khoori, S. M., Shaheen, H., & Thomas, L. (2001). Knowledge and practice of contraception in United Arab Emirates women. *Journal of Family Planning and Reproductive Health Care*, 27(4), 212–216. https://doi.org/10.1783/147118901101195786.

American College of Obstetricians and Gynecologists. (2014). Guidelines for women's health care, a resource manual. Available at https://www.acog.org/advocacy/facts-are-important/abortion-is-healthcare.

Husain, Y., Alalwan, A., Al- Musawi, Z., Abdulla, G., Hasan, K., & Jassim, G. (2019). Knowledge towards human papilloma virus (HPV) infection and attitude towards its vaccine in the Kingdom of Bahrain: Cross-sectional study. *BMJ Open*, 9(9), e031017. https://doi.org/10.1136/bmjopen-2019-031017.

Hussain, A. N., Alkhenizan, A., McWalter, P., Qazi, N., Alshmassi, A., Farooqi, S., & Abdulkarim, A. (2016). Attitudes and perceptions towards HPV vaccination among young women in Saudi Arabia. *Journal of Family & Community medicine*, 23(3), 145–150. https://doi.org/10.4103/2230-8229.189107.

Jassim, G., Obeid, A., & Al Nasheet, H. A. (2018). Knowledge, attitudes, and practices regarding cervical cancer and screening among women visiting primary health care centres in Bahrain. *BMC Public Health*, 18(1), 128. https://doi.org/10.1186/s12889-018-5023-7.

Karim, S. I., Irfan, F., Rowais, N. A., Zahrani, B. A., Qureshi, R., & Qadrah, B. H. A. (2015). Emergency contraception: Awareness, attitudes and barriers of Saudi Arabian women. *Pakistan Journal of Medical Sciences*, 31(6), 1500–1505. https://doi.org/10.12669/pjms.316.8127.

Lenfest, Y. (2018). From bioethics to medical anthropology to humanities and back: A year in review. Available at https://blog.petrieflom.law.harvard.edu/about/.

Livni, E. (2019). Saudi Arabia's abortion laws are more forgiving than Alabama's [Press release]. Available at https://qz.com/1628427/saudi-arabias-abortion-laws-are-more-forgiving-than-alabamas/.

News, A. (2022). A women's well-being app builds on Saudi Arabia's health-tech success [Press release]. Available at https://www.arabnews.com/node/1953276/middle-east.

Ortashi, O., Raheel, H., Shalal, M., & Osman, N. (2013). Awareness and knowledge about human papillomavirus infection and vaccination among women in UAE. *Asian Pacific Journal of Cancer Prevention*, 14(10), 6077–6080. https://doi.org/10.7314/apjcp.2013.14.10.6077.

Ott, M. A., & Santelli, J. S. (2007). Abstinence and abstinence-only education. *Current Opinion in Obstetrics and Gynecology*, 19(5), 446–452. https://doi.org/10.1097/GCO.0b013e3282efdc0b.

Regitz-Zagrosek, V. (2012). Sex and gender differences in health. Science & Society Series on Sex and Science. *EMBO Reports*, 13(7), 596–603. https://doi.org/10.1038/embor.2012.87.

Rehnström Loi, U., Gemzell-Danielsson, K., Faxelid, E., & Klingberg-Allvin, M. (2015). Health care providers' perceptions of and attitudes towards induced abortions in sub-Saharan Africa and Southeast Asia: A systematic literature review of qualitative and quantitative data. *BMC Public Health*, 15(1), 139. https://doi.org/10.1186/s12889-015-1502-2.

Saadeh, R., Alfaqih, M., Odat, A., & Allouh, M. Z. (2021). Attitudes of medical and health sciences students towards abortion in Jordan. *BioMed Research International*, 2021, 6624181. https://doi.org/10.1155/2021/6624181.

Shaikh, B. T., Azmat, S. K., & Mazhar, A. (2013). Family planning and contraception in Islamic countries: A critical review of the literature. *Journal of Pakistan Medical Association*, 63(4 Suppl 3), S67–72.

Smerecnik, C., Schaalma, H., Gerjo, K., Meijer, S., & Poelman, J. (2010). An exploratory study of Muslim adolescents' views on sexuality: Implications for sex education and prevention. *BMC Public Health*, 10(1), 533. https://doi.org/10.1186/1471-2458-10-533.

So, V.H. T., Channon, A.A., Ali, M.M., Merdad, L., Al Sabahi, S., Al Suwaidi, H., et al. (2018). Uptake of breast and cervical cancer screening in four Gulf Cooperation Council countries. *European Journal of Cancer Prevention: The Official Journal of the European Cancer Prevention Organisation (ECP)*, 28(5), 451-456. https://doi.org/10.1097/CEJ.0000000000000466.

Stein, K., Lewendon, G., Jenkins, R., & Davis, C. (2005). Improving uptake of cervical cancer screening in women with prolonged history of non-attendance for screening: A randomized trial of enhanced invitation methods. *Journal of Medical Screening*, 12(4), 185–189. https://doi.org/10.1258/096914105775220741.

Maffi, I. & Tønnessen, L. (2019). EDITORIAL: The limits of the law: Abortion in the Middle East and North Africa [Press release]. Available at https://cdn1.sph.harvard.edu/wp-content/uploads/sites/2469/2019/12/Editorial-MENA.pdf.

Trim, K., Nagji, N., Elit, L., & Roy, K. (2012). Parental knowledge, attitudes, and behaviours towards human papillomavirus vaccination for their children: A systematic review from 2001 to 2011. *Obstetrics and Gynecology International*, 2012, 921236. https://doi.org/10.1155/2012/921236.

UNICEF. (2018). Immunization Regional Snapshot 2018 Middle East and North Africa. Retrieved from file:///C:/Users/gjassim/Downloads/Immunization-regional-snapshots-MENA-2020.pdf

United Nations. (2019). Contraceptive use by method 2019: Data booklet. Available at https://digitallibrary.un.org/record/3849735?ln=en.

WHO (World Health Organization) (2016). World Health Statistics 2016: Monitoring health for the SDGs Sustainable Development Goals. Geneva: WHO.

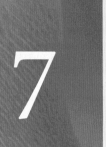

7

FEMALE INCONTINENCE IN THE MIDDLE EAST
Revisiting a Priority in Women's Health

DIAA E. E. RIZK

In modern medicine especially, we see clearly that medicine is and must be a reflection of contemporaneous culture.

Emerson, 2020

INTRODUCTION

This chapter will review the prevalence and consequences of female urinary incontinence (UI) and faecal incontinence (FI) in the Middle East and the perceptions, health seeking behaviour and barriers to care of both conditions. Some of the regional challenges in providing quality incontinence services and the strategies to improve the delivery of incontinence care for women will also be discussed. The definition, risk factors, underlying mechanism, diagnosis, health burden and management of female incontinence will be described briefly here, as a detailed account of the topic is beyond the scope of this book.

URINARY INCONTINENCE AND FAECAL INCONTINENCE: DEFINITION

UI is defined as any involuntary loss of urine irrespective of the consequences (Sussman et al., 2020; Vaughan & Markland, 2020). The most accepted definition of FI is the involuntary loss of liquid or solid stools causing social or hygienic inconvenience. Anal incontinence denotes any involuntary leakage, whether of gas or faeces, through the anus (ACOG, 2019; Freeman & Menees, 2016). UI and FI in women are embarrassing and debilitating symptoms that represent a significant women's health problem because of the prevalence, the impairment of health-related quality of life and the associated adverse psychosocial and economic consequences. Although UI is considered of lesser impact and importance than FI, UI may constitute a greater problem for affected women and is more frequently seen than FI (Vaughan & Markland 2020; Islam et al., 2019). The association of UI and FI in women, double incontinence, is common and can be explained by the same underlying risk factors (Sussman et al., 2020; Vaughan & Markland, 2020; Freeman & Menees, 2016; ACOG, 2019).

BACKGROUND

Female incontinence should not be narrowly seen as a health problem but must be addressed from a broader outlook that takes into consideration the impact on women's lives both in terms of cause and effect and is therefore one case that falls under the health status/roles of women (Rizk & El-Safty, 2006). The health status of any society cannot be understood separately from the cultural factors that determine the individuals' attitudes towards health and their behaviour in seeking care. Culture embodies the values that constitute the background to individuals' health attitudes and behaviours. The important biological influences of sociodemographic, economic, genetic and environmental factors on women's health are well recognised. Moreover, the impact of sophisticated and often competing anthropologic and societal variables such as ethnicity, race, culture, religion, spirituality, geopolitical orientation, indigenous psychology, personality and gender identity on an individual's realisation of health role, experience of health and illness, and utilisation of health services is, however, less appreciated in women's health research, particularly incontinence studies (Mostafaei et al., 2020).

Importantly, the Middle East is a pronatal society with an average total fertility rate of >4 and a female life expectancy at birth of >70 years in most countries. Thus a high prevalence of both UI and FI is expected in women from this region since the two most important risk factors for incontinence—repeated vaginal births and long postmenopausal life span—are common. In fact, pooled prevalence rates of UI and FI in community-dwelling women of 30% and 8%, respectively, were reported from the Middle East (Mostafaei et al., 2020; Rizk et al., 2001a, 2001b). Incontinent

women in the Middle East, however, rarely seek medical help because of several reasons and barriers (Rizk & El-Safty, 2006; Rizk et al., 2001a, 2001b; Rizk, 1999, 2009a, 2009b, 2017). The perceptions, healthcare seeking behaviour and consequences of female incontinence are also unique in the Middle East (Rizk & El-Safty, 2006; Rizk et al., 2001a, 2001b; Rizk, 1999).

EVIDENCE BASE: GLOBAL AND REGIONAL

Comparison of results from various studies estimating the prevalence of UI and FI in women is limited by differences in the definition of incontinence, particularly its onset (current or past), severity (whether or not it poses a social or hygienic problem) and frequency (daily or episodic). Other factors are the type of patient population studied, whether community dwelling or institutionalised and whether they were seeking care or not; the ethnic group examined; and the study design including sampling techniques and standards and methods of data collection (Freeman & Menees, 2016; Islam et al., 2019; Rizk & El-Safty, 2006; Mostafaei et al., 2020; Rizk et al., 2001a, 2001b; Rizk, 2017). Therefore available results vary widely but comparable studies of community-dwelling women from other parts of the world have shown prevalence rates of 44%–57% for UI and 1%–15% for FI (Islam, et al., 2019; Mostafaei et al., 2020). This is not significantly different from the overall prevalence rates observed in Middle Eastern women.

Female incontinence is affected by racial/ethnic factors with a greater risk of developing incontinence in Whites than in other populations including Middle Eastern women (Rizk et al., 2004; Rizk, Abadir, et al., 2005; Hallock & Handa, 2016). Although this could be the result of more frequent symptom reporting or of diagnosis, it is likely that differences in parity, body mass index, obstetric practice, lifestyle factors such as diet, occupation, smoking and athletic exercise, position at delivery, micturition or defaecation, life expectancy and collagen metabolism could be responsible. It could also be due to the considerable genetic variation in the topography of the female pelvis. The maternal bony pelvis is an important factor influencing the degree of maternal soft tissue damage and nerve injury during parturition and consequent pelvic floor weakness.

The larger bony pelvis in White women compared to Middle Eastern women allows greater transmission of intra-abdominal pressure to the pelvic floor. In addition, the more horizontal pelvic inclination in Whites enhances the direct effect of intra-abdominal vector forces on the pelvic floor that are normally deflected anteriorly during increased intra-abdominal pressure (Vaughan & Markland, 2020; Rizk et al., 2004).

URINARY INCONTINENCE AND FAECAL INCONTINENCE: AN OUTLINE OF THE CONDITION

The causes of UI in women are manifold: difficult or traumatic vaginal birth, advancing age, a chronic increase in intra-abdominal pressure due to obesity, obstructive airway diseases and chronic constipation as well as diseases of the nervous system such as stroke, multiple sclerosis and diabetes mellitus (Vaughan & Markland, 2020; Freeman & Menees, 2016). Obstetric risk factors include parity, forceps delivery, episiotomy, large birth weight, short maternal stature, occiput-posterior position of the foetus and prolonged labour, particularly of the second stage (Rizk, Abadir, et al., 2005; Rizk & El-Safty, 2006). The causes of female FI are similar and additionally include surgical operations on the anus and rectum (ACOG, 2019). UI and FI are more common in women than in men particularly after the menopause when the sex ratio shows a female to male preponderance of 8:1 (Rizk et al., 2001a, 2001b).

Female UI develops when the urethra descends below the pelvic floor because of weakness of anatomical structures that normally supports the urethra to maintain continence. This causes an unequal pressure transmission ratio between the bladder and urethra during increased intra-abdominal pressure with a greater gradient in the bladder resulting in *stress UI*. Compression of the pudendal nerve that supplies the urethral sphincter mechanism and pelvic floor muscles against the ischial spines by the foetal head can occur during labour leading to de-enervation and impaired urethral resistance and subsequent stress UI. An idiopathic decrease in bladder compliance to store urine or abnormal neurogenic control of micturition because of medical disorders like diabetes mellitus and multiple sclerosis causes *overactive bladder syndrome* that presents with frequency, nocturia and urgency with or without urge UI (Rizk, Abadir, et al., 2005; Vaughan & Markland, 2020; Freeman & Menees, 2016).

Female FI is caused by traumatic injuries to the anal sphincter and pelvic floor muscles during vaginal birth, the so-called *obstetric FI*, or during surgical operations on the rectum and anal canal (Freeman & Menees, 2016; ACOG, 2019). Hormonal changes after the menopause and progressive tissue weakness with advancing age softens the collagen framework in the urethral and anal canal submucosa and the endopelvic fascia that contribute to their ability to control micturition and defaecation (Rizk & Fahim 2008; Rizk et al., 2018).

Female UI and FI are not life-threatening disorders but both are disabling conditions causing significant physical and psychological morbidity in women of all ages (Sussman et al., 2020; Vaughan & Markland, 2020; Freeman & Menees, 2016; ACOG, 2019; Islam et al., 2019). Sufferers give up many aspects of their usual life with obvious detriment to their social and family interactions. Important aspects of quality of life affected are the need to wash frequently because of smell, to wear protective perineal pads, to change underwear regularly, to map the presence of available toilets, to drink and eat less and to restrict social, sport and work-related activities. Incontinence in women also causes avoidance of sexual activity and sexual dysfunction and has a negative impact on long-term interpersonal and sexual relationships, career progression and emotional well-being (Vaughan & Markland, 2020; Freeman & Menees, 2016; ACOG, 2019).

Diagnosis and identification of the cause of female UI in clinical practice requires expert gynaecological and/or urological assessment through history taking, physical examination and evaluation of the function of the bladder and urethra by urodynamic tests such as cystometry and uroflowmetry, cystoscopy and imaging with ultrasound or magnetic resonance (Vaughan & Markland, 2020). The clinical approach to FI is the same when anorectal manometry and pudendal nerve conduction studies are used to investigate the function of the anal canal and rectum and the clinician involved is a gynaecologist or a colo-proctologist (Freeman & Menees, 2016; ACOG, 2019).

Treatment of female incontinence depends on the underlying cause and includes several modalities that begin with modification of lifestyle (Sussman et al., 2020; Vaughan & Markland, 2020; Freeman & Menees, 2016; ACOG, 2019). This includes dietary manipulation to lose weight, minimising fluids that cause diuresis, such as alcohol and carbonated beverages, foods that cause excessive softening of stools, and/or regulating bowel habits to avoid chronic constipation and smoking cessation. Ensuring timed urination and evacuation to empty the bladder and rectum regularly and biofeedback techniques to reinforce the nervous control of bladder and rectum can significantly reduce the severity of UI and FI. Biofeedback is a neurophysical procedure that involves using visual or auditory feedback to teach incontinent women how to recognise and control autonomic functions including bladder and bowel control and pelvic floor muscle tension. Pelvic floor muscle training is the next step of management.

There is strong contemporary evidence that an 8- to 12-week programme of pelvic floor muscle training supervised by a physiotherapist is effective not only in treating but also in preventing postnatal UI and FI with a greater treatment effect following more intensive regimes (Rizk, 2009a, 2009b). Efforts to improve women's compliance with training are required because the long-term effects of physiotherapy are disappointing without rigorous patient compliance. If conservative measures fail, specific therapy to address incontinence is indicated. Stress UI is treated by surgical intervention to restore the urethra to its normal pelvic position or improve urethral sphincter function. Overactive bladder syndrome is treated by drugs that inhibit contraction of the bladder detrusor muscle like anticholinergics, β3-stimulants and trans-cystoscopic botulinum toxin injection or by neuromodulation of sacral nerves that supply the lower urinary tract (Sussman et al., 2020; Vaughan & Markland, 2020). Neuromodulation is also used to treat FI while surgical treatment aims to increase the integrity, repair or strengthen the anal sphincter (Freeman & Menees, 2016; ACOG, 2019).

There is a significant financial burden of incontinence in affected women because of the costs involved (Vaughan & Markland, 2020; Freeman & Menees, 2016; ACOG, 2019). These can be categorised into diagnostic cost: particularly of urodynamic or manometry studies; treatment cost: whether surgery or physiotherapy; routine care cost: disposable garments and laundry; consequence cost: falls and fractures in the elderly, infections, comorbidities and hospital admissions; indirect cost: lost productivity and absenteeism of women and their caregivers; intangible cost: pain, suffering and decreased health-related quality of life. The costs will still be incurred if incontinent women do not seek medical attention because routine care, consequence, indirect and intangible costs are not affected.

REGIONAL ASPECTS AND SPECIFIC CHALLENGES

Middle Eastern women are as individualistic as anywhere else in the world, although their lifestyle and social norms might be different and are principally dictated by their religious faith—Islam in the vast majority (El-Safty, 2004). Praying is a daily and ritually prescribed activity in Muslim women, which involves kneeling and that may precipitate incontinence because of increased intra-abdominal pressure requiring ablution after urination or defaecation for cleansing. Interference with praying alone because of incontinence can severely impair the quality of life of incontinent Muslim women in the Middle East and highlights the cross-cultural and ethnic differences in women's attitudes towards incontinence (Rizk & El-Safty, 2006; Rizk et al., 2001a, 2001b; Rizk, 1999).

The specific nature of the male-dominated Middle Eastern culture, *patriarchy*, where religion also plays an important role, represents a strong factor in shaping the health behaviour of women in the region (El-Safty, 2004). Furthermore, attitudes towards pregnancy, childbirth and the whole issue of women's health are necessarily rooted in the broader milieu of culture. Studies in the field of sociology/anthropology covering Middle Eastern countries have also revealed that the formal health services may be bypassed and underutilised, even when available, when the major healthcare provider is the traditional public system. This attitude tends to prevail in all areas of healthcare and is more common in women's health including incontinence services (Rizk, 2009a, 2009b). Scientific reports and social monographs consistently point to the persistence of the inverse healthcare law among women from these countries because of inequities in healthcare access, utilisation and delivery—the availability of good quality healthcare, women's health included, is inversely related to the women who need it (El-Safty, 2004; Baessler & Rizk 2020). This factor seriously limits women's access to incontinence services in low-resource countries of the region.

Intrinsic barriers to female incontinence care seeking in the Middle East are social traditions, cultural beliefs and inadequate public knowledge (Rizk & El-Safty, 2006; Rizk, 2009a, 2009b, 2017). It is common that women continue to live silently with incontinence because of lack of awareness due to inadequate knowledge and embarrassment in admitting incontinence, even when they are aware that it may be related to childbirth or ageing (Rizk & El-Safty, 2006; Rizk et al., 2001a, 2001b; Rizk, 1999). Discomfort and uneasiness are likely to be common feelings which the woman tries to tolerate silently especially when in public. It is interesting that UI and/or FI is also perceived by most women in the Middle East as a neurological or senile disorder rather than a gynaecological condition caused by childbirth or menopause/ageing, emphasising the gap between lay and biomedical knowledge of female incontinence (Rizk & El-Safty, 2006; Rizk et al., 2001a, 2001b; Rizk, 2009a, 2009b, 2017). The external barriers to incontinence care in Middle Eastern countries are limited access to and/or inadequate healthcare facilities, inconvenience of consultation because most primary healthcare centres are not clientele-friendly due to patient volume and long waiting lists, low expectations from healthcare, fear of medical encounters, particularly gynaecological examination, incurred service cost and limited availability of toilets in most clinics (Rizk & El-Safty, 2006).

The socioeconomic affluence and concomitant development of healthcare delivery infrastructure, as well as availability of free healthcare with almost universal coverage of the whole population in some Middle Eastern countries, tend to balance the traditional barriers to incontinence care seeking. Incontinent women in these countries, however, rarely seek care because of another important barrier—'public misinformation' (Rizk, 2017). Almost 23% of urinary incontinent women in one study were unaware that there is a need for medical help because UI is considered normal in old age and/or preferred to discuss their problem with relatives or friends because UI may resolve spontaneously (Rizk, 2009a, 2009b). This finding underscores

the global differences in women's medical knowledge and suggests that individual health awareness is another important intrinsic barrier item to incontinence care seeking in the Middle East (Rizk, 2017).

The intimate and sensitive nature of gynaecological disorders like female incontinence in a predominantly strict and conservative socioreligious environment like the Middle East significantly influences a preference for same-sex physician–patient dyad higher than that reported in Western studies (Rizk & El-Safty, 2006). Most women in the Middle East thus feel more comfortable in consulting a female incontinence provider because of the embarrassment of a pelvic examination and sexual or reproductive counselling within the context of their religious beliefs and sociocultural values (Rizk, El-Zubeir, et al., 2005).

Modesty, shyness and bashfulness are major attributes of the Middle Eastern woman's personality which she internalises through the process of socialisation (El-Safty, 2004). This observation may adversely affect the involvement of male providers in female incontinence care and consequently in acquisition of clinical skills for incontinence practice by male trainees. In turn, there will be an important impact on the future structure of the medical workforce, service delivery and postgraduate training for female incontinence in Middle Eastern countries (Rizk & El-Safty, 2006). Preference for a male provider is, however, associated with recognition of his role as professional/expert (Rizk, El-Zubeir, et al., 2005). It is, therefore, likely that when expertise is perceived as required, such as in incontinence care, Middle Eastern women may have less concern about a provider's sex. In fact, gender stereotyping places male providers in the traditionally accepted role of the expert practitioner (El-Safty, 2004; Rizk, El-Zubeir, et al., 2005). When professional expertise is required outside the sensitive field of gynaecology, same-sex preference is superseded by other priorities. The paradox here is that Middle Eastern women do not have female sex preferences for medical providers involved in intimate procedures and examinations of nonreproductive diseases such as breast surgeons, cardiologists and dentists (Rizk, El-Zubeir, et al., 2005).

Perceptions and experiences of childbirth are different for Middle Eastern women (Rizk et al., 2001a, 2001b). Popular beliefs consider pregnancy and childbirth as natural processes or episodes in the female's life (El-Safty, 2004). Such an attitude helps explain the absence of antenatal care as well as the common utilisation of traditional health practitioners rather than health professionals in delivery as well as postnatal care in most women. Same-sex preference is another factor that cannot be underestimated here, represented by the female midwife/obstetric nurse.

The inherent desire for spontaneous labour and resistance to any interference with the process of delivery results in relatively lower rates of caesarean delivery compared to Western data (Rizk & El-Safty, 2006; Rizk et al., 2001a, 2001b). Most women in one study from the Middle East strongly believed that caesarean is worse than vaginal delivery whatever the reason and should be performed only for compelling medical indications (Rizk et al., 2001a, 2001b). Such an attitude is especially pertinent where traditional values prevail as in the rural and Bedouin sectors (El-Safty, 2004). Hence, caesarean delivery does not represent a socially accepted option based on the traditional perceptions of pregnancy and childbirth as natural processes that do not need any intervention. This observation has an important bearing on counselling of Middle Eastern women about the benefit/risk ratio of elective caesarean delivery versus vaginal birth on subsequent pelvic floor supportive function and prevention of incontinence (Rizk, 2009a, 2009b; Serati et al., 2016).

A disappointing finding from some incontinence studies in the Middle East is that routine medical assessment of most women by their physician, whether a family practitioner or a specialist, does not include inquiry about the presence of UI or FI (Rizk et al., 2001a, 2001b; Rizk, 1999). Although few patients complain spontaneously of UI or FI, this problem can be elicited easily during history taking and on physical examination. Detection and management of incontinent women by their healthcare providers, therefore, remains suboptimal in the Middle East.

SPECIFIC INTERVENTIONS

The misconceptions about the causes and available treatment of female incontinence and the reluctance of affected women to seek medical advice despite the negative influence on their practice of religious faith and quality of life are aggravated by the high prevalence of these disorders in the Middle East. Expert medical advice to these women is therefore necessary to correct the myth about UI and FI being normal or untreatable (Rizk & El-Safty, 2006). Education of more health professionals from the region about normal pelvic floor function and mechanism of urinary and faecal continence is also required. On a broader societal level, a constructive way is needed to disseminate information to Middle Eastern women about health matters in general, and incontinence in particular, because of their adverse effect on the quality of life (Rizk & El-Safty, 2006; Rizk et al., 2001a, 2001b; Rizk, 1999). The message that UI and/or FI is always abnormal, interferes with a Muslim woman's daily activities with respect to prayer and is a source of frustration unless she seeks proper medical care and does not shy away from the situation, needs to be transmitted. Current medical practice must also change to respond to incontinent women's demands for scientific information about their symptoms, possible diagnosis and management options. Most incontinent women in the Middle East will accept medical intervention and welcome comprehensive clinical assessment if they understand the underlying cause and receive explanation about the available treatment modalities and their success rates (Rizk et al., 2001a, 2001b; Rizk, 1999). Patient decision aids like fact boxes are a very useful and simple tool in this context (Baessler & Rizk, 2020).

National health policies should be formulated to improve delivery of care, accessibility, cost and public image of female incontinence services particularly in low-resource countries of the Middle East (Rizk & El-Safty, 2006; Rizk, 2009a, 2009b, 2017). Health promotion clinics in a primary care setting may be an efficient means of improving incontinence care in women, particularly if effort is made to allow a detailed and pointed discussion about incontinence and make the clinic as user friendly as possible to the clientele, with ample washroom facilities (Rizk et al., 2001a, 2001b). Alternative recruitment policy initiatives and planning strategies for delivering the anticipated increased demand for community- and hospital-based incontinence services in the region should allow for women's preference for a female incontinence provider (Rizk & El-Safty, 2006; Rizk, El-Zubeir, et al., 2005). Birth attendants in the Middle East should endeavour to minimise obstetric pelvic floor injury during childbirth since most mothers will strongly disagree to have elective caesarean for the sole reason of reducing the likelihood of incontinence (Rizk & El-Safty, 2006; Rizk, 2009a, 2009b; Serati et al., 2016; Rizk, El-Zubeir, et al., 2005).

In view of the expected increase in prevalence of female incontinence in the Middle East, a growing demand for curative services is anticipated. The need may be higher than the reported prevalence rates since most women in the region do not seek healthcare. The most pragmatic and short-term solution to restore the demand/supply equilibrium in these countries is to reinforce the preventive perspective of health practice (Rizk, 2009a, 2009b). The goal is to transcend artificial trans-specialty boundaries of women's health and pursue the time-honoured public health idiom in incontinence care 'prevention is better than cure'. This novel approach involves raising awareness among maternity care givers about childbirth-induced incontinence and disseminating information about the safe and evidence-based labour practices using available electronic literature resources such as the WHO Reproductive Health Library: Pregnancy and Childbirth, Care during childbirth (https://apps.who. int/iris/handle/10665/206006) that is updated annually (Rizk, Abadir, et al., 2005). Birth attendants should communicate to women the prophylactic benefits of routine pelvic floor muscle training during pregnancy and after delivery especially when targeted to specific groups like those who had prolonged or traumatic vaginal delivery. Capacity building of a cadre of career champions in pelvic floor physiotherapy backed up with modern equipment should be brought to the attention of health policy makers and other stakeholders as an urgent manpower and funding priority.

Women healthcare providers in the Middle East must also assume a greater responsibility in counselling women about the risks of incontinence after delivery to improve the health literacy of the target population and actively involve women in understanding the mechanisms of childbirth-induced injuries, self-manage their reproductive and birthing choices and comply with prophylactic measures (Serati et al., 2016; Rizk, Abadir, et al., 2005). The provider's responsibility also includes participation in public health education programmes aiming to modify the potential lifestyle risk factors that increase the effect of pelvic floor trauma during labour such as constipation,

smoking and obesity and supporting government strategies and community outreach programmes that promotes women's education, emancipation, reproductive rights and engagement in incontinence care. Patient and public involvement has become an integral part of health systems and services including incontinence care (Ismail & Rizk, 2015). The emphasis is on including and empowering individuals and communities in shaping, running and monitoring services and ensuring that resources are allocated according to patient needs. It is meant to guarantee the development of quality incontinence services that are effective, responsive, accessible and accountable to its users.

There is a paucity of published literature in the field of ethnicity and female incontinence because determination of ethnicity is difficult, is not dichotomous, has no scientific definition and depends on social class, location and nationality (Rizk, 2008). More robust analysis of future epidemiological studies from multiethnic populations of incontinent women including the Middle East must include qualitative ethnographic research to improve our understanding of the poorly studied interrelationship between the risk of incontinence and ethnic differences in healthcare seeking behaviour, lifestyle, reproductive capacity, social activities, genetic constitution, childbirth practices and anatomy of the pelvis (Rizk et al., 2004; Rizk, 2008).

THINKING GRID

- What do you think could be done to change obstetric practice in Middle Eastern countries to minimise pelvic floor trauma during labour?
- What are the possibilities and challenges in developing a culturally competent health promotion campaign to inform Middle Eastern women about incontinence? What would it look like? Content? Method?
- How would you develop a culturally competent and religiously sensitive social package that would reduce the barriers to seeking incontinence care for Middle Eastern women?
- Identify women healthcare providers who could act as 'champions' of female incontinence. How would you engage them in your health promotion campaign and how might you evaluate such an intervention?

SUMMARY AND TAKEAWAY POINTS

1. The principal two risk factors of UI and FI in Middle Eastern women are vaginal delivery causing pelvic floor damage especially with nonevidence based and harmful obstetric practices and advancing age resulting in progressive weakness of the supportive connective tissue of pelvic organs.

2. Female incontinence is becoming a women's health priority in the Middle East because of rising prevalence, significant impairment of health-related quality of life particularly interference with praying and sexual dysfunction and adverse economic consequences on women's productivity and healthcare systems.

3. The main barriers to incontinence care seeking in Middle Eastern women is inadequate knowledge, misconceptions and misinformation about the causes and treatment options of incontinence, inconvenience of medical consultation because of sociocultural reluctance to see a male practitioner about an intimate condition and lack of public health facilities.

4. A novel approach to cope with the expected increasing demand for female incontinence care in the Middle East is to reinforce prevention through promoting evidence-based obstetric care, training health professionals to understand and detect female incontinence and improving women's compliance with prophylactic pelvic floor muscle training during pregnancy and after vaginal delivery.

5. There is an ethnic influence on female incontinence with a proposed lower risk in Middle Eastern women than in White populations possibly because of differences in obstetric, genetic, biological and environmental factors. Until further research data are available, it is not clear whether there is a real difference or whether this is caused by genetic or environmental factors.

6. Women healthcare providers in the Middle East are the perfect professionals to lead public health efforts to reduce the burden and impact of female incontinence by pioneering knowledge transfer, advocating health promotion and soliciting national support to develop incontinence services.

REFERENCES

ACOG (The American College of Obstetricians and Gynecologists). (2019). ACOG Practice Bulletin No. 210, Summary: Fecal incontinence. *Obstetrics and Gynecology, 133*(4), 837–839.

Baessler, K., & Rizk, D. E. E. (2020). Factors influencing patient decision making in urogynecology: You are what you know. *International Urogynecology Journal, 31*, 1057–1058.

El-Safty, M. (2004). Women in Egypt: Islamic rights vs. cultural practices. *Sex Roles: A Journal of Research, 51*, 273–281.

Emerson, C. (2000). The historical method of teaching clinical medicine. Round Table Conference: 37th Annual Meeting, Cleveland, October 26, 1926. *Academic Medicine, 75*, 351.

Freeman, A., & Menees, S. (2016). Fecal incontinence and pelvic floor dysfunction in women: A review. *Gastroenterology Clinics of North America, 45*, 217–237.

Hallock, J. L., & Handa, V. L. (2016). The epidemiology of pelvic floor disorders and childbirth: An update. *Obstetrics and Gynecology Clinics of North America, 43*, 1–13.

Islam, R. M., Oldroyd, J., Rana, J., Romero, L., & Karim, N. (2019). Prevalence of symptomatic pelvic floor disorders in community-dwelling women in low and middle-income countries: A systematic review and meta-analysis. *International Urogynecology Journal, 30*, 2001–2011.

Ismail, S., & Rizk, D. E. E. (2015). Patient and public involvement in urogynecology: A pause for reflection before taking a leap. *International Urogynecology Journal, 26*, 625–627.

Mostafaei, H., Sadeghi-Bazargani, H., Hajebrahimi, S., Salehi-Pourmehr, H., Ghojazadeh, M., Onur, R., et al. (2020). Prevalence of female urinary incontinence in the developing world: A systematic review and meta-analysis-A Report from the Developing World Committee of the International Continence Society and Iranian Research Center for Evidence Based Medicine. *Neurourology & Urodynamics, 39*, 1063–1086.

Rizk, D. E. E. (2008). Ethnic differences in women's knowledge level and other barriers to care seeking and the true incidence and/or prevalence rate of female pelvic floor disorders. *International Urogynecology Journal, 19*, 1587–1588.

Rizk, D. E. E. (2009a). Measuring barriers to urinary incontinence care seeking in women: The knowledge barrier. *Neurourology & Urodynamics, 28*, 101.

Rizk, D. E. E. (2009b). Minimizing the risk of childbirth-induced pelvic floor dysfunctions in the developing world: "preventive" urogynecology. *International Urogynecology Journal, 20*, 615–617.

Rizk, D. E. E. (2017). Towards a more scientific approach for measuring barriers to seeking health care in women with fecal incontinence: The BCABL Questionnaire. *International Urogynecology Journal, 28*, 505–506.

Rizk, D. E. E., Abadir, M. N., Thomas, L. B., & Abu-Zidan, F. (2005). Determinants of the length of episiotomy or spontaneous posterior perineal lacerations during vaginal birth. *International Urogynecology Journal, 16*, 395–400.

Rizk, D. E. E., Al-Kafaji, G., Jaradat, A. A., Al-Tayab, D., Bakhiet, M., & Salvatore, S. (2018). Circulating matrix metalloproteinases and their tissue inhibitors as markers for ethnic pelvic floor tissue integrity. *Biomedical Reports, 9*, 233–240.

Rizk, D. E. E., Czechowski, J., & Ekelund, L. (2004). Dynamic assessment of pelvic floor and bony pelvis morphologic condition with the use of magnetic resonance imaging in a multi-ethnic, nulliparous, and healthy female population. *American Journal of Obstetrics and Gynecology, 191*, 83–89.

Rizk, D. E. E., & El-Safty, M. M. (2006). Female pelvic floor dysfunction in the Middle East: A tale of three factors; Culture, religion and socialization of health role stereotypes. *International Urogynecology Journal, 17*, 436–438.

Rizk, D. E. E., El-Zubeir, M. A., Al-Dhaheri, A. M., Al-Mansouri, F. R., & Al-Jenaibi, H. S. (2005). Priorities and determinants of women's choice of their obstetrician and gynecologist provider in the United Arab Emirates. *Acta Obstetricia et Gynecologica Scandinavica, 84*, 48–53.

Rizk, D. E. E., & Fahim, M. A. (2008). Ageing of the female pelvic floor: Towards treatment "a la carte" of the "geripause". *International Urogynecology Journal, 19*, 455–458.

Rizk, D. E. E., Hassan, M. Y., Shaheen, H., Cherian, J. V., Micallef, R., & Dunn, E. (2001a). The prevalence and determinants of health care-seeking behavior for fecal incontinence in United Arab Emirates women. *Diseases of the Colon & Rectum, 44*, 1850–1856.

Rizk, D. E. E., Nasser, M., Thomas, L., & Ezimokhai, M. (2001b). Women's perceptions and experiences of childbirth in United Arab Emirates. *Journal of Perinatal Medicine, 29*, 298–307.

Rizk, D. E. E., Shaheen, H., Thomas, L., Dunn, E., & Hassan, M. Y. (1999). The prevalence and determinants of health-care seeking behavior for urinary incontinence in United Arab Emirates women. *International Urogynecology Journal, 10*, 160–165.

Serati, M., Rizk, D. E. E., & Salvatore, S. (2016). Vaginal birth and pelvic floor dysfunction revisited: Can cesarean delivery be protective? *International Urogynecology Journal, 27*, 1–2.

Sussman, R. D., Syan, R., & Brucker, B. M. (2020). Guideline of guidelines: Urinary incontinence in women. *BJU International, 125*, 638–655.

Vaughan, C. P., & Markland, A. D. (2020). Urinary incontinence in women. *Annals of Internal Medicine, 172*(3). https://doi.org/10.7326/AITC202002040.

FURTHER READING

https://www.ucsfhealth.org/education/faq-incontinence.

https://patients.uroweb.org/other-diseases/urinary-incontinence/.

https://www.nhs.uk/conditions/urinary-incontinence/.

https://www.mayoclinic.org/diseases-conditions/urinary-incontinence/symptoms-causes/syc-20352808.

https://www.mayoclinic.org/diseases-conditions/fecal-incontinence/symptoms-causes/syc-20351397.

https://www.niddk.nih.gov/health-information/digestive-diseases/bowel-control-problems-fecal-incontinence/treatment.

https://my.clevelandclinic.org/health/diseases/14574-fecal-bowel-incontinence.

https://www.moh.gov.sa/en/HealthAwareness/EducationalContent/wh/Pages/0021.aspx.

8 MENTAL HEALTH AND WELL-BEING

JANE LEANNE GRIFFITHS ▪ NABEEL AL YATEEM ▪ RACHEL ROSSITER

INTRODUCTION

Descriptions of fragmented, inadequate and at times absent care and treatment for those experiencing mental illness continue to be reported across the globe. Multiple factors contribute to this continuing situation including an artificial divide between the provision of health services designed to address various human ailments such as acute infections, physical injuries and chronic physical conditions and those designed to respond to people experiencing psychological distress and mental illnesses. A further contributor to inadequate care is the shame associated with mental illness (Carla Abi et al., 2019; Zolezzi et al., 2018) with stigma being particularly relevant to this region. The stigma associated with mental health illness will be discussed further in this chapter but stigma, post-traumatic stress disorder (PTSD) due to ongoing conflict in the Middle East and the high rates of displaced persons, significantly impacts on the burden of mental health illness.

Concurrently, epidemiological research reports an increasing global burden of mental illness (James et al., 2018), while high rates of PTSD, anxiety and depression have been reported in child and adolescent refugee populations and asylum seekers (Blackmore et al., 2020). Studies have identified that 94% of young people with mental health problems do not get help (Maalouf, 2019).

To address the widespread inequities, the 2030 Agenda for Sustainable Development outlines 17 sustainable development goals (SDGs) (United Nations, 2015) providing a globally relevant roadmap aimed at improving the well-being of humans in all nations. SDG 3 includes a focus on addressing the burden of disease related to mental disorders (United Nations, 2015):

'SDG3: Ensure healthy lives and promote well-being for all at all ages

- Target 3.4: By 2030, reduce by one third premature mortality from non-communicable diseases through prevention and treatment and promote mental health and well-being

- Target 3.8: Achieve universal health coverage, including financial risk protection, access to quality essential healthcare services and access to safe, effective, quality and affordable essential medicines and vaccines for all
- Indicator 3.4.2: Suicide mortality rate'.

The emergence of coronavirus disease (COVID-19) and the resultant pandemic has been identified as halting or reversing progress that was underway in promoting well-being for all and 'exposed and intensified inequalities within and among countries' (United Nations, 2021, p. 3). In the past, such catastrophic events have been a catalyst for change. The Under-Secretary-General for Economic and Social Affairs, Liu Zhenmin highlights the resilience, adaptability and innovation that have emerged in many parts of the world, drawing attention to the way in which the 'pandemic has sped up the digital transformation of Governments and businesses, profoundly changing the ways in which we interact, learn and work' (United Nations, 2021, p. 3).

It is against this backdrop that this chapter provides the opportunity to broaden your knowledge of mental health and well-being, the regional and cultural challenges that impact people's mental health and to examine the evidence-base for interventions to promote mental health well-being and support those experiencing mental ill-health. This approach is also relevant when dealing with the physical ailments of patients you will encounter in the region.

DEFINING MENTAL HEALTH

The World Health Constitution first signed in 1946 defines health as 'a state of complete physical, mental and social-well-being and not merely the absence of disease or infirmity' (World Health Organization (WHO), 2020). However, this definition from the WHO does not capture the complexity and multifaceted nature of human functioning. To effectively explore the topic of mental health and well-being, it is essential to consider mental health from the perspective of overall health.

The Transdomain Model of Health (Fig. 8.1) (Manwell et al., 2015) provides a useful schematic representation of the way in which physical, social and

mental health each contribute to a person's overall health and well-being. Other researchers have focussed on specifically defining mental health with Galderisi et al. (2015, 2017) suggesting that mental health is the ability of an individual to demonstrate social skills, cope with adverse events and manage their own emotions.

This definition also references the 'universal values of society' although positive mental health needs also require to be defined 'in terms that are culturally sensitive and inclusive' (Vaillant, 2012, p. 94).

MENTAL ILL-HEALTH

The WHO describes mental disorders as 'generally characterized by a combination of abnormal thoughts, perceptions, emotions, behaviour and relationships with others' and identify the following as mental disorders: anxiety, depression, bipolar disorder, schizophrenia and other psychoses, dementia and developmental disorders including autism' (WHO, 2019a).

Two major classification systems are currently available for both diagnostic and research purposes.

1. Diagnostic and Statistical Manual of Mental Disorder (DSM-V).
   a. This version was published in 2013.
   b. Primarily used in the United States by clinicians and psychiatrists (American Psychiatric Association, 2013).
2. International Classification of Diseases 11th Revision (ICD-11), https://icd.who.int/en
   a. Replaces ICD-10.
   b. Recently approved by the World Health Assembly.
   c. For implementation globally from January 2022.
   d. Described as an important advance in the field of psychiatric classification.

It is beyond the scope of this chapter to examine the ongoing questions and controversies associated with either of these two classification systems.

Fig. 8.2 provides a brief overview of anxiety disorders and depressive disorders. Although these common disorders are sometimes dismissed as inconsequential, the impact on a person's functioning and ability to achieve their potential and maintain healthy relationships is significant.

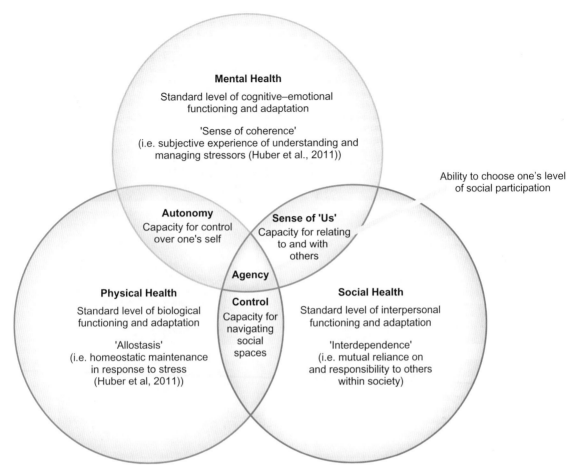

Fig. 8.1 ▪ Transdomain model of health. (With permission from Manwell, L. A., Barbic, S. P., Roberts, K., Durisko, Z., Lee, C., Ware, E., et al. (2015). What is mental health? Evidence towards a new definition from a mixed methods multidisciplinary international survey. *BMJ Open, 5*(6), e007079. https://doi.org/10.1136/bmjopen-2014-007079. See also Huber, M., et al. (2011). How should we define health? *BMJ, 343*, d4163. doi:10.1136/bmj.d4163.)

While bipolar disorder and psychotic disorders (including schizophrenia) occur much less frequently, these disorders require specialist psychiatric intervention and long-term treatment and support (Fig. 8.3).

GLOBAL PREVALENCE AND THE BURDEN OF MENTAL DISORDERS

Globally, mental disorders (specifically anxiety and depressive disorders) rank among the top 25 contributors to the health-related burden. Neither global prevalence nor burden has reduced since 1990, although extensive research describes positive outcomes from evidence-based interventions.

Depressive disorders, for example, have been identified as one of the causes of health loss worldwide in younger people aged 10–49 years (GBD 2019 Diseases and Injuries Collaborators, 2020). The COVID-19 pandemic resulted in extraordinary efforts to implement 'social distancing' impacting social connectedness, access to support and the shutdown of day-to-day activities (Galea et al., 2020). This further increased both the prevalence and burden of anxiety and depressive disorders. In most contexts, mental healthcare services were already fragmented and under resourced and the pandemic resulted in 'an increased urgency to strengthen mental health systems in most countries' (Santomauro et al., 2021,

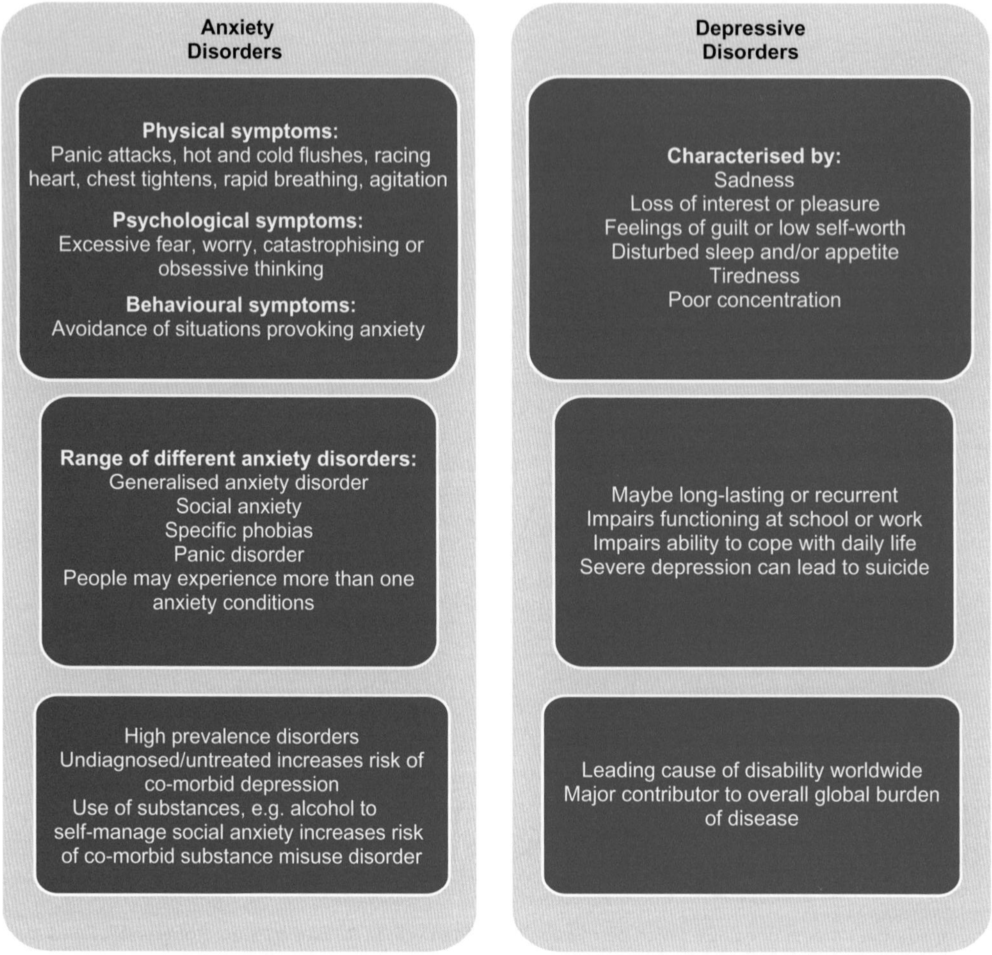

Anxiety Disorders

Physical symptoms:
Panic attacks, hot and cold flushes, racing heart, chest tightens, rapid breathing, agitation

Psychological symptoms:
Excessive fear, worry, catastrophising or obsessive thinking

Behavioural symptoms:
Avoidance of situations provoking anxiety

Range of different anxiety disorders:
Generalised anxiety disorder
Social anxiety
Specific phobias
Panic disorder
People may experience more than one anxiety conditions

High prevalence disorders
Undiagnosed/untreated increases risk of co-morbid depression
Use of substances, e.g. alcohol to self-manage social anxiety increases risk of co-morbid substance misuse disorder

Depressive Disorders

Characterised by:
Sadness
Loss of interest or pleasure
Feelings of guilt or low self-worth
Disturbed sleep and/or appetite
Tiredness
Poor concentration

Maybe long-lasting or recurrent
Impairs functioning at school or work
Impairs ability to cope with daily life
Severe depression can lead to suicide

Leading cause of disability worldwide
Major contributor to overall global burden of disease

Fig. 8.2 ■ Anxiety and depressive disorders.

p. 1700). It is, therefore, essential that treatments be implemented to address anxiety and depressive disorders within our societies.

REGIONAL PREVALENCE

The current and lifetime prevalence of both mental and substance disorders, and particularly high incidence of anxiety and depression, in the Eastern Mediterranean Region (15 countries) has been reported as high (Wakim et al., 2021). Factors contributing to the increased prevalence of depression, anxiety and stress-related disorders in the region include 'the experience of war, conflict, population displacement, infrastructure damage and unem-

ployment' (Zuberi et al., 2021, p. 1035). Existing research undertaken in the Gulf Cooperation Council (GCC) specific to depressive disorders has been described as limited and lacking rigour (Alzahrani, 2020). However, a broader review of mental illness research in the GCC suggests that the sociocultural context impacts people's experiences when engaging with mental health services (Hickey et al., 2016). Gaps in data specific to suicide, eating disorders and substance use in research focussing on the mental health and well-being of university students in 22 Arab countries has recently been identified (Sweileh, 2021).

A review of mental disorders research across the countries of the Organisation of Islamic Cooperation

Bipolar Disorder	Schizophrenia	Psychotic Disorders
Abnormally upbeat, jumpy or wired	Hallucinations Delusions Disorganised thinking	Abnormal thinking and perceptions Losing reality
Acute mania Mixed mood state (manic or depressed) Acute depressive episodes Maintenance	Social withdrawal Decreased emotional expression Apathy	Disturbed thoughts Confused thoughts Delusions Suspicious

Fig. 8.3 ■ Bipolar, schizophrenia and psychotic disorders.

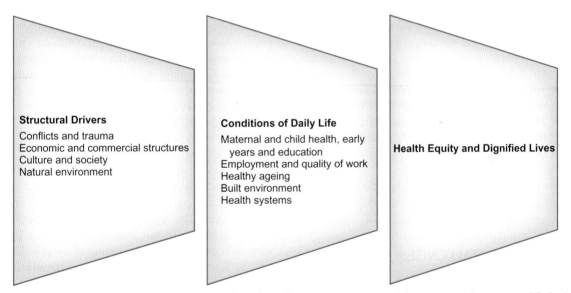

Structural Drivers
Conflicts and trauma
Economic and commercial structures
Culture and society
Natural environment

Conditions of Daily Life
Maternal and child health, early years and education
Employment and quality of work
Healthy ageing
Built environment
Health systems

Health Equity and Dignified Lives

Fig. 8.4 ■ Taken from the social determinants of health in the EMR. *EMR*, Eastern Mediterranean Region. (Modified with permission from Commission on Social Determinants of Health in the Eastern Mediterranean Region. (2021). Build back fairer: Achieving health equity in the Eastern Mediterranean Region–Report of the Commission on Social Determinants of Health in the Eastern Mediterranean Region (Report). WHO Regional Office for the Eastern Mediterranean, p. 11.)

(OIC) (many of which lie within the Eastern Mediterranean Region) identified significant variation in published research. Figs 8.3 and 8.4 provide insight into the disease process and the impact of societal influences on mental health outcomes. The review recommended greater international collaboration with researchers and noted that suicide and self-harm were seriously under-researched. The impact of stigma associated with mental disorders was identified as a potential contributor to the paucity of research from some of the OIC countries (Al-Adawi et al., 2002; Lewison et al., 2021).

The findings from a large-scale methodologically rigorous mental health epidemiological study undertaken in Saudi Arabia were released in full in 2020. The data are described as a 'rich picture of mental health in a region that is undergoing very rapid transitions, while experiencing conflicts that in some cases have resulted in large scale displacements of populations' (Chatterji, 2020, p. 1). Some of the key points from this study include:

- Lifetime prevalence of mental disorders is 34.2%, with anxiety disorders the most prevalent at 23.2% and mood disorders at 9.3%. Onset typically in childhood, adolescence or early adulthood (Altwaijri et al., 2020b).
- Twelve-month prevalence and severity of mental disorders are reported as high compared to similar high-income countries (Altwaijri et al., 2020a).
- 'Unmet need for treatment of lifetime mental disorders is a major problem in the Kingdom of Saudi Arabia. Interventions to ensure prompt help-seeking are needed to reduce the burdens and hazards of untreated mental disorders' (Al-Subaie et al., 2020).
- For wealthy women, depression is in the top two contributors to death or disability (WHO, 2022).
- For high-income men, depression is rated as the fourth leading cause of early death or disability (WHO, 2022).

As a health professional, it is important to take the time to access prevalence data specific to the context in which you are practicing.

REGIONAL CHALLENGES

Mental health services in the region have tended to focus on custodial care. The stigma of psychiatric illness is hidden within the community and is often confused with drug and alcohol disorders. Ongoing treatment options are only available to the local population as the management is different for the expatriate population who are medicated through the acute stage of their illness and then deported. Mental health services are fragmented and scattered, with unregulated private clinics providing the bulk of mental healthcare. Most nurses working in the psychiatric units do not have formal education or a specialisation in mental

health nursing (Chowdhury, 2016, p. 1665). The rapid modernisation and growth within the region has arguably resulted in increasing the stress levels of residents, while the stigma of mental health which prevails within the culture has resulted in a general lack of understanding of mental illness and an ever-increasing burden of mental health problems.

Inequities in the social determinants of health across the region require urgent attention to enable all members of each community to achieve overall health and well-being (Commission on Social Determinants of Health in the Eastern Mediterranean Region, 2021). The impact of the COVID-19 pandemic has further intensified existing inequities.

While most of the countries in the Gulf region meet the criteria for 'very high human development', Iran, Egypt, Lebanon, Libya and Jordan meet the 'high human development criteria'. Iraq is classified at medium and Yemen at low human development scores (Commission on Social Determinants of Health in the Eastern Mediterranean Region, 2021). Although differences in health and life expectancy reflect differences in structural drivers and conditions of people's everyday lives, inequitable access to healthcare services in those countries is described as having very high human development impacting ill-health and mortality.

In each of the countries comprising the Gulf and the Middle East, there are multiple contextual factors to consider when planning and delivering mental health services (Patel et al., 2018).

Policies and practices related to widespread labour immigration in this region are beyond the scope of this chapter. However, in the Arab States region, migrant workers comprise a large percentage of the population, with 2019 reports indicating that there were 30 million international immigrants (31% women) in the GCC, Jordan and Lebanon (International Labour Organization (ILO), 2021). Many of these workers are separated from family and social networks of care and support that are protective for mental well-being (Baldassar & Wilding, 2019) while also carrying a huge burden of responsibility for their families in their country of origin who are reliant upon the monies they send home.

Refugees and Stateless

The 'Arab Spring' and long-standing conflicts in Palestine, Iraq, Syria and Yemen have resulted in millions of people fleeing their homelands and seeking refuge in other countries. This has not only affected the refugees but also has impacted on the health and financial resources of the surrounding countries as these refugees are now reliant upon the new country for food, education, housing and healthcare. This has a knock-on effect on the local populations as finite resources are re-directed to fund refugees.

Populations That Are Stateless

Populations that are now considered 'stateless' include Palestine, Yemen and other countries involved in conflict, as these populations may have passports from their home countries, but such travel documents are likely to restrict their movements. These individuals are vulnerable to changes in internal politics and face the prospect of deportation with nowhere to go, which causes these stateless people to become affected mentally (depressed) as they face uncertain future solutions. These refugees may have limited access to physical healthcare but are denied access to mental healthcare.

Trauma and Distress

Many of those arriving in refugee camps are evidencing symptoms of stress, emerging mental illness as well as physical injuries. This is an outcome of dislocation resulting from rapid change that has occurred over the past 50 years. This upheaval in their social and economic structure is markedly different from their previously self-sufficient and sustainable lifestyle. Previously most of these people had families, friends, homes, jobs, comfortable lifestyles, money and security. When the conflicts occurred, this lifestyle was destroyed and individuals/families were either removed or escaped from the offensive situation.

The challenge for healthcare staff is the divide between patients' cultural identity and the evidence-based knowledge of health professionals. Healthcare professionals struggle with their local culture and history versus evidence-based practice when dealing with displaced/refugee clients.

Other sections of society who face mental health problems in this region are expatriate workers, such as maids/carers, who have problems with attachment due to their differing backgrounds. These maids/carers have left their own families behind in their home countries and this new family may bring emotional attachments. This becomes both a mental health and physical issue if they then face abuse or neglect from their employer. Expatriate industrial workers also face significant mental health issues as they are often young, come from remote villages in their home countries and are isolated for the first time due to working abroad.

The cultural background of this region with a strong focus on 'family' can mean the extended family bringing differing parenting styles. This 'idea' of family is further explored in Chapter 2.

Religious and/or Cultural Beliefs

- It is important to differentiate between cultural beliefs and religious beliefs. The religious mindset and cultural background significantly influence perceptions of mental illness and how/who/where to seek assistance. Several studies have identified the different attitudes of Arabic society towards mental illness and treatment.
- Cultural beliefs may attribute mental illness to 'jinn possession' (see Chapter 13) or being under the influence of the devil and therefore requiring isolation from society (Al-Adawi et al., 2002). Consequently, mental health problems may be identified as punishment for wrongdoing by the person or their family.
- Stigma and fear: 49% of patients identified stigma in attending mental health services or fear of being treated by mental health professionals. The preference for counselling in 30% of the cohorts was focussed on their Iman (religious leader) or friends of the family (Chowdhury, 2016).
- Taboo subject—mental illness: seeking mental health assistance is still considered a sign of 'weakness and failure' across the Arabic population.
- There is limited research on suicide and self-harm but what is known is (Wakim et al., 2021):
  - Shame is associated with suicide
  - Suicide is a sinful act
  - Many countries in this region also deem suicide to be a criminal act.
- Gender inequality.

This region is very patriarchal with fathers and brothers largely having control over the family. Nevertheless, this approach is slowly changing and different countries in the Middle East are giving women independence and involvement in decision-making processes about themselves, their families and even their countries. However, this male dominance patently affects the ability of healthcare providers to treat female patients. Patient confidentiality and individual consultations can be a challenge when treating female patients particularly when dealing with mental health issues.

MENTAL HEALTH SERVICES: PROMOTING PERSON-CENTRED AND RIGHTS-BASED APPROACHES

The WHO has called for all services to move away from an 'entrenched overreliance on the biomedical model in which the predominant focus of care is on diagnosis, medication and symptom reduction while the full range of social determinants that impact people's mental health was overlooked' (WHO, 2021). The rising burden of mental ill-health as a consequence of COVID-19 requires focussed attention on prevention and an upscaling of mental healthcare services for those who are unwell (Carbone, 2020). It is therefore essential that these services are evidence-based and respect human rights.

These services must ensure inclusion of those with lived experience in planning and delivery of services. Changes in policy and society will only occur if people who suffer from mental health illnesses or are supporting family and friends with these diseases are included in the decision-making process. This will ensure that the challenges mental health clients face and the needs they have will be addressed (WHO, 2021).

The following section draws your attention to the continuum of approaches required to enable all global citizens to receive person-centred care that meets international human rights standards.

PROMOTING MENTAL HEALTH AND WELL-BEING/PREVENTING MENTAL ILLNESS

To promote and support mental health and well-being, it is essential to recognise the social and ecological determinants specific to the context and culture that are impacting the community. Rather than focussing health promotion activities solely on the individual, creating an environment that is conducive to well-being is essential.

Growing research evidence is demonstrating the positive impacts of community interventions in promoting mental health and social equity.

EARLY INTERVENTION

Research reveals that mental illness frequently begins during adolescence, sometimes in late childhood. Approximately half of mental illness emerges by 14 years of age, with three-quarters beginning by 24 years of age (Fusar-Poli et al., 2021). Without early and effective intervention, mental illness is likely to persist, adversely impacting the young person's ability to complete their education and achieve other age congruent milestones. Overall, life expectancy is reduced by 10–20 years (Chan et al., 2021).

The splitting of mental healthcare services into paediatric and adult services (between ages 15–18 years) coincides with the period of high-risk for the development of mental illness. 'Psychopathology and brain maturation see no abrupt transition among adolescence and early adulthood' (Fusar-Poli et al., 2021, p. 200). This 'splitting' of services results in missed opportunities to provide continuity of care for young people, resulting in many adolescents and young adults not receiving the early intervention that is needed

Key to effective early intervention is the provision of services delivered in the community and in primary healthcare centres. Globally, a number of models are emerging to facilitate a shift from stand-alone psychiatric facilities (Wakida et al., 2018). For example, stepped care (Table 8.1) is designed to 'support an early intervention approach where people with mental health problems and mental illness have their needs addressed early, rather than waiting until the problems worsen and require more intensive intervention' while 'allocating resource in accordance with population need' (Australian Government Department of Health, 2019, p. 7).

TREATMENT

Traditionally, addressing mental health illnesses in this region has been undertaken in 'custodial care' environments or with patients being 'locked away' from society by their families. Culturally safe and responsive care includes the following thinking grid.

TABLE 8.1	
Stepped Care	
Grade	Condition
1	Well population
2	At-risk groups—early symptoms, previous illness
3	Mild mental illness
4	Moderate mental illness
5	Severe mental illness

Note: The numbers define the grades of mental health in individuals from 1 (healthy mental health) through to 5 (significant mental health disease).

THINKING GRID

Therapeutic communication

- Self-awareness
  - Ask yourself—What would it be like to be in this person's situation?
  - Put aside biases and assumptions
  - Non-judgemental stance
- Ask
- Listen

The integration of mental health services into primary healthcare has been carried out by various countries and thus integrated treatment is now being promoted in this region (Wakida et al., 2018).

COMMUNITY-BASED MENTAL HEALTH SERVICES

The stigma associated with mental health illnesses and the reluctance of patients to present to traditional healthcare facilities has encouraged the development of community-based services. Community-based services are designed to provide mental healthcare in the community to serve the most vulnerable population suffering from serious mental illnesses in their own environment (Fig. 8.5). The primary goal is to prevent psychiatric crisis and further complications. This type of service is designed to meet the community needs within a culturally relevant context. It promotes community education to increase public awareness and to decrease the stigma of mental illnesses. Potential clients are assessed and diagnosed by a psychiatrist who

refers the patient to the community team. Consent is obtained from the patient or their carer. An assessment of the patient's home is undertaken to ensure the safety of the team. Once on the programme the patient is regularly assessed and a care plan implemented. Strict inclusion and exclusion criteria apply to all patients. Refer to Case Study 8.1.

CRISIS INTERVENTIONS

Crisis intervention is initiated by the family/care giver (if at home) or by the police or ambulance if in public. Mental health services need to have a crisis intervention team that can respond either within a health facility (code black) or on outreach. The crisis intervention team responds to the acute crisis in the community and manages the crisis in collaboration with the authorities. Assessment is undertaken by the team including an environmental assessment in conjunction with the police. De-escalation will be implemented by counselling from the intervention team. The patient will be transported to hospital for ongoing assessment and treatment. Crisis intervention is usually required because of a suicide attempt, aggressive or violent behaviour or homicidal or destructive behaviour.

FUTURE DIRECTIONS

The United Arab Emirates (UAE) has produced a national approach and guidelines to address Mental health issues concerning public health aspects of mental and behavioural disorders. This also provides comprehensive information for the policymakers,

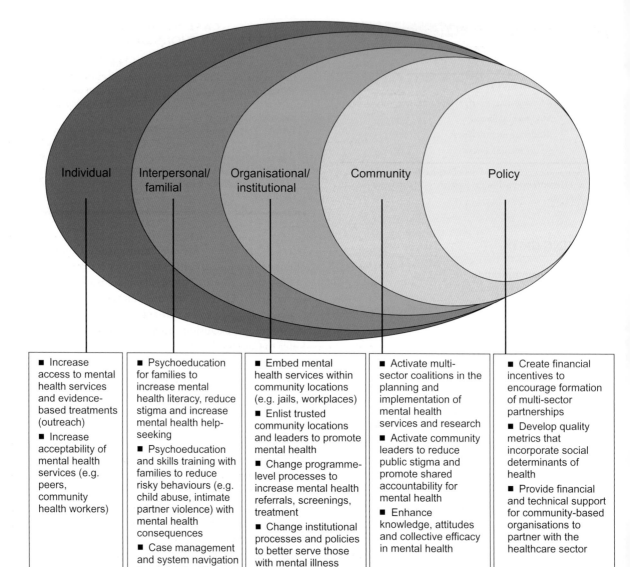

Fig. 8.5 ■ Overview of community intervention processes by social-ecological level. (Adapted with permission from McElroy, K. R., Bibeau, D., Steckler, A., & Glanz, K. (1988). An ecological perspective on health promotion programs. *Health Education Quarterly*, 15, 351–377. In Castillo, E. G., Ijadi-Maghsoodi, R., Shadravan, S., Moore, E., Mensah, M. O., 3rd, Docherty, M., et al. (2019). Community interventions to promote mental health and social equity. *Current Psychiatry Reports*, 21(5), 35. https://doi.org/10.1007/s11920-019-1017-0.)

and it can also be utilised as an awareness-raising tool. This approach is the result of a huge effort that brings together a pool of research studies conducted in the UAE in mental and behavioural disorders. It is designed to facilitate and inspire commitment, innovation and cooperation in preventing mental and behavioural disorders and to offer the best care possible given the circumstances (United Arab Emirates Ministry of Health and Prevention, 2019).

THINKING GRID

- Access the WHO special initiative for mental health (2019–2023).
- Access the Mental Health Gap Action Programme (mhGAP), https://www.who.int/teams/mental-health-and-substance-use/treatment-care/mental-health-gap-action-programme.
- Review the assumptions for the success of this initiative:
  - How do mental health services in your community and region meet up to these assumptions?
  - What gaps have you been able to identify?
  - What actions could you share with your colleagues to better ensure quality services for all members of your community?
  - What actions could you identify to improve acceptance of mental health services for all members of your community?

SUMMARY AND TAKEAWAY POINTS

COVID-19 has highlighted the need for strong mental help globally. The pandemic identified that mental health issues can arise when people are socially isolated and hence the importance of timely and appropriate support. Hopefully the pandemic has/will continue to remove the social and cultural stigmas associated with mental health problems. It is essential that this opportunity is not wasted in this region. The following 'take home messages' therefore need to be supported.

- It is crucial that psychiatrists and mental health professionals play a key role in prompting policymakers to develop well-tailored mental health policies, boost the priority afforded to mental health, as well as support implementation of culturally appropriate policies. Other issues to

be addressed include laws and regulations to address suicide or self-harm.

- Implementation of child protection laws and policies including a focus on children and adolescents and improved perinatal or obstetric care to prevent birth trauma, given its association with physical and mental disabilities.
- A focus on professional and public awareness of these disorders raised through local and global initiatives and campaigns targeting neurologists, general practitioners, specialists in public health, psychiatrists, media, health economists, health planners and most importantly the general population (United Arab Emirates Ministry of Health and Prevention, 2019).
- Mental Health Gap Action Programme (mhGAP) from WHO is focussed on increasing services for mental, neurological and substance use disorders, especially for countries with low and middle income. This is crucial for this region (WHO, 2019b).
- Implementation of basic training and educational interventions for caregivers, patient information programmes and self-help groups to facilitate and encourage patients and families. Involvement of carers, families and patients in policymaking and service planning. These stakeholders need to be represented in the media and in the implementation and development of services and policies for people with mental health illnesses (Stein et al., 2020).

REFERENCES

Al-Adawi, S., Dorylo, A., Al-Ghafry, D., Al Noobi, B., Al-Salmi, A., Burke, D., et al. (2002). Perception of and attitude towards mental illness in Oman. *International Journal of Social Psychiatry*, 48(4), 305–317.

Al-Subaie, A. S., Altwaijri, Y. A., Al-Habeeb, A., Bilal, L., Almeharish, A., Sampson, N. A., et al. (2020). Lifetime treatment of DSM-IV mental disorders in the Saudi National Mental Health Survey. *International Journal of Methods in Psychiatric Research*, 29(3), e1837. https://doi.org/10.1002/mpr.1837.

Altwaijri, Y. A., Al-Habeeb, A., Al-Subaie, A. S., Bilal, L., Al-Desouki, M., Shahab, M. K., et al. (2020a). Twelve-month prevalence and severity of mental disorders in the Saudi National Mental Health Survey. *International Journal of Methods in Psychiatric Research*, 29(3), e1831. https://doi.org/10.1002/mpr.1831.

Altwaijri, Y. A., Al-Subaie, A. S., Al-Habeeb, A., Bilal, L., Al-Desouki, M., Aradati, M., et al. (2020b). Lifetime prevalence and age-of-onset distributions of mental disorders in the Saudi National Mental

Health Survey. *International Journal of Methods in Psychiatric Research*, *29*(3), e1836. https://doi.org/10.1002/mpr.1836.

Alzahrani, O. (2020). Depressive disorders in the Arabian Gulf Cooperation Council countries: A literature review. *The Journal of International Medical Research*, *48*(10). https://doi.org/10.1177/0300060520961917. 300060520961917.

American Psychiatric Association. (2013). *Diagnostic and statistical manual of mental disorders* (5th ed.). American Psychiatric Publishing.

Australian Government Department of Health. (2019). PHN Mental Health Flexible Funding Pool Programme Guidance: Stepped Care. Australian Government Department of Health. Available at https://www1.health.gov.au/internet/main/publishing.nsf/Content/2126B045A8DA90FDCA257F6500018260/$File/1.%20PHN%20Guidance%20-%20Stepped%20Care%20-%202019.pdf. Accessed 30 August 2022.

Baldassar, L., & Wilding, R. (2019). Migration, aging, and digital kinning: The role of distant care support networks in experiences of aging well. *Gerontologist*, *60*(2), 313–321. https://doi.org/10.1093/geront/gnz156.

Blackmore, R., Gray, K. M., Boyle, J. A., Fazel, M., Ranasinha, S., Fitzgerald, G., et al. (2020). Systematic review and meta-analysis: The prevalence of mental illness in child and adolescent refugees and asylum seekers. *Journal of the American Academy of Child & Adolescent Psychiatry*, *59*(6), 705–714. https://doi.org/10.1016/j.jaac.2019.11.011.

Carbone, S. R. (2020). Flattening the curve of mental ill-health: The importance of primary prevention in managing the mental health impacts of COVID-19. *Mental Health & Prevention*, *19*, 200185. https://doi.org/10.1016/j.mhp.2020.200185.

Carla Abi, D., Haddad, C., Sacre, H., Salameh, P., Akel, M., Obeid, S., et al. (2019). Knowledge, attitude and behaviors towards patients with mental illness: Results from a national Lebanese study. *PLoS One*, *14*(9), e0222172. https://doi.org/10.1371/journal.pone.0222172.

Chan, M. F., Al Balushi, R., Al Falahi, M., Mahadevan, S., Al Saadoon, M., & Al-Adawi, S. (2021). Child and adolescent mental health disorders in the GCC: A systematic review and meta-analysis. *International Journal of Pediatrics and Adolescent Medicine*, *8*(3), 134–145. https://doi.org/10.1016/j.ijpam.2021.04.002.

Chatterji, S. (2020). The Saudi National Mental Health Survey: Filling critical gaps in methodology and data in mental health epidemiology. *International Journal of Methods in Psychiatric Research*, *29*(3), e1852. https://doi.org/10.1002/mpr.1852.

Chowdhury, N. (2016). Integration between mental health care providers and traditional spiritual healers: Contextualising Islam in the twenty first century. *Journal of Religion and Health*, *55*, 1665–1671.

Commission on Social Determinants of Health in the Eastern Mediterranean Region. (2021). Build back fairer: Achieving health equity in the Eastern Mediterranean Region: Report of the Commission on Social Determinants of Health in the Eastern Mediterranean Region [Report]. WHO Regional Office for the Eastern Mediterranean.

Fusar-Poli, P., Correll, C. U., Arango, C., Berk, M., Patel, V., & Ioannidis, J. P. A. (2021). Preventive psychiatry: A blueprint for improving the mental health of young people. *World Psychiatry*, *20*(2), 200–221. https://doi.org/10.1002/wps.20869.

Galderisi, S., Heinz, A., Kastrup, M., Beezhold, J., & Sartorius, N. (2015). Toward a new definition of mental health. *World Psychiatry: Official Journal of the World Psychiatric Association (WPA)*, *14*(2), 231–233. https://doi.org/10.1002/wps.20231.

Galderisi, S., Heinz, A., Kastrup, M., Beezhold, J., & Sartorius, N. (2017). A proposed new definition of mental health. *Psychiatric Policy*, *51*(3), 407–411. https://doi.org/10.12740/pp/74145.

Galea, S., Merchant, R. M., & Lurie, N. (2020). The mental health consequences of COVID-19 and physical distancing: The need for prevention and early intervention. *JAMA Internal Medicine*, *180*(6), 817–818. https://doi.org/10.1001/jamainternmed.2020.1562.

GBD 2019 Diseases and Injuries Collaborators. (2020). Global burden of 369 diseases and injuries in 204 countries and territories, 1990-2019: A systematic analysis for the Global Burden of Disease Study 2019. *Lancet*, *396*(10258), 1204–1222. https://doi.org/10.1016/s0140-6736(20)30925-9.

Hickey, J. E., Pryjmachuk, S., & Waterman, H. (2016). Mental illness research in the Gulf Cooperation Council: A scoping review. *Health Research Policy and Systems*, *14*(1), 59. https://doi.org/10.1186/s12961-016-0123-2.

International Labour Organization (ILO). (2021). *Labour Migration*. ILO. https://www.ilo.org/beirut/areasofwork/labour-migration/lang--en/index.htm

James, S. L., Abate, D., Abate, K. H., Abay, S. M., Abbafati, C., Abbasi, N., et al. (2018). Global, regional, and national incidence, prevalence, and years lived with disability for 354 diseases and injuries for 195 countries and territories, 1990–2017: A systematic analysis for the Global Burden of Disease Study 2017. *The Lancet*, *392*(10159), 1789–1858. https://doi.org/10.1016/S0140-6736(18)32279-7.

Lewison, G., Sullivan, R., & Kiliç, C. (2021). Mental health disorders research in the countries of the Organisation of Islamic Cooperation (OIC), 2008-17, and the disease burden: Bibliometric study. *PLoS ONE*, *16*(4), e0250414. https://doi.org/10.1371/journal.pone.0250414.

Manwell, L. A., Barbic, S. P., Roberts, K., Durisko, Z., Lee, C., Ware, E., et al. (2015). What is mental health? Evidence towards a new definition from a mixed methods multidisciplinary international survey. *BMJ Open*, *5*(6), e007079. https://doi.org/10.1136/bmjopen-2014-007079.

Maalouf, F., Alamiri, B., Atweh, S., Becker, A., Cheour, M., Darwish, H., et al. (2019). Mental health research in the Arab region: Challenges and a call for action. *Lancet Psychiatry*, *6*, 961–966.

Patel, V., Saxena, S., Lund, C., Thornicroft, G., Baingana, F., Bolton, P., et al. (2018). The Lancet Commission on global mental health and sustainable development. *The Lancet*, *392*(10157), 1553–1598. https://doi.org/10.1016/S0140-6736(18)31612-X.

Santomauro, D. F., Mantilla Herrera, A. M., Shadid, J., Zheng, P., Ashbaugh, C., Pigott, D. M., et al. (2021). Global prevalence and burden of depressive and anxiety disorders in 204 countries and territories in 2020 due to the COVID-19 pandemic. *The Lancet*, *398*(10312), 1700–1712. https://doi.org/10.1016/S0140-6736(21)02143-7.

Stein, D. J., Szatmari, P., Gaebel, W., Berk, M., Vieta, E., Maj, M., et al. (2020). Mental, behavioral and neurodevelopmental disorders in the ICD-11: An international perspective on key changes and controversies. *BMC Medicine*, *18*(1), 21. https://doi.org/10.1186/s12916-020-1495-2.

Sweileh, W. M. (2021). Contribution of researchers in the Arab region to peer-reviewed literature on mental health and well-being of university students. *International Journal of Mental Health Systems*, *15*(1), 50. https://doi.org/10.1186/s13033-021-00477-9.

United Arab Emirates Ministry of Health and Prevention. (2019). Mental health. Published Work on Mental Health in the United Arab Emirates—1992–2019. Available at www.mohap.gov.ae.

United Nations. (2015). *Transforming our World: The 2030 Agenda for Sustainable Development*. United Nations.

United Nations. (2021). *The Sustainable Development Goals Report 2021*. United Nations.

Vaillant, G. E. (2012). Positive mental health: Is there a cross-cultural definition? *World Psychiatry*, *11*(2), 93–99. https://doi.org/10.1016/j.wpsyc.2012.05.006.

Wakida, E. K., Talib, Z. M., Akena, D., Okello, E. S., Kinengyere, A., Mindra, A., et al. (2018). Barriers and facilitators to the integration of mental health services into primary health care: A systematic review. *Systematic Reviews*, *7*(1), 211. https://doi.org/10.1186/s13643-018-0882-7.

Wakim, E., El Hage, S., Safi, S., El Kareh, A., El Masri, J., & Salameh, P. (2021). Insights in neuropsychiatry: Suicide and self-mutilation in the Mena Region- a bibliometric quantitative and co-occurrence medline-based analysis. *Cureus*, *13*(10), e18680. https://doi.org/10.7759/cureus.18680.

WHO (World Health Organization). (2019a). *Fact sheet: Mental disorders*. Available at https://www.who.int/news-room/fact-sheets/detail/mental-disorders. Accessed on 8 December 2021.

WHO. (2019b). *The WHO special initiative for mental health (2019-2023): Universal health coverage for mental health*. World Health Organization.

WHO. (2020). *Basic documents: forty-ninth edition (including amendments adopted up to 31 May 2019)*. World Health Organization.

WHO. (2021). *Guidance on community mental health services: Promoting person-centred and rights-based approaches*. World Health Organization.

WHO. (2022). *Mental health and psychosocial support*. World Health Organization.

Zolezzi, M., Alamri, M., Shaar, S., & Rainkie, D. (2018). Stigma associated with mental illness and its treatment in the Arab culture: A systematic review. *International Journal of Social Psychiatry*, *64*(6), 597–609. https://doi.org/10.1177/0020764018789200.

Zuberi, A., Waqas, A., Naveed, S., Hossain, M. M., Rahman, A., Saeed, K., et al. (2021). Prevalence of mental disorders in the WHO Eastern Mediterranean Region: A systematic review and meta-analysis. *Frontiers in Psychiatry*, *12*(1035). https://doi.org/10.3389/fpsyt.2021.665019.

9 INFECTION

JANE LEANNE GRIFFITHS

INTRODUCTION

2020 caught the world and healthcare providers by surprise. It has been more than 100 years since the world has faced a pandemic impacting on every country. Technology and healthcare have changed significantly since the 1900s and the COVID-19 pandemic forced us to rapidly review how we protect our communities and provide healthcare.

Governments, heath systems and the community were not prepared for this catastrophic event and air travel resulted in a rapid spread of the virus to all corners of the earth. Moreover, the extensive use of social media providing instantaneous (but not necessarily accurate) information, meant everyone had a different opinion of how to address this deadly disease, as well as whether the virus was actually real and life-threatening. Unfortunately, some people preferred conspiracy theories, others opted to believe personal opinions whilst the scientific evidence did its very best to keep up and respond effectively and in a timely manner to the rapid spread.

Different healthcare systems have had to identify a medical care response and processes to address the immediate clinical needs on their doorstep. Without doubt, healthcare professionals stepped in and stepped up to meet the challenge. Simultaneously, it seemed like the rest of healthcare was placed on pause while prospective patients had to get involved in some clinical decision-making about when, how or where to seek help, and/or how to manage their conditions differently.

The pandemic has significantly affected our communities. To try and control the pandemic, the focus of healthcare has been on protecting our society but at what cost? Healthcare budgets are limited and diverting funds to address the pandemic resulted in a reduction in funding for other clinical activities. 'Locking down' populations increased mental health anxieties which resulted in the escalation of suicide rates amongst our young (Dolgin, 2021). The cancelling of elective surgery and screening processes caused a surge in the rates of cancer and saw an increase in disabilities amongst our older populations (https://www.thelancet.com). Healthcare professionals dealt with the problems of the infection and the myriad other issues that arose as a consequence of the infection, often leading to stress, exhaustion and burnout (Chang, 2022).

The pandemic has forced changes in both care delivery and in the development and implementation of technology to support patient care. Hopefully, the future will not be the same and the importance of mental health for patients, the community and our staff is something that needs to remain current and be addressed. We need to use data, e-health and patient applications to focus on addressing the clinical and mental health issues that are dormant in our communities.

The pandemic has been a focus of all our lives for the last few years. However, it is only one of many infectious diseases affecting the world and this region. This chapter will explore the significant infections that affect the world and this region (Bahrain, Iran, Jordan, Kuwait, Lebanon, Oman, Qatar, Saudi Arabia, the UAE, Yemen, North Africa), the methodologies used to control/contain these diseases, the impacts on the communities affected as well as the importance of infection control practices to keep our healthcare workers safe.

> ### *The fundamentals of infection*
>
> Microorganisms or microbes are tiny living things that are too small to be seen. They live in us and around us and most work for us or with us. Conversely, pathogens are microorganisms that have the potential to cause disease (infectious disease) and account for approximately 1% of all microorganisms. Pathogens comprise viruses, bacteria, protozoa, fungi and helminths.

BACKGROUND

The tracking of the global burden of infectious diseases has been in place since 1996. Prior to this formal tracking, ad hoc collections of information occurred at a national level including data collections on malaria, poliomyelitis, influenza and tuberculosis (TB) from the mid-1950s (Michaud, 2009). In this first study in 1996, causes of death from infectious diseases were categorized as infectious and parasitic diseases. These infectious diseases are now categorized as group I and consist of 14 infectious and parasitic diseases and 3 respiratory infections that are outlined in Box 9.1 (Michaud, 2009).

GLOBAL IMPACTS

In 2001, 14.2 million deaths occurred globally from infectious diseases (Michaud, 2009, p. 448). The leading causes of death from infectious diseases included HIV, diarrheal disease, TB and malaria. Many of these deaths were from countries deemed to be low

BOX 9.1

Risk Factors for Infectious Diseases

- Malnutrition
- Unsafe sex
- Poor water supply
- Tobacco
- Lack of Sanitation
- Alcohol
- Hygiene
- Pollution

or middle income. There is a higher prevalence of communicable diseases from sub-Sahara Africa and Asia, with many of these diseases occurring in equatorial and semi-tropical climates (Emad et al., 2021, p. 7). These high rates of disease are also impacted by the risk factors identified in Box 9.1 (Michaud, 2009 p. 453).

Several countries within the Middle East have faced conflict for many years. People have been displaced and now face a life without effective sanitation, safe water supply and food. This places them at greater risk of contracting several of the infectious diseases outlined in Box 9.2. The significant number of expatriate workers located in the Gulf Cooperative Council (GCC) countries also face these hazardous problems being situated in overcrowded labour camps, with minimal access to healthcare. The expatriate workers located in these labour camps may be sharing rooms with up to 16 workers in double bunk beds and shared bathrooms. An obvious consequence of this multiple close quarter occupancy is the rapid spread of infectious diseases (Amnesty International, 2020).

The COVID-19 pandemic resulted in 611 million cases and 6.54 million deaths globally (WHO, 2022a). The virus can spread from an infected person's mouth or nose in small liquid particles when they cough, sneeze, speak, sing or breathe. These particles range from larger respiratory droplets to smaller aerosols (National Center for Immunization and Respiratory Diseases, 2019).

People can be infected by breathing in the virus if they are near someone who has COVID-19 or by touching a contaminated surface and then their eyes, nose or mouth. The virus spreads more easily indoors and in crowded settings. Prior to the rapid development of vaccines, individuals were forced

BOX 9.2

Group I Infectious Diseases

A. INFECTIOUS DISEASES
1. Tuberculosis
2. Sexually transmitted diseases, excluding HIV
   a. Syphilis
   b. Chlamydia
   c. Gonorrhoea
3. HIV/AIDS
4. Diarrheal diseases
5. Childhood cluster diseases
   a. Pertussis
   b. Poliomyelitis
   c. Diphtheria
   d. Measles
   e. Tetanus
6. Bacterial meningitis and meningococcaemia
7. Hepatitis B and hepatitis C
8. Malaria
9. Tropical-cluster causes
   a. Trypanosomiasis
   b. Chagas' disease
   c. Schistosomiasis
   d. Leishmaniasis
   e. Lymphatic filariasis
   f. Onchocerciasis
10. Leprosy
11. Dengue
12. Japanese encephalitis
13. Trachoma
14. Intestinal nematode infections
    a. Ascariasis
    b. Trichuriasis
    c. Ancylostomiasis and necatoriasis
B. RESPIRATORY INFECTIONS
1. Lower respiratory infections
2. Upper respiratory infections
3. Otitis media

Based on WHO (World Health Organization). (2022a). Health emergency dashboard. Available at https://extranet.who.int>publicemergency.

to protect themselves by wearing masks, washing hands frequently and socially distancing. Many countries were also 'locked down' preventing people from travelling outside of their homes (Greyling et al., 2021). Initially all domestic and international flights were grounded; however, by that stage of the pandemic, the virus had already travelled internationally. Between the end of 2020 and September 2022, there have been 12.6 billion vaccines administered globally (WHO, 2022a).

The fundamentals of infection

An infection is where pathogens invade a host (human) and multiply. An infection does not always result in disease. Infection occurs at a portal of entry either percutaneously (across the skin) or mucocutaneously (via the mucous membrane: eye, nose, mouth, genital area). The respiratory tract (mouth and nose), gastrointestinal tract (mouth, oral cavity) and urogenital tract are key portals of entry. Infection requires three key aspects to be present for infection to *potentially* occur:

Pathogen + infectious fluid + portal of entry

Note: Not all fluids are infectious. Some fluids may have a pathogen such as virus present in it, but not in sufficient numbers to cause harm.

REGIONAL IMPACTS

This section will specifically discuss three infectious diseases that have significant impact on the Middle Eastern region. These diseases are: COVID-19, TB and meningococcal meningitis.

The first case of COVID-19 in the Middle East was identified at the beginning of 2020. Since then, 23 million cases of COVID-19 have been reported from the Eastern Mediterranean countries up to September 2022 (WHO, 2022a) (Table 9.1). As with all infectious diseases, it is essential that adequate, timely and accurate reporting is undertaken. This is a problem that all public health services face in trying to track, trace and identify the spread of diseases.

Contact tracing is a corner stone in defeating any communicable disease. Preventive measures include prophylaxis, vaccination, contact screening and monitoring during the incubation period (Ministry of Justice, 2020).

TABLE 9.1
COVID-19 Statistics 2020–2022

Country	Deaths	Reported Positive Cases
Jordan	14,116	1.75 million
Lebanon	10,666	1.21 million
UAE	2342	1.02 million
Saudi Arabia	9902	81,600
Bahrain	1520	678,000
Kuwait	2563	659,000
Egypt	24,797	516,000
Qatar	682	446,000
Oman	4628	398,000

Based on WHO (World Health Organization. (2022a). Health emergency dashboard. Available at https://extranet.who.int>publicemergency.

The Middle East and Arabic region has a mixture of low-, medium- and high-income societies. This amalgam of cultures and economies impacts on the infectious disease risks to the Eastern Mediterranean region which reports results for the Middle East and Arabic region. The other issue for this region is that it is centrally located to the rest of the world. Qatar and the UAE have become transport hubs connecting the rest of the world. People from Africa, Asia, the Pacific and Europe fly through this region to link to other countries. Dubai airport handled 86.4 million passengers in 2019 and expects to return to these numbers by 2023. Dubai is the world's busiest airport for international travel and has held that title for 8 years (Griffiths, 2002). The challenge for this region is that these passengers are coming from countries that have high rates of infectious diseases and therefore potentially bring with them unwanted 'gifts'.

In GCC countries, 80% of the workforce are expatriate workers who hail from Africa, Asia and Eastern Europe with visa screening of infectious diseases a pre-requisite for work permits and/or residency. This measure is designed to identify potential infectious diseases before they can spread through the community. This screening reviews the HIV, pulmonary TB, leprosy and hepatitis B and syphilis status of potential employees (Ministry of Justice, 2020). These tests are undertaken on all expatriates and further tests may be required dependent on the job role.

TB is one of the most significant contagious pathogens internationally and is the leading cause of death from infectious diseases generally, especially for patients with HIV (Habous et al., 2020). TB was beginning to be controlled but has re-emerged more virulently, largely thanks to antimicrobial resistance. Thus, the prevention, diagnosis and treatment of TB has been compromised due to the resistance of the usual TB drugs. This resistance is mainly caused by following improper treatment of patients. In the past, patients were started on TB medication but did not complete the full course due to lack of available medication or travelling to another country. Patients also 'shared' their medication with other ill members of their family. This led to the growth of drug-resistant strains of the disease (Habous et al., 2020, p. 391). Patients with TB may also suffer from malnourishment, diabetes, excessive alcohol, smoking and HIV. While the Western world has mainly been exposed to pulmonary TB, this region has tended to be exposed to other forms of TB such as meningeal TB. Expatriate workers from countries with a high prevalence of TB contribute to the occurrence of new cases and are the largest group of carriers for TB. Consequently, it would be helpful to develop appropriate policies to monitor and manage expatriates and refugees in this region and thus control the infection.

CASE STUDY 9.1
HAJJ EXPOSURE

In 2000–2001, over 2 million Muslims undertook the pilgrimage to Mecca/Medina in Saudi Arabia for a month. Of the 2 million plus pilgrims attending Hajj, 500,000 contracted meningococcal disease. Furthermore, once they returned home, 18 to 28/100,000 of the pilgrims' unvaccinated household contacts also contracted this disease. A total of 185,000 people from across the world died because of this infection, accounting for a 37% case fatality rate.

As a result of this catastrophic event, mandated meningococcal vaccination of all pilgrims now occurs together with a recommendation that the pilgrims' household contacts are also vaccinated. Visas to attend Hajj are now dependent on proof of vaccination.

Source: Based on Wilder-Smith, A., Goh, K. T., Barkham, T., & Paton, N. I. (2003). Hajj-associated outbreak strain of *Neisseria meningitidis* serogroup W135: estimates of the attack rate in a defined population and the risk of invasive disease developing in carriers. *Clin Infect Dis*, 36(6), 679–683.

Unfortunately, 27% of patients with TB are also known to be HIV-positive (Habibzadeh, 2012).

Meningococcal disease refers to any illness caused by bacteria called *Neisseria meningitidis*. These illnesses are often severe, can be deadly, and include infections of the lining of the brain and spinal cord (meningitis) and bloodstream. This disease is particularly prevalent in this region because of the Hajj and Umrah pilgrimages by Muslims to Mecca and Medina in Saudi Arabia. While the annual Hajj pilgrimage involves >2 million pilgrims from over 185 countries, two thirds of these arrive from 13 countries, chiefly from across South-East Asia, the Middle East and North African (MENA) regions (Badur et al., 2022). Case Study 9.1 describes the outbreak that occurred during Hajj 2000–2001.

REGIONAL CHALLENGES

The focus of infection control in this region is early detection, timely prevention and control of communicable diseases. This is mandated by law in many of the Middle East countries. 'Communicable diseases must be reported. Failure to do so will make the person liable to penalties including jail or fine or both' (Ministry of Justice, 2020).

Tables 9.2–9.4 outline the reportable diseases.

One of the reportable diseases unique to this region is Middle East respiratory syndrome (MERS). This is a viral respiratory illness that was first identified in Saudi Arabia in 2012. Most people infected with MERS-CoV developed severe respiratory illness, including

TABLE 9.2				
Immediately Reportable Diseases				
Immediately Reportable Communicable Disease (0–8 hours)				
Acute flaccid paralysis (AFP)	Anthrax	Botulism	Cholera	Measles
Diphtheria	Food poisoning	Enterohemorrhagic Escherichia coli	Avian influenza	Plague
Middle East respiratory syndrome (MERS)	Novel coronavirus disease COVID-19 (SARS-CoV-2)	Monkeypox	Nipah virus	Smallpox
Poliomyelitis	Rabies	Rubella	Severe acute respiratory syndrome (SARS)	
Typhus	Viral haemorrhagic fever (Ebola, Lassa, etc.)	Yellow fever	Any unusually/emerging disease	

Based on DHA Health Regulation Department. 2022. Communicable Disease Notification Policy. DHA/HRS/HPSD/HP-10 Version 2.1, pp. 6–7.

TABLE 9.3				
Reportable Diseases Within 24 Hours				
Immediately Reportable Diseases Within 24 Hours				
Haemophilus influenza invasive disease	Hepatitis A	Hepatitis E	Human immunodeficiency virus (HIV)/AIDS	Legionellosis
Salmonellosis	Shigellosis	Meningitis Specify aetiology: bacterial or viral	Influenza A H1N1	Dengue fever
Leprosy (Hansen disease)	Malaria	Pertussis	Tetanus (including neonatal)	Tuberculosis (pulmonary)
Tuberculous meningitis (extra pulmonary)				

Based on DHA Health Regulation Department. 2022. Communicable Disease Notification Policy. DHA/HRS/HPSD/HP-10 Version 2.1, pp. 6–7.

TABLE 9.4

Reportable Diseases Within 5 Working Days

Weekly Reportable Communicable Disease (Within 5 Working Days)

Ascariasis	Cytomegalovirus	Influenza
Amoebiasis	Encephalitis or bacterial or viral	Invasive pneumo-coccal disease (IPD)
Brucellosis	Foodborne illness Specify: amoebic dysentery or bacillary dysentery	Listeriosis
Chickenpox (Varicella)	Giardiasis	Mumps
Conjunctivitis	Infectious mononucleosis	Relapsing fever
Scabies	Scarlet fever	Streptococcal disease, invasive, group A or B · Streptococcal pneumonia invasive disease (other than meningitis)
Sexually transmitted infections (STIs): chlamydia, gonorrhoea, syphilis (early & late), chancroid, genital warts, herpes simplex, trichomoniasis	Typhoid/paratyphoid	Vital hepatitis (B, C, D)
Trachoma	Other protozoal intestinal diseases	Other zoonotic bacterial diseases not classified elsewhere
Other unspecified infectious diseases		

Based on DHA Health Regulation Department. 2022. Communicable Disease Notification Policy. DHA/HRS/HPSD/HP-10 Version 2.1, pp. 6–7.

fever, cough and shortness of breath. MERS spread to Bahrain, Iran, Jordan, Kuwait, Lebanon, Oman, Qatar, Saudi Arabia, UAE and Yemen. Thereafter, it progressed internationally via travellers to their home countries, infecting not just humans but camels and bats. In every 10 patients confirmed with the disease, 3–4 have died

CASE STUDY 9.2
MANAGEMENT OF COVID-19

It was identified quickly that the existing healthcare facilities would not be able to cope with the expected influx of patients suspected of or infected with COVID-19. Consequently, hospitals were closed to elective surgery and many outpatient clinics were suspended. A rapid response saw 17,689 additional beds added to the existing 2000 hospital beds. These beds were for quarantine and isolation purposes with the acute hospital beds focussed on very ill patients or those requiring intensive care. Drive-through screening sites were built to allow potential patients to be tested with minimal contact. The use of PPE was a challenge both from a supply perspective and ensuring staff were familiar with the safe and effective use of PPE. The existing pilot telemedicine programmes were further developed and rolled out to include access for both citizens and expatriate residents. Pre-COVID, between 100 to 200 patients each month used this consultation service, during COVID 7500 patients per month were checked using this system.

This pandemic had a significant impact on healthcare staff. Learning to deliver care for entire shifts whilst encased in PPE, fear of catching the disease, seeing their colleagues die from the infection and working in unfamiliar clinical areas re-focussed the importance of following infection control policies and procedures for all staff.

Source: Based on Griffiths, J. 2020. Impact of COVID-19 on nursing. Compassion, clinical effectiveness and burnout. Essential strategies for nurse leadership. Dubai: Obix/Informa, p. 6.
The Lancet Rheumatology (2021). Too long to wait: The impact of COVID-19 on elective surgery (Editorial). *The Lancet Rheumatology, 3*(2), e83. https://doi.org/10.1016/S2665-9913(21)00001-1.

The fundamentals of infection

The spread of microbes is called transmission. Different pathogens have different modes of transmission. The main routes of transmission are 'touch', i.e., person-to-person contact, contaminated blood or body fluids (sexual intercourse, injecting drugs, needlestick injury), saliva (kissing), airborne (coughing, sneezing, droplets), foodborne (Salmonella, *E. coli* 157), waterborne (typhoid, cholera), insects (e.g., malaria) or fomites, i.e., non-living objects such as bedding or towels (fungi).

with many of these patients being healthcare professionals (Centers for Disease Control and Prevention, 2019). 'From April 2012 till August 2022, a total of

2591 laboratory-confirmed cases of Middle East respiratory syndrome (MERS) were reported globally, with 894 associated deaths at a case-fatality ratio (CFR) of 34.5%. Most of these cases were reported from Saudi Arabia, with 2184 cases and 813 related deaths (CFR: 37.2%)' (WHO, 2022b; WHO Eastern Mediterranean, 2022).

SPECIFIC INTERVENTIONS

Given the high risk of infectious diseases and the challenges of managing disparate factors such as hosts, migrating populations, vulnerabilities, war and famine, the Middle East has made considerable strides over the past 20 years in investing in fundamental infection control practices. This has included, but is not limited to, rigorous hand washing techniques and the wearing of personal protective equipment (PPE) (e.g., gowns, gloves, disposable N95 respirator, eye protection) by healthcare staff. Accredited infection control education programmes have included staff orientation, annual re-certification of infection control practices and various ad hoc training programmes, in addition to the implementation of 'bundles' in clinical areas such as Intensive Care as well as for patients with various arterial lines (Alothman et al., 2020).

Infections, whether acquired in hospitals or in the community, are a major public health problem internationally. The WHO estimates that 10 in every 100 patients in this region will acquire at least one healthcare-associated infection or hospital-acquired infection (HAI) in comparison with 7 out of every 100 in the Western world. HAIs significantly impact on the length of hospital stay, long-term disability and increased antimicrobial resistance.

Historically, community-acquired infections (CAIs) are known to have better outcomes, but the increase in antimicrobial resistance due to virulent strains of organisms remains a significant public health concern with the most common infections being urinary tract, pneumonias, skin and soft tissue, and gastrointestinal. The CAI results from WHO differ significantly from the outcomes from the European Union which range from 2.3% to 10.8% (depending on the country). The differences between European and Middle Eastern results may be from variations in healthcare systems, hospital

TABLE 9.5
Point Prevalence Study

Regional Countries

Egypt

Oman

Bahrain

Kingdom of Saudi Arabia

Kuwait

UAE

Lebanon

Based on Alothman, A., Al Thaqafi, A., Al Ansary, A., Zikri, A., Fayed, A., Khamis, F., et al. (2020). Prevalence of infections and antimicrobial use in the acute-care hospital setting in the Middle East: Results from the first point-prevalence survey in the region. *Int J Infect Dis, 101*, 249–258.

type/characteristics, seasons and the prevalence of diabetes in the Middle Eastern population. The European results also identified a lower use of antimicrobials. There is an emphasis in Europe of a controlled use of antimicrobials to reduce antimicrobial resistance. The Middle East commonly overuses antimicrobials as they are readily available 'over the counter' in pharmacies and there is a paucity of antimicrobial stewardship programmes in the region (Alothman et al., 2020). Refer to Chapter 14 for further details.

CAIs and HAIs are associated with significant morbidity and mortality. In 2018, a point prevalence study was conducted in seven Middle Eastern countries as outlined in Table 9.5.

The study was conducted by the Infection Control and Infectious Diseases teams of the local hospitals. On a nominated date, these teams reviewed all inpatients who were deemed to fit the criteria. Of those inpatients who were part of the study, the overall infection prevalence was 28.3%. The outcomes were broken down to HAIs of 11.2% and CAI of 16.98%. This meant that 11.2% of infected patients acquired their infection whilst in hospital, while 16.98% of those patients identified with an infection acquired it from the community. Of these, 98.2% of patients were receiving antimicrobial therapy with significant levels of resistance to the antimicrobials used. These findings of an increased use of antimicrobials represent a considerable public health threat (Alothman et al., 2020).

HAI transmission can be reduced/controlled by several basic methods which include hand hygiene, isolation precautions for infected or colonized patients and rigorous environmental cleaning (Talbot, 2012). Moreover, 50% of antibiotic usage in hospitals is deemed inappropriate. Accordingly, the international focus on antimicrobial stewardship programmes is designed to prevent overuse of antibiotics and reduce multiresistant organisms. HAIs and their associated costs can be markedly reduced by (1) identifying pathogens prior to prescribing, (b) reducing the use of broad-spectrum antibiotics and (c) prohibiting the use of antibiotics for viral or non-infectious diseases (Talbot, 2012).

These preventative measures are more likely to be successful in healthcare facilities that have the capability to undertake testing but are less likely to succeed in countries in conflict who struggle with refugees, stateless populations and minimal healthcare facilities. Thus, countries such as Yemen, Syria, Iraq and Palestine who have faced, and are potentially still facing years of hostilities with limited healthcare facilities, sanitation and starvation, are most at risk.

One of the methods used by several Middle Eastern countries to ensure quality, evidence-based healthcare practices is to engage external accreditation agencies to regularly survey healthcare facilities to ensure they comply with international standards. There are several different accreditation agencies used within the Middle East and although these companies are different, their methods and standards are similar. For example, education programmes must be in place for all staff with regular updates and reviews including use of PPE (Joint Commission International (JCI) 6th Edition, 2017).

Accrediting bodies place considerable weight on standards aimed at reducing, mitigating or eliminating risks of (transmitting or acquiring) infections amongst healthcare facilities staff, patients, workers, visitors or the community. These standards are expected to be implemented for all healthcare activities but will differ according to the clinical care provided, geographical locations and numbers of staff and patients with any corresponding infection control programme identifying the risks to the organization of any likely infection, community changes and global developments.

COVID-19 was obviously a specific and unexpected challenge to healthcare facilities that needed to be addressed quickly and effectively. Case study 9.2 outlines the specific challenges in a GCC country.

A number of risk management strategies need to be put into place to prevent infection including the management and isolation of patients suspected/confirmed of having a contagious disease. For example, negative pressure rooms need to be available for patients with airborne infections (JCI 6th Edition, 2017). Further, a plan is required for emergency preparedness to respond to any global communicable disease essentially because communicable diseases rapidly spread from one country to another with the ease of travel opportunities. Moreover, it is essential for staff to be educated in the early identification of potential infectious diseases and for all staff (including frontline clerical staff) to be familiar with signs and symptoms of these various diseases to reduce time to diagnosis, isolation and treatment (JCI 6th Edition, 2017).

It is also important that any data relating to infectious diseases is shared with global surveillance entities such as the World Health Organization. This sharing of international data acknowledges early identification of potential infectious diseases which then allows these diseases to be tracked, notified early and the required preparedness to manage an outbreak implemented in the relevant countries.

The fundamentals of infection

How do you protect yourself against infection? Think about how pathogens are spread or transmitted.

- Good hygiene: wash hands thoroughly before and after, cover your face when coughing, do not share personal items
- Good food hygiene: wash foods prior to preparation, wash hands before and after touching raw meat, store correctly, cook thoroughly
- Vaccinate: children, adults, travellers
- Travel precautions: insect precautions, e.g., DEET, use bottled water only, do not eat uncooked vegetables and only eat fruit you have peeled yourself
- Sexual transmission: safer sex should be practiced, so – no sex, sex only with your own partner or using barrier precautions
- Animal control: stay clear of wild animals, use pesticides, seal holes, keep areas clean and tidy

The following thinking grid is included for the reader to consider how their clinical practice will be impacted by working in this region.

THINKING GRID

- What infection control processes are the most critical in the Middle East?
  - Why?
  - How would you change staff perceptions to comply?
- Why are little known infectious diseases more common in the Middle East?
  - What would you need to do to identify these infectious diseases?
  - What would you need to do if your patient had one of these infectious diseases?

SUMMARY

COVID-19 has identified the need to streamline clinical information and data and to collaboratively provide healthcare globally during a health crisis. Knowledge and frontline care are evolving rapidly, and we need to be able to react and respond faster in the future. Public health has historically taken a backseat in health and the COVID-19 pandemic has demonstrated just how important protecting our populations from disease can be if health care data can be monitored and tracked. The role of contact tracing and use of evidence-based treatments are essential in providing not only care for patients suffering from infectious diseases but also understanding rapidly the risk of outbreaks.

The final 'take home point' of this chapter is about the need to protect yourself. There are fundamentals of infection and these have been outlined throughout this chapter. Be sensible and logical and apply universal precautions. Working in healthcare has always been a stressful and risky profession. It is essential you ensure you are protected against any infection you may encounter. Pay attention at the infection control education sessions, learn how to wear PPE correctly and focus on the signs and symptoms your patients display. Never be complacent as your life may depend on it.

REFERENCES

Alothman, A., Al Thaqafi, A., Al Ansary, A., Zikri, A., Fayed, A., Khamis, F., et al. (2020). Prevalence of infections and antimicrobial use in the acute-care hospital setting in the Middle East: Results from the first point-prevalence survey in the region. *International Journal of Infectious Diseases*, 101, 249–258.

Amnesty International. (2020). Qatar: Migrant Workers in Labour Camps. March 202.

Badur, S., Khalaf, M., Öztürk, S., Al-Raddadi, R., Amir, A., Farahat, F., et al. (2022). Meningococcal disease and immunization activities in Hajj and Umrah pilgrimage: A review. *Infectious Diseases and Therapy*, 11(4), 1343–1369.

Centers for Disease Control and Prevention. (2019). Middle East syndrome (MERS). Available at https://www.cdc.gov/coronavirus/mers.

Chang, B. P. (2022). The health care workforce under stress-Clinician heal thyself. *JAMA Netw Open*, 5(1), e2143167.

Department of Health. (2018). *Communicable Disease Bulletin*. Vol 9: Issue No. 3. Abu Dhabi.

Dolgin, R. (2021). Impact of COVID-19 on suicide rates. *PsyCom*, 14. May.

Emadi, M., Delvari, S., & Bavarti, M. (2021). Global socioeconomic inequality in the burden of communicable and non-communicable diseases and injuries: An analysis on global burden of disease study 2019. *BMC*, 1–7. September.

Greyling, T., Roussou, S., & Adhikari, T. (2021). The good, the bad, and the ugly of lockdown during COVID-19. *PLOS ONE, January*, 22.

Griffiths, P. (2002). Dubai Airport sees pre-pandemic monthly passenger volumes by end 2023. Reuters. August. p1.

Habibzadeh, F. (2012). Tuberculosis in the Middle East. Editors Page. *The Lancet*, Vol 38, December.

Joint Commission International. (2017). *Joint Commission International Standards for Hospitals 6th Edition*. July. Illinois. pp1-362.

Habous, M., Elimam, M., AlDabal, L., Chidambaran, B., & AlDeesi, Z. (2020). Pattern of primary tuberculosis drug resistance and associated risk factors at Dubai health authority in Dubai. *Int J Mycobacteriol*, 9(4), 391–396.

Ministry of Justice. (2020). *Federal Law No. 14 of 2014*. March 24. Abu Dhabi.

Michaud, C. (2009). Global burden of infectious diseases. *Encyclopedia of Microbiology*, 2009, 444–454.

National Center for Immunization and Respiratory Diseases. (2019). *Middle East Respiratory Syndrome (MERS)*. USA: Centre for Disease Control.

Talbot, T. (2012). Module one healthcare organisation infection prevention and control programs. Joint Commission Resources. *Illinois*, 1–53.

WHO (World Health Organization) (2022a). *Health Emergency Dashboard*. Available at https://extranet.who.int/publicemergency. Accessed 19 September 2023.

WHO. (2022b). *Middle East respiratory syndrome*. Regional Office for the Eastern Mediterranean. Available at https://www.emro.who.int/health-topics/mers-cov/mers-outbreaks.html. Accessed 6 October 2023.

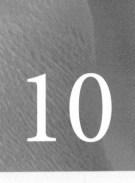

10

UPPER AND LOWER RESPIRATORY CONDITIONS

ORLA MERRIGAN

CHAPTER OUTLINE

INTRODUCTION

Geographically, the Middle East region is an area covered by large desert mass, with very hot and humid temperatures in the summer months and low temperatures in the winter. Multiple respiratory diseases are prevalent in the Middle East due to several factors, ranging from extreme weather conditions, environmental and social factors, to smoking and genetic conditions. Respiratory disease is an umbrella term for a variety of pathogenic conditions that affect the respiratory system. All of these respiratory diseases affect the lung's ability to function effectively, such as reducing its ability to absorb oxygen and release carbon dioxide. In addition to reduced lung function, respiratory disease can also affect the functioning of the heart. The Middle East region has seen a dramatic rise in obesity and smoking among the population which has resulted in increasing numbers of patients being diagnosed and treated with lung disease; this is creating an additional burden on the current medical system in the Gulf.

Respiratory disorders were listed as the fifth highest cause of death in Saudi Arabia in 2014, and more recently 57% of all deaths in Saudi Arabia were attributed to chronic lung disease, in particular asthma and interstitial lung disease (Lenze et al., 2020). However, Idrees et al. (2012) reported that respiratory disease in the Middle East region remains underdiagnosed and underestimated. The Ministry of Health in Saudi Arabia has recognised these concerns and has sought to address these through measures such as access to healthcare for lung disease and staff development (Saudi Vision 2030, 2016). In Saudi Arabia, the first guidelines for airway disease management have been established as an attempt to reduce the morbidity and mortality of patients with respiratory disorders in the region.

The challenge is a lack of respiratory care in the Middle East, and this is evidenced by Aldhahir et al. (2021) who reported on the lack of pulmonary rehabilitation programmes available in the Middle East, and also a lack of trained competent staff in the field of respiratory care. As a result of the unavailability of respiratory specialised services in the region to meet the growing number of patients with respiratory disease, the burden of respiratory disease in the Middle East is exacerbated. Other challenges to the management of respiratory conditions in the Middle East are factors such as cultural practices, religious beliefs, healthcare costs and failure to follow evidence-based standards (Alsubaiei et al., 2018). All these factors highlight the drive to develop effective strategies to address this healthcare burden.

BACKGROUND

Pathology in the Middle East

This chapter will discuss the spectrum of lung disease prevalent in the Middle East region. Lung diseases in the Middle East are a result of multiple factors which range from environmental, occupational exposure, exposure to warfare and social factors. The chapter will discuss the most common lung diseases in the Middle East and other lung diseases that are prevalent due to genetic conditions.

Environmental and Occupational

The Middle East is an area largely covered with desert, with changes in weather ranging between hot and humid in summer to cold temperatures in winter. Factors such as weather variances and dusty desert particles particularly exacerbate chronic lung disease in susceptible individuals, most predominantly patients with asthma. Additionally, allergens, low parental education, low birth weight, family history of asthma and cigarette smoking and house dust mites are all contributing factors and have all been attributed to the growing number of people in the region with asthma (Al-Kubaisy et al., 2005; Alsowaidi et al., 2010.). Sandstorms, which are common in the region, are known to cause sudden heavy exposure to dust and sand that precipitate pulmonary alveolar proteinosis and silicosis (Sattar et al., 2003). Both second-hand smoking and inhalation of fuel fumes are on the rise and are further contributing factor to lung diseases in the Middle East. Alsubaie et al. (2018) highlight that additional variables such as biomass fuel, dusts, gases and outdoor air pollution are also commonly contributing to the increased burden of chronic obstructive pulmonary disease (COPD) in Saudi Arabia and elsewhere in the Middle East.

Smoking

Multiple social factors contribute to respiratory disorders in the Middle East region. Tobacco use is very popular in all age groups in the region, with cheap tobacco available in shops. Unlike the rest of the world where tobacco and smoking are declining, unfortunately in the Middle East smoking and tobacco use is on the rise, particularly among teenagers and young adults. Smoking a water pipe, or shisha, is increasing globally. It is part of tradition and culture in the Middle East region; however, there are general misconceptions regarding the side effects and health effects of the pipes. Traditional values often lead to water pipe use in women and children (Al-Damegh et al., 2004). The research has indicated that smoking water pipes is linked to a variety of life-threatening conditions, including pulmonary disease, coronary heart disease and pregnancy-related complications (Maziak et al., 2004)

Several studies conducted in Saudi Arabia since the early 1930s reveal that smoking is on the rise, especially among men and women in their 20s (Al Ghobain et al., 2015; Al Moamary et al., 2012). A study in 2013 found that the overall prevalence of smoking was 12.2%, and men were more likely to smoke than women (21.5% vs. 1.1%) (Moradi-Lakeh et al., 2015). More recent statistics from the United Arab Emirates (UAE) National Health Survey (2017–2018) reported that 9.1% of adults currently smoke (15.7% of males, 2.4% of females) and that the average age of smoking commencement was 20.2 years. Among smokers of the age group 18–27, 43.6% were smoking e-cigarettes, while 14.5% smoked regular cigarettes, 12.6% smoked water pipes and 57.3% smoked medwakh. These statistics indicate the significant increase in the use of tobacco products, shisha and e-cigarettes. The increase in e-cigarette use or vaping is as a result of the belief among the younger Middle Eastern population that vaping is less harmful than traditional tobacco. A further interesting finding from this survey was the most common reason that these young people commenced vaping was because they were introduced to it either by a friend or family member who 'vaped' (Abbasi et al., 2022). It is important to note that e-cigarettes may also be a precursor for the use of regular cigarettes and other types of nicotine-containing products (Ibrahim et al., 2021). The fact that e-cigarettes have different flavours has also shown to be an important reason for the initiation of vaping among young adults (Glantz & Bareham, 2018).

Incense

Incense burning is a common practice and part of traditional social practice in the Middle East with it being burnt both in shopping malls and in homes; however, there has been documented cases in the Middle East where inhalation of these fumes can trigger an asthma attack (Al-Rawas et al., 2009).

Wars

The term 'Persian Gulf Syndrome' arose following the Gulf War in 1991. The combination of fine desert dust with released chemicals caused 'desert storm pneumonitis' (Taeger et al., 2008). Some authors suggest that that these symptoms are associated with the inhalation of depleted uranium dust which was frequently used during the Gulf War. However, back in 2011, research questioned whether long-term exposure to uranium can cause lung malignancy, noting that previous research on German uranium miners did identify a risk (Taeger et al., 2008).

Mass Gatherings

Mass gatherings are also a common practice in the Middle Eastern region, and this can range from either family gatherings to religious weekly gatherings at the mosque for Friday prayer or the annual Haj which attracts millions of visitors to do this annual pilgrimage. Large increased numbers of tuberculosis infections have been linked to Haj visits due to overcrowding and unsanitary practices (Wilder-Smith et al., 2005). During Haj, tuberculosis was reported as the most common presenting cause of pneumonia that required hospital admissions (Alzeer et al., 1998).

Immigrants and Labour Camps

There is a large diverse population in Middle Eastern countries, with many people choosing to migrate to work in the region for financial reasons. Many of these immigrants travel from countries with high rates of multidrug-resistant tuberculosis and very low rates of immunisation and vaccinations, such as the Indian subcontinent, South East Asia, Africa and Russia (Chemtob et al., 2002; Farnia et al., 2006). The large working migrant population tends to live in substantial labour camps in very close proximity in the Middle East, thus becoming a breeding ground for infectious diseases, particularly respiratory in origin. However, it is very difficult to acquire any recent statistics that capture the figures on this.

Infections

Community-acquired pneumonia (CAP) has increased over the years in the Middle East region, with the mortality rate for CAP at 13% (Al-Muhairi et al., 2006). Similarly, methicillin-resistant pneumococcal pneumonia (MRSA) is highly prevalent in the regional hospitals causing severe mortality and morbidity. Two problems with medications have been widely observed in the Middle East. First, non-compliance with medication is commonly seen with patients in the Middle East, with a large proportion of patients who either fail to take their medication or stop medication prematurely (Erdem et al., 2008). Reportedly, drug resistance is twice as high in Middle Eastern patients who have in the past received antituberculous therapy (Walsh et al., 2019). Second, there is the problem of the overuse of antibiotics which occurred due to the easy availability of antibiotics which, up until recently, could be purchased over the counter without a prescription in the Middle East. However, due to multiresistance to antibiotic treatment, some countries like Bahrain have stopped this practice, and now a medical prescription is necessary to acquire antibiotics from a pharmacy. See Case Study 10.1 outlining a migrant worker with CAP.

Chronic Disease

Chronic respiratory disorders are chronic diseases that affect the airways and other areas of the lungs. The most common chronic respiratory disorders include asthma, lung cancer, COPD and emphysema. It is estimated that approximately 40 million individuals suffer from respiratory disease in the Middle East region, and the most common ones are COPD, emphysema, asthma and lung malignancies. Certain genetic factors within the Middle Eastern population contribute to respiratory conditions such as sickle cell disease (SCD), cystic fibrosis (CF) and sleep disorders linked to obesity.

COPD is an umbrella term for a variety of respiratory diseases which cause breathlessness, and it can develop over many years in the absence of any symptoms; therefore it can remain undetected for a long period of time. Emphysema is a debilitating form of respiratory disease, which is another form of COPD. Emphysema is mainly caused by smoking and presents as difficulty is expelling air from the lungs. There is no cure for this disease, however quitting smoking, shisha and vaping can help to slow its progression. Asthma is another very common respiratory condition that is caused by inflammation of the airways causing difficulty in breathing. Triggers for asthma attacks are infections, pollutions and allergic reactions, and symptoms of an attack include wheezing, dry cough, shortness of breath and chest tightness (Case Study 10.2). Unfortunately, in the Middle East,

CASE STUDY 10.1
COMMUNITY-ACQUIRED PNEUMONIA (CAP)

A middle-aged expatriate lady from the UK, non-smoker, reasonably fit and well, except for medications for hypertension. Several weeks ago, she fell and broke her fifth metatarsal and was largely immobile, causing her to spend long periods on the sofa, lying in a recumbent position, watching television and reading. Within 7–10 days post fracture, she started experiencing symptoms of cough, some mild pleuritic pain and feeling generally unwell, with no fever. She elected to see a family medicine practitioner who did not exam her at all (as is often the case due to cultural mores) but prescribed her a course of antibiotics, which she duly completed. However, she remained unwell and her cough worsened as did her pleuritic chest pain. She presented at the local hospital and was fully examined and had a chest x-ray (CXR). Her diagnosis was CAP with pleural effusion and atelectasis. She was prescribed a further, more appropriate course of antibiotics and duly completed these, and eventually recovered. She was aware of several colleagues who were much younger and fitter than she was, but who had been hospitalised and treated with nebulizers, intravenous antibiotics and oxygen therapy due to CAP.

KEY ASPECTS
- The symptoms of CAP are not always obvious and can be slow and insidious
- CAPs can affect all ages, sex and people with no pre-existing conditions
- CAPs are often most prevalent in case of season change or dust storms when pathogens are inhaled via sand vectors
- Early recognition of symptoms prevents hospitalisation and reduces the need for aggressive intervention
- People with underlying conditions such as SCD, asthma and COPD are at greatest risk

CASE STUDY 10.2
ASTHMA

Mohammed was a 23-year-old migrant worker living in sub-optimal, close-quarter living conditions which were shared by fellow workers. Mohammed worked in construction and was used to working outside in dusty conditions for 12 hours a day. He had no previous ill health of note and was the main earner for his extended family back in Bangladesh. He knew he was unwell but continued to work as he was concerned about losing his employment. He collapsed whilst at work and was rushed to ED. He was fully examined and had a full blood work-up plus CXR. He was noted to have a low peak flow rate and was diagnosed asthmatic. This diagnosis had implications for his future employment.

KEY ASPECTS
- Migrant workers are at greatest risk of ill health and are less likely to present early and access health services due to cost and long working hours
- In most scenarios, migrant workers tend to cover their nose and mouth with a scarf, but these are often unchanged for long periods of time and can harbour microorganisms
- When the season changes and there are sandstorms, people who work in dusty conditions often experience excess wax and nasal and aural congestion. It is advised to use seawater (or saline) to flush the nose to prevent accumulation. Failure to do so can result in pathogens reproducing and causing upper respiratory tract infections which can then develop further into lower respiratory tract infections
- Migrant workers, especially in the hotter months, may not attend to self-care or eat nutritious meals and properly hydrate during the day. Consequently, they may be somewhat immunocompromised
- Migrant workers may suffer from a failure to articulate their concerns appropriately due to language barriers
- Healthcare workers should recognize that migrant workers are economic migrants and may be less inclined to follow healthcare advice that may compromise their employment. Healthcare workers should ensure they communicate effectively about compliance with therapies, especially antibiotics

asthma care varies from country to country; Alqathani et al. (2022) suggest that access to asthma care is variable in the region from one country to another and does not guarantee a good outcome. Chronic bronchitis is another type of COPD which presents as a chronic cough. The main feature of chronic bronchitis is that people tend to cough up large amounts of sputum, particularly in the mornings. Episodes of acute bronchitis are an infectious problem treated with antibiotics.

Lung Malignancies
Lung cancer can develop in any part of the lungs, therefore making it difficult to detect. It primarily develops in the main area of the lungs, which presents as tumours that interfere with normal lung function. Symptoms such as chronic coughing, coughing up blood, changes in voice and harsh breathing sounds may go unnoticed for many years. Lung cancer is the most common listed form of cancer in the Middle East and is ranked first of all malignancies in male and second among Bahraini females (Alsubaiei et al., 2018).

Unfortunately, it has been reported that the incidence of lung cancer is steadily rising and both cigarette smoking and shisha are the main risk factors for this condition (Aldhahir et al., 2021).

Cystic Fibrosis

The number of patients diagnosed with CF in the Middle East region has been growing since 2010, with new mutations for this pathology being identified. Most recent data from the Middle East region purport that the incidence of CF in the Middle East varies according to the ethnic background and the degree of consanguinity. The expected rates of CF in these Middle Eastern countries range from 1 in 2560 to 1 in 15,876 (Ahmed et al., 2020). Management of CF has greatly improved over the last few years, particularly in areas of life longevity and survival rate. The most important factors that contribute to prolonged life span are dependent on early diagnosis, understanding and treatment of the disease and being under the care of a respiratory multidisciplinary team (Bell et al., 2020). In the United States and Europe, CF is diagnosed before 6 months of age in comparison with the Middle East where it is diagnosed at 18–24 months (Mackenzie et al., 2014). International evidence for best practice (Proesmans, 2017) advocates care for CF to include prenatal diagnosis, genetic counselling and future screening. Patients with CF face barriers to treatment options such as lung transplantation which is not widely available in the Middle East.

Prevalence of Sickle Cell Disease Contributing to Respiratory Conditions

The Middle East has had one of the highest consanguinity rates in the world (Akbayram et al., 2009), with high rates of both SCD and thalassemia having a significant impact on lung health. SCD is particularly common in the Middle East population, with an incidence of ~1:200 births (Seaton, 2008). Patients with SCD are at high risk of sickle cell crisis secondary to hypoxic conditions resulting in respiratory and organ infarction. It has been highlighted that the risk of hypoxia in patients with SCD in the Middle East is high due to the large numbers of immigrant population who frequently travel by air (Waness et al., 2011). These patients are at very high risk of recurrent chest infections, pulmonary infarcts and pulmonary embolism during pregnancy. Al Bukar et al. (2019) cited that 79% of SCD hospital admissions developed sickle

cell chronic lung disease and acute respiratory complications. Treatment for SCD consists of pain management, antibiotic care, maintaining adequate oxygenation, blood transfusion, exchange transfusion and respiratory support and sometimes invasive mechanical ventilation in acute cases. Chronic lung disease occurs with SCD and presents on chest x-ray as interstitial abnormalities or impaired pulmonary function testing, and in many SCD case presentations both restrictive and obstructive patterns have been found (Waness et al., 2011). In its most severe form, SCD can manifest in the form of pulmonary hypertension. It is difficult to identify the number of respiratory causes of death with SCD in the Gulf region as religious and cultural practice demand people are buried before the next prayer and postmortems ascertaining the cause of death are rarely undertaken.

Sleep Disorders Linked to Obesity

Sleep disorders have become a new area of medical specialty in the Middle East region since 1990s, secondary to the increasing rise in obesity in the region (Waness et al., 2011). There is a need to increase services in this field, in areas such as clinical services, patient education, training of staff and hospital administration services. Unfortunately, there appears to be a lack of knowledge and awareness relating to sleep disorders in the Middle East region. This is evidenced by results of a survey of primary healthcare physician's in Riyadh which reported that 43% of primary care physicians did not know of the existence of sleep medicine as a specialty, 40% felt that sleep disorders were not common and 38% did not know of to whom they should refer their patients (Al-Rasheedi et al., 2022). This was the first study to assess the prevalence of sleep apnoea (SA) using the validated Berlin questionnaire among any Arab population, indicating that SA was predominant in females (39%) compared with males (33%) in Saudi Arabia. This rate appears higher in females from Saudi Arabia than in those from other Middle Eastern countries. The high SA statistic for females can possibly be directly attributed to the high prevalence of obesity in the female population of Saudi Arabia, with 50% of females in Saudi between 40 and 49 years having a body mass index over $30\,kg/m^2$ (Al-Nozha et al., 2005). Further data from the regions reported the polysomnography per capita rate of only 7.1 per 100,000 people per year, in comparison with 18–427 in developed countries (BaHammam & Aljafen, 2007). This study did highlight the lack of staff such as trained sleep technicians and a lack of facilities such as beds and sleep labs. Lack of staff and resources was a major obstacle for the establishment of a sleep medicine service in 80% of the surveyed hospitals. In the past, there was a limited number of beds designated for sleep studies per 10,000 people in Saudi Arabia at 0.06 beds, significantly lower than statistics (0.3–1.5) designated per population in developed countries.

Treatment for SA is usually the use of non-invasive mechanical continuous positive airway (CPAP) or bi-level positive airway pressure (BIPAP) ventilators to facilitate breathing at night.

MERS and COVID-19

Middle East Respiratory Syndrome (MERS) is a viral respiratory condition which was first identified in Saudi Arabia in 2012, and the Middle East accounted for 87% cases of MERS, with a high mortality rate of 35%. Presenting symptoms of MERS were cough, fever and shortness of breath with some patients proceeding to acquire pneumonia and require mechanical ventilation. Transmission of MERS occurred in healthcare facilities and from patient to patient in the clinical area. Treatment for MERS comprised intravenous fluid therapy and oxygenation therapy. In 2020, there was an outbreak of the worldwide pandemic caused by the COVID-19 virus, once again causing high mortality rates globally due to respiratory failure. However, because of the rapid strategic response in the Middle East, with a combination of early national lockdowns and rapid rollout of COVID vaccination programmes, the mortality rates were low in the Middle East in comparison with worldwide statistics.

HISTORY TAKING AND ASSESSMENT

Due to the complexity of respiratory diseases in the Middle East, a full medical assessment must include a genetic history and diagnosis of patients via a variety of respiratory related tests such as arterial blood gases, chest x-rays, lung function testing and pulse oximetry.

TREATMENT AND CARE

Treatment depends on the type of respiratory disease. If a person is a smoker or exposed to secondhand smoke,

the solution is to quit smoking. This can successfully be achieved with smoking cessation programmes and prescribed medication to aid smoking cessation such as Champix or Zyban. If an individual is exposed to air pollutants or triggering substances, wearing a filtered mask approved by workplace health and safety regulation is advisable. Other treatments include deep breathing exercises, spirometry, nebulizers to clear airways and gentle exercise to promote gaseous exchange.

The physician or respiratory nurse can devise a pulmonary rehabilitation programme which is individualised based on the severity and type of illness. Medications can be administered to treat respiratory symptoms such as coughing, wheezing, infection and high blood pressure. Supplemental oxygen may be required for some patients following testing to assess this need. Regular exercise can help with a variety of lung conditions; and it has been proven that regular exercise, such as walking, improves lung function in patients with chronic obstructive disease (Demeyer et al., 2016).

BIPAP and CPAP

Some patients require some assistance with respiratory function with non-invasive treatment. Both BiPAP and CPAP are treatments used to improve respiratory function. However, if the patient is unable to tolerate these non-invasive treatments, mechanical invasive ventilation is required.

Palliative Care for Respiratory Patients

A new area for patients with chronic respiratory condition is end-of-life care for their condition. Palliative care is a new concept in the Middle East and requires further development. At present there are minimal palliative care or hospice facilities across the Middle East, and end-of-life care is in its infancy. There is a great need for advanced nurse practitioners in respiratory care to manage the care for this patient group.

SUMMARY AND TAKEAWAY POINTS

From a Middle Eastern perspective when it comes to respiratory disease, the following key points are worth noting:

- Respiratory disorders are a major cause of death in the Middle East, with chronic lung disease such as asthma and interstitial lung disease being reported. It is estimated that approximately 40 million individuals are suffering from respiratory disease in the Middle East region. However, it remains underdiagnosed and underestimated, and therefore may be a much larger health problem than reported.

■ There is a general lack of respiratory care in the Middle East, as well as a lack of pulmonary rehabilitation programmes and associated trained competent staff in the field of respiratory care.

■ The management of respiratory conditions in the Middle East may be affected by factors such as cultural practices, religious beliefs, healthcare costs and failure to follow evidence-based standards.

■ Unlike the rest of the world where tobacco and smoking rates are declining, smoking, tobacco use and vaping are on the rise in the Middle East, particularly among teenagers and young adults.

■ The large working migrant population tends to live in large labour camps in the Middle East, therefore becoming a breeding ground for infectious diseases, particularly those which are respiratory in origin (i.e., tuberculosis).

■ CAP has increased over the years in the Middle East region, with the mortality rate for CAP at 13%. Similarly, MRSA is highly prevalent in the regional hospitals, causing severe mortality and morbidity.

■ The numbers of patients diagnosed with CF in the Middle East region has been increasing over the last 10–15 years, with new mutations for this pathology being identified.

■ The Middle East has one of the highest consanguinity rates in the world, with high rates of both SCD and thalassemia having a significant impact on lung health.

■ Governments and Health Departments across the Middle East are aware of the burden of disease attributed to respiratory infections and chronic lung disorders and have plans in place to reduce their rates.

Respiratory problems and needs in the Middle East are complex and very specific to the region and population and they are rising across a variety of lung disorders. This can be partly attributed to ongoing environmental issues in the region, smoking, a rise in obesity and sedentary lifestyle and the increasing immigrant population. In addition to the rise in obesity in the region and the high numbers of the population who smoke tobacco and shisha and the increased number of vaping, this will place additional pressure on the medical services within the region.

A strong focused public awareness campaign is required to address these concerns, and a strategic approach from health authorities is required across the region to address the challenges from these environmental and cultural issues in order to implement a robust plan for effective management. Investment in respiratory care, smoking cessation and laws on smoking in public areas (which have successfully worked around the world) to reduce smoking are warranted. The introduction of the concept of palliative care in both medical education programmes and in clinical areas is required and explored further in Chapter 16. To address the rising incidence of respiratory illness across the region, there needs to be an increase in the numbers of medical and nursing specialists trained in this field, an increase in diagnostics such as sleep labs and the availability of accessible sleep lab beds in line with best practice recommendations per population.

REFERENCES

Abbasi, Y., Van Hout, M., Faragalla, C., & Itani, L. (2022). Knowledge and use of electronic cigarettes in young adults in the United Arab Emirates, particularly during the COVID-19 pandemic. *International Journal of Environmental Research and Public Health, 19*(13).

Ahmed, S., Cheok, G., N Goh, A. E., Han, A., Hong, S. J., Indawati, W., Lutful Kabir, A., Kabra, S. K., et al. (2020). Cystic fibrosis in Asia. *Pediatric Respirology and Critical Care Medicine, 4*, 8–12.

Akbayram, S., Sari, N., Akgun, C., et al. (2009). The frequency of consanguineous marriage in eastern Turkey. *Genetic Counseling, 20*, 207–214.

Al-Damegh, S. A., Saleh, M. A., Al-Alfi, M. A., et al. (2004). Cigarette smoking behaviour among male secondary school students in the Central region of Saudi Arabia. *Saudi Medical Journal, 25*, 215–219.

Aldhahir, A. M., Alghamdi, S. M., Alqahtani, J. S., Alqahtani, K. A., Al Rajah, A. M., Alkhathlan, B. S., et al. (2021). Pulmonary rehabilitation for COPD: A narrative review and call for further implementation in Saudi Arabia. *Annals of Thoracic Medicine, 16*(4), 299–305.

Al Ghobain, M., Alhamad, E. H., Alorainy, H. S., Al Kassimi, F., Lababidi, H., & Al-Hajjaj, M. S. (2015). The prevalence of chronic obstructive pulmonary disease in Riyadh, Saudi Arabia: A BOLD study. *The International Journal of Tuberculosis and Lung Disease, 19*(10), 1252–1257.

Al-Kubaisy, W., Ali, S. H., & Al-Thamiri, D. (2005). Risk factors for asthma among primary school children in Baghdad, Iraq. *Saudi Medical Journal, 26*, 460–466.

Al Moamary, M. S., Al Ghobain, M. O., Al Shehri, S. N., Gasmelseed, A. Y., & Al-Hajjaj, M. S. (2012). Predicting tobacco use among high school students by using the global youth tobacco survey in Riyadh, Saudi Arabia. *Annals of Thoracic Medicine, 7*(3), 122–129. https://doi.org/10.4103/1817-1737.98843.

Al-Muhairi, S., Zoubeidi, T., Ellis, M., et al. (2006). Demographics and microbiological profile of pneumonia in United Arab Emirates. *Monaldi Archives for Chest Disease, 65*, 13–18.

Al-Nozha, M. M., Al-Mazrou, Y. Y., Al-Maatouq, M. A., et al. (2005). Obesity in Saudi Arabia. *Saudi Medical Journal, 26*, 824–829.

Alqathani, M., Pavela, G., Lein, D. L., Vilcassim, R., & Hendricks, P. S. (2022). The influence of mental health and respiratory symptoms on the association between chronic lung disease and e-cigarette use in adults in the United States. *Respiratory Care, 67*(7), 814–822.

Al-Rasheedi, A. N., Thirunavukkarasu, A., Almutairi, A., Alruwaili, S., Alotaibi, H., Alzaid, W., et al. (2022). Knowledge and attitude towards obstructive sleep apnea among primary care physicians in northern regions of Saudi Arabia: A multicenter study. *Healthcare (Basel), 10*(12), 2369.

Al-Rawas, O. A., Al-Maniri, A. A., & Al-Riyami, B. M. (2009). Home exposure to Arabian incense (bakhour) and asthma symptoms in children: A community survey in two regions in Oman. *BMC Pulmonary Medicine, 9*, 23.

Alsowaidi, S., Abdulle, A., & Bernsen, R. (2010). Prevalence and risk factors of asthma among adolescents and their parents in Al-Ain. *Respiration, 79*, 105–111.

Alsubaiei, M. E., Cafarella, P. A., Frith, P. A., McEvoy, R. D., & Effing, T. W. (2018). Factors influencing management of chronic respiratory diseases in general and chronic obstructive pulmonary disease in particular in Saudi Arabia: An overview. *Annals of Thoracic Medicine, 13*(3), 144–149.

Alzeer, A., Mashlah, A., Fakim, N., et al. (1998). Tuberculosis is the commonest cause of pneumonia requiring hospitalization during Hajj (pilgrimage to Makkah). *The Journal of Infection, 36*, 303–306.

BaHammam, A. S., & Aljafen, B. (2007). Sleep medicine service in Saudi Arabia. A quantitative assessment. *Saudi Medical Journal, 28*, 917–921.

Bell, S. C., Mall, M. A., Gutierrez, H., Macek, M., Madge, S., Davies, J. C., et al. (2020). The future of cystic fibrosis care: A global perspective. *The Lancet Respiratory Medicine, 8*, 65–124.

Bukar, A. A., Sulaiman, M. M., Ladu, A., Abba, A. M., Ahmed, M. K., Marama, G. T., et al. (2019). Chronic kidney disease amongst sickle cell anaemia patients at the University of Maiduguri Teaching Hospital, Northeastern Nigeria: A study of prevalence and risk factors. *The Mediterranean Journal of Hematology and Infectious Diseases, 11*(1), e2019010. https://doi.org/10.4084/MJHID.2019.010.

Chemtob, D., Leventhal, A., & Weiler-Ravell, D. (2002). Tuberculosis in Israel—Main epidemiological aspects. *Harefuah, 141* 226–232, 316.

Demeyer, H., Donaire-Gonzalez, D., Pons, I. S., Anto, J. M., & Garcia-Aymerich, J. (2016). The importance of being physically active on functional decline in patients with COPD. *European Respiratory Journal, 48*, OA1522. https://doi.org/10.1183/13993003.congress-2016.OA1522.

Erdem, I., Ozgultekin, A., Sengoz Inan, A., et al. (2008). Incidence, etiology, and antibiotic resistance patterns of gram-negative microorganisms isolated from patients with ventilator-associated pneumonia in a medical-surgical intensive care unit of a teaching hospital in Istanbul, Turkey (2004–2006). *Japanese Journal of Infectious Diseases, 61*, 339–342.

Farnia, P., Masjedi, M. R., Mirsaeidi, M., et al. (2006). Prevalence of Haarlem I and Beijing types of *Mycobacterium tuberculosis* strains in Iranian and Afghan MDR-TB patients. *The Journal of Infection, 53*, 331–336.

Glantz, S. A., & Bareham, D. W. (2018). E-cigarettes: Use, effects on smoking, risks, and policy implications. *Annual Review of Public Health, 39*, 215–235.

Ibrahim, S., Habiballah, M., Sayed, I. E. (2021). Efficacy of electronic cigarettes for smoking cessation: A systematic review and meta-analysis. *American Journal of Health Promotion : AJHP, 35*, 442–455.

Idrees, M., Koniski, M. L., Taright, S., Shahrour, N., Polatli, M., Ben Kheder, A., et al. (2012). Management of chronic obstructive pulmonary disease in the Middle East and North Africa: Results of the BREATHE study. *Respiratory Medicine, 106*(Suppl 2), S33–S44.

Lenze, E. J., Mattar, C., Zorumski, C. F., et al. (2020). Fluvoxamine vs placebo and clinical deterioration in outpatients with symptomatic COVID-19: A randomized clinical trial. *The Journal of the American Medical Association, 324*(22), 2292–2300.

MacKenzie, T., Gifford, A. H., Sabadosa, K. A., Quinton, H. B., Knapp, E. A., Goss, C. H., et al. (2014). Longevity of patients with cystic fibrosis in 2000 to 2010 and beyond: Survival analysis of the Cystic Fibrosis Foundation patient registry. *Annals of Internal Medicine, 161*, 233–241.

Maziak, W., Ward, K. D., Afifi Soweid, R. A., et al. (2004). Tobacco smoking using a water pipe: A re-emerging strain in a global epidemic. *Tobacco Control, 13*, 327–333.

Moradi-Lakeh, M., El Bcheraoui, C., Tuffaha, M., Daoud, F., Al Saeedi, M., Basulaiman, M., et al. (2015). Tobacco consumption in the Kingdom of Saudi Arabia, 2013: Findings from a national survey. *BMC Public Health, 15*, 611.

Proesmans, M. (2017). Best practices in the treatment of early cystic fibrosis lung disease. *Therapeutic Advances in Respiratory Disease, 11*(2), 97–104. Feb.

Sattar, H. A., Mobayed, H., al-Mohammed, A. A., et al. (2003). The pattern of indoor and outdoor respiratory allergens in asthmatic adult patients in a humid and desert newly developed country. *European Annals of Allergy and Clinical Immunology, 35*, 300–305.

Saudi Vision 2030. (2016). Available at https://www.vision2030.gov.sa/media/rc0b5oy1/saudi_vision203.pdf. Accessed 29 September 2023.

Seaton, A. (2008). Pulmonary manifestations of systemic disease (5th ed., pp. 1380–1403). In A. Seaton, D. Seaton, & A. G. Leitch (Eds.),

Crofton and Douglous' Respiratory Diseases (Vol. 2, pp. 1380–1403). Oxford: Blackwell Science Ltd.

Taeger, D., Krahn, U., Wiethege, T., et al. (2008). A study on lung cancer mortality related to radon, quartz, and arsenic exposures in German uranium miners. *Journal of Toxicology and Environmental Health, Part A, 71*, 859–865.

UAE National Health Survey Report 2017–2018. United Arab Emirates Ministry of Health and Prevention. (2018). Available at https://cdn.who.int/media/docs/default-source/ncds/ncd-surveillance/data-reporting/united-arab-emirates/uaenational-health-survey-report-2017-2018.pdf?sfvrsn=86b8b1d9_1&download=true.

Walsh, K. F., Souroutzidis, A., Vilbrun, S. C., Peeples, M., Joissaint, G., Delva, S., et al. (2019). Potentially high number of ineffective drugs with the standard shorter course regimen for multidrug-resistant tuberculosis treatment in Haiti. *The American Journal of Tropical Medicine and Hygiene, 100*(2), 392–398.

Waness, A., El-Sameed, Y. A., Mahboub, B., Noshi, M., Al-Jahadali, H., Vats, M., & Mehta, A. C. (2011). Respiratory disorders in the Middle East: A review. *Respirology, 16*(5), 755–766.

Wilder-Smith, A., Foo, W., Earnest, A., et al. (2005). High risk of *Mycobacterium tuberculosis* infection during the Hajj pilgrimage. *Tropical Medicine and International Health, 10*, 336–339.

11

COMMUNICATION AND CARING IN CULTURALLY DIVERSE SETTINGS

MAY MCCREADDIE ■ SANDRA GOODWIN ■ CATHERINE ABOU'ZAID

INTRODUCTION: COMMUNICATION, CARE AND DIVERSITY

This chapter reviews four key aspects relevant to all the chapters presented within this text: communication, caring, diversity and cultural competency. The first two aspects—communication and caring—are fundamental to modern healthcare and are longstanding tenets of safe, effective, quality care. However, the remaining two speak to an evolving world where people have, arguably, become more enlightened about the complexities of the human race: learning to embrace peoples' differences, that is, diversity, and hopefully being able to do so effectively, that is, being culturally competent. Unfortunately, the art of communication is often somewhat dismissed as a given, even in the more 'mundane' and fundamen-

tal aspects of healthcare which make-up over 80% of all healthcare provision (e.g. taking blood pressure or venesection). Such 'tasks' may be routine (e.g. short, repetitive; a sequence of actions regularly taken: Lillrank, 2002) but they are also more likely to become problematic interactions (and/or complaints: McCreaddie & Benwell, 2021, 2018) simply because the participants have failed to attend to the basics of human interaction such as building rapport or active listening.

For example, communication can be key to ensuring patients understand instructions, guidance and advice, from how to take daily medications to following general postoperative instructions—both examples being potentially routine and presumably, therefore, relatively nonproblematic (Benwell & McCreaddie,

2016). Yet both the aforementioned scenarios are in themselves, vibrant, complex and potentially challenging. Healthcare workers—whether breaking bad news or providing relatively simple instructions—need to be able to communicate effectively with the relevant protagonists while being mindful of the context, the prior experiences (of both parties) and the visceral emotions that may be evident.

From the outset, therefore, we think it is best to consider 'communication' as being performative: something to be accomplished and not just delivered. Communication is a nuanced art full of subtle little rules; it is not just about *what* is being said, it is about *how* it is being said, to *whom*, *where* in the conversation and to *what* end? It is therefore not a passive traditional act involving one person 'informing' the other (Hargie, 2019). It is much more complex than that. As such, communication is dynamic, complex and situated—no matter how routine or otherwise.

COMMUNICATION PER SE

Have you ever interviewed someone for a job—especially a healthcare post or even an applicant for nursing or medical training—and the applicant invariably presents themselves as having 'good' or even 'excellent' communication as part of their curriculum vitae? It is customary, if not de rigeur, to claim to be a competent if not highly effective communicator, especially in a service industry such as healthcare. You cannot work with people—especially sick, vulnerable and potentially cognitively impaired people—and not be an excellent communicator. Yet, unfortunately, many students and staff simply lack self-awareness with regard to their attitudes, knowledge, abilities, assumptions and skills (Gude et al., 2017). If you do not understand yourself, then you are extremely unlikely to be able to listen to and understand others, their perceptions and their frames of reference.

Take a look at Box 11.1, outlining examples of healthcare communication. New students or staff members tend to look at these examples and then slowly turn a lighter shade of pale. Suddenly, their 'excellent' communication skills slowly fade away, back to being just ink on the page.

THINKING GRID

- What would *you* do? What exactly would you say?
- How would *you* manage the myriad challenges evident in each scenario?
- What aspects are *common* to all scenarios?
- How do you think you would *feel* in each scenario as the healthcare worker?
- And how might this *impact* your subsequent 'communication'?
- Are you experienced or skilled enough to be able to manage all of the above successfully?
- And how would you know if you had communicated effectively?

BOX 11.1

Examples of Healthcare 'Communication'

- You walk into a patient's room, and they ask you, 'does this cancer thing mean I'm going to die?'
- A son is angry that his elderly Indian mother has fallen in your unit. He berates you in front of staff and visitors.
- A fellow healthcare worker—a local member of staff—has asked you to take over their workload for the remainder of the shift, as well as your own. You are really busy and it is your first day in the unit.
- An Arab women's husband has just had a severe psychotic episode and she is extremely upset and inconsolable.
- A daughter is struggling to care for her mother who has dementia at home; you are asked to speak to her about considering long-term care as an option.
- A grandmother has just learned that her 10-year old grandson, her only grandchild, has died playing 'chicken' on the road. You are asked to 'comfort' her.

Carefully review each scenario and consider how you would respond. Use the 'thinking grid' shown earlier to help guide your responses.

Note: 'Chicken' is a dangerous 'game' played by children who run out in front of cars as a dare.

Learning to interact effectively with patients and their relatives, as well as with your peers, is not something that can be learned in days, weeks or months. It takes years. Years of practice, experience, development and reflection—and even then, you still make mistakes.

THE ARABIAN GULF AND GREATER MIDDLE EAST

The Arabian Gulf and Greater Middle East is a veritable mosaic of ethnicities, religions and cultures. Neither the patient cohorts nor the healthcare teams are homogenous—they come from across the globe. Consequently, various languages are spoken, with different local nuances or dialects, based upon ethnicities, cultural attitudes, values and beliefs and all this in the acute and emotive setting of healthcare where life-changing situations may prevail.

More than two out of three migrant workers are concentrated in high-income countries with the Arab States currently hosting an incredible 24 million migrant workers (ILO, 2021). The majority of these migrant workers come from developing countries with high unemployment rates such as Asia and Africa—increasingly from East Africa— and are sent abroad to earn remittances to provide for families at home. In turn, the Arab states, specifically the Gulf Cooperation Council (GCC), are largely reliant upon non-nationals (average of 70.4%) to provide a variety of labours, for example, care and construction work—with over 124 billion USD earned or remitted abroad in 2017 (IOM, 2020). The healthcare working environment in the Arabian Gulf and Greater Middle East is probably the most diverse, challenging and evolving in the world. It is also a fantastic place to live, work and *learn*.

HIGH CONTEXT AND LOW CONTEXT ASPECTS OF COMMUNICATION

Communication involves numerous diverse elements including healthcare literacy, attitudes, emotions, listening, rapport, verbals, nonverbals, cultural competency, language, etc.—the list is not exhaustive (Hargie, 2019; Littlejohn & Foss, 2009). All of these aspects need to be 'read' and appropriately responded to. Yet, many of these aspects are culture-specific.

It would underplay the nuances of communication to suggest that cultures are either considered high context or low context, rather a spectrum exists and nations and ethnicities vary accordingly. A seminal text in this area is that of Edward T. Hall (1959), an anthropologist who outlined cultural distinctions such as 'proxemics' (the notion of personal space for 'comfort' in different cultures) and high culture and low culture contexts. In short, a low-context culture (e.g. UK, Australia, Scandinavia, Dutch, German) is a 'direct' communication context, decoding the content or words and acting on the pragmatics and/ or facts of what is being said with a preference for quick, fast-paced communication and larger personal space. Conversely, a high-context culture (Japanese, Korean, Middle Eastern, Russian) is more indirect and places greater bearing on nonverbals or other associated aspects, emphasising relational aspects and groups or tribal/family, embracing shorter personal space, as well as being prepared to take much longer to conclude the discussion.

Low culture contexts focus on words and meaning whereas high context cultures tend towards gestures. While temporality (time) is a commodity in Western or low context cultures, in high context cultures it is simply perceived as a natural process that belongs to others. Thus where family discussions are required about important issues then these may take some considerable time as it is important to include all (Mobeireek et al., 2008). Moreover, given the focus on the relational aspects, for example, family and tribe, in high context cultures, there is a greater propensity for offence. Conversely, in low context 'individual' cultures, disagreement is viewed as just that—a different viewpoint—rather than a focus for discord.

The above factors have been broadly summarised in Table 11.1, but it would be wrong to 'stereotype' races on that basis, rather these aspects hark back to how tribes and peoples have emerged and survived through centuries. For example, through building complex tribal networks that keep families safe in harsh desert environments or conversely, in seeking to find new lands, necessitating the complex building of hardy ships and the concomitant practicalities of feeding large crews for months at a time.

However, that is not to say that nations in either contexts are unable or incapable of being 'relational' or indeed 'practical'—it is simply important to appreciate how their past influences their present and, in turn, how this is likely to impact how they perceive your attempts to communicate. Box 11.2 provides some

TABLE 11.1
High-context Cultures Versus Low-context Cultures

High-context Cultures	Low-context Cultures
For example, Japan, Korea, the Middle East, Russia	For example, the UK, Australia, Scandinavia, Germany
Indirect	Direct
Focus on relational aspects: health, well-being	Focus on the task at hand—pragmatic, what needs to be done
Focus on building rapport and relationships	Focus on decoding the words of the discussion
Takes time to build conversations	Time-efficient, shorter
Proxemics: less personal space	Larger personal space

BOX 11.2

Some Examples of Good and Bad 'Communication' In the Arabian Gulf

1. Email communication: Always try to make some personal time and request after a person or their families' well-being prior to getting to the matter at hand. Without this 'personal' relational touch, such communication in high-culture contexts can appear 'cold' and discourteous. In-person communication should follow the same process.

2. A local colleague wrote a long email to a senior manager in the local hospital. It was prefaced by the usual enquiry as to her well-being, etc. and thereafter went on to explain the arrangements for some training. The senior manager—who should have known better—simply replied with one word 'Fine'. My local colleague was apoplectic at her taciturn response and the perceived lack of courtesy.

3. Other social aspects such as bringing or accepting food and drinks (cakes, savouries) are considered important in setting the scene for any meeting as hospitality is a key feature of this region and not to do so would be considered impolite, if not insulting. Indeed, I have been at important meetings where the vast majority of the time is spent determining coffee orders

and savouries. Having taken time to 'invest' in this aspect, business matters can be speedily concluded.

4. Another local colleague proceeded to tell me in a very verbose way (in my opinion) about a specific member of staff who (in his opinion) was always being overly sycophantic with the institution's hierarchy, praising them at every opportunity, being obsequious and taking every chance he could to ingratiate himself to them. My colleague described these behaviours in some detail using marked hand gestures, pacing the room and emphatically nodding his head at the same time. I watched and listened patiently. His detailed description and accounts must have taken about 5–7 minutes at least before he at last paused and looked at me for a response. I nodded and said 'Ah, (pause) you mean he is a brown nose'. He looked shocked and confused for a few seconds and initially I thought my response might have been a bit too rude. But no, once he had decoded the distilled meaning and realised the inference he erupted into uproarious laughter, so much so he was actually physically doubled over. He kept laughing and repeated the phrase over and over again. And every time we met each other after that, he would just laugh and repeat the phrase again. We had transcended a classic communication clash between two context cultures and built rapport, albeit in a slightly more low-context way.

authentic examples of 'communication' experienced in this region by the authors and how different protagonists may have perceived their intent.

Example 4 in Box 11.2 demonstrates three key aspects in communication differences between high- and low-context cultures. First, the differences of temporality (time taken to discuss), the broad descriptions and vivid examples versus the short distillation (brown nose) in conjunction with the preponderance of gestures and physicality versus the seated, quiet stare. Second, it also demonstrates that you can both, theoretically at any rate, be speaking the same language but if it is not your native language then there are likely to be silences or 'gaps' in the conversation, especially when idioms or slang terms are used. Consequently, such terms are unlikely to be immediately transferrable to someone's native language, and the non-native speaker may therefore take some time to decode what is being said and/or to be able to attribute similar meaning. Third, example 4 ably demonstrates the power of humour in any conversation, with humour being a very under-researched and appreciated aspect of communication (Martin & Ford, 2018). Humour is a complex, dynamic phenomenon that can bring people together through a shared understanding and laugh (McCreaddie & Wiggins, 2008). However, humour can be a risky business and a sense of humour varies across cultures and continents (Davies, 2002; McCreaddie & Payne, 2012).

INTERDISCIPLINARY AND MULTICULTURAL COMMUNICATION IN HEALTHCARE

The health ecosystems of the Arabian Gulf and Greater Middle East are patently maturing in terms of international best practices and associated accreditation. Effective communication is crucial to these developments as they improve patient outcomes, help educate and train healthcare workers, enhance staff and patient satisfaction, improve health literacy and create positive interactions with patients and families.

That said, there is a limited evidence base with regard to the impact of multiculturalism on communication in the region (Almutairi & McCarthy, 2012). One area that is therefore perhaps worth exploring in more detail is that of the patient handover or handoff where critical information is exchanged among staff to ensure the safe and effective management of the patient in recovery. In this region, such handovers are likely to involve participants from different disciplines and diverse cultures and their peculiarities. Consequently, this may give rise to numerous communication challenges that need to be overcome.

THE EXAMPLE OF THE HANDOVER

Poor quality handover communication has been shown to result in serious adverse events and is a key area of healthcare quality irrespective of the context or culture

(Australian Commission, 2008). Greater risks are noted to accrue when handovers involve relatively inexperienced staff, no paper documentation to back up verbal handovers (Kardex, Recovery Chart), different professional groups (nurses, doctors, orderlies), interdepartmental communication (theatre, ward) and where boundaries (accountability) and role expectations (responsibility) are unclear (Australian Commission, 2008; Desmedt et al., 2021; Raesi et al., 2019). Moreover, the handover is acknowledged as being predicated on more than technical information and hence, positive interpersonal behaviours between coworkers are also key (Balka et al., 2013). However, consider the challenges of the handover in the clinical settings of the Arabian Gulf and Greater Middle East where intercultural communication—defined by Koester and Lustig (2015, p. 20) as 'an interaction amongst persons from two or more differing cultural backgrounds'—predominates. Imagine the myriad factors present in intercultural handover in this region (Table 11.2).

In healthcare environments with rapid turnovers such as the perioperative setting, it is generally expected that participating staff will be knowledgeable, efficient and competent. The types of handover communication in these settings, therefore, tends to be direct, brief and delivered with a specific purpose and it also tends to presume understanding on the part of the recipient. However, if you consider the linguistic aspects (Table 11.2) of such handovers alone—especially in a multicultural context—then there are numerous aspects that may not be clear or explicit. What about esoteric terms, differences in terminology, abbreviations (Hull, 2016), accents, speech rate, fluency, pitch and volume? What if you then add in the nonverbals such as head shaking, gestures, posture, facial expressions? There is an incredible propensity for 'communication' to be misinterpreted, ignored or simply not recognised. And that is but one aspect or complex 'difference(s)' between the protagonists.

One of the authors spent some considerable time working and teaching in Eastern Europe, India as well as the Arabian Gulf. These diverse settings all have different challenges, whether it is trying to make 'small talk' (Benwell & McCreaddie, 2016) with an Eastern European colleague while trying to overlook their perceived brusqueness or understanding that an Indian colleague's continual shake of the head in a side-to-side fashion in conversations actually means agreement

TABLE 11.2

Potential Differences Among the Handover Team

Factor	Example
Countries and cultures	Western: the UK, Ireland, Scandinavia, Australia, etc. (low context).
	Eastern: Indian, Filipino, Bangladeshi, Arab (various) (mix of low context and high context).
Genders	Tendency towards very gendered roles in this region, e.g. men = doctors, women = nurses.
Role expectation	Western nurses tend to be more autonomous and more used to working in a complementary manner with other disciplines. Western nurses are also more likely to question aspects of care irrespective of the discipline involved.
	Eastern nurses tend to be more subservient and obey doctors' orders.
Hierarchies	Many organisations in the Arabian Gulf region, including healthcare, tend to be very hierarchical and disciplinary in nature. Complaints about care and treatment will be dealt with quickly.
Education and training	Westerners tend to be better educated and trained in terms of qualifications and experience, e.g. MSc, BSc.
Castes/race/ethnicity perceptions	Given the history of the region, westerners (the UK, the USA, etc.) tend to be more coveted than non-westerners and are also likely to be on higher salaries.
Language/linguistics	English is the language used in most healthcare settings but most staff will not be native English language speakers. Thus there may be considerable variation and differences in linguistics such as content, terminology, idioms (verbals) and paralinguistics (accents, rate, fluency, pitch, volume) and other nonverbals (head nodding, head shaking, gestures, facial expression, posture)—all of which may be misinterpreted or simply not recognised.

rather than disagreement. None of those examples are stereotypes or stereotypical—as in an oversimplified conception or belief—rather these are cultural generalisations or general applications. Everyone from X region is not the same. There are dominant cultural patterns, subcultures, idiocultures with varying values, attitudes, norms and behaviours—and many of those are not necessarily the same as the dominant culture and, likewise, the dominant culture may not necessarily be the 'majority' culture. Accordingly, there are also cultural patterns for religions, ages and genders. In short, diversity transcends borders, characteristics and cultures.

Some of the *explicit* aspects outlined above such as verbals or nonverbals can be learned or perhaps, better understood to reduce misunderstandings, create better outcomes for patients and enhance staff co-operation and satisfaction. However, there are *implicit* aspects outlined in Table 11.2 that are arguably more entrenched and much more challenging to unravel. Thus, where handovers are not clear, direct and understandable, what factors may mitigate against staff members seeking clarification? For example, Parrone et al. (2008) suggested that any attempt to request further information, seek clarification or question instructions in handovers may be perceived as team member incompetence. And

no-one wants to be perceived as incompetent—especially not if your family is dependent upon your remittances. While practical aspects such as reducing speech rate, better enunciation, no abbreviations and back-up documentation can improve the process and outcome of the handover, they invariably fail to address the more *implicit* 'human' aspects of interactions such as feeling disempowered (e.g. hierarchy, gender, role expectation, race/ethnicity) with many of these predicated, to a certain extent, on culture or ethnicity. Moreover, handover 'tools' such as SBAR (situation, background, assessment, recommendation) provide a framework for communication between members of the healthcare team about a patient's condition but are again dependent upon numerous other relational factors (Shahid & Thomas, 2018). While an Australian nurse may happily challenge an anaesthetist over their postoperative opioid prescription, would a Filipino nurse be prepared to do the same? And if they did what might the outcome be?

CULTURAL DIVERSITY AMONG STAFF

The predominant ethnicities among healthcare staff in the Arabian Gulf and Greater Middle East are Indians and Filipinos with Arabs and Western expatriates being relative minorities in comparison. A total of 221,344 nurses from the Philippines and 70,471 nurses from India work in the Organisation for Economic Co-operation and Development Countries (OECD) with the GCC thought to be, by far, the largest recipient countries with approximately one-third of the nursing workforce (Buchan et al. 2022; OECD, 2019). Filipino nurses hail from a strong collectivist culture of service and are taught to respect teachers and experienced staff. While stating that Filipino nurses and perhaps, to a lesser extent, Indian nurses are subservient is perhaps an overstatement, they certainly both tend to avoid conflict, especially with hierarchy. Filipino and Indian nurses have been broadly educated along the traditional biomedical approach that follows 'doctors' orders' and where, in turn, nurse–doctor ratios are much different to those in the West or GCC. That said, Filipino staff appear more oriented to a 'caring hands-on' approach rather than the more concrete logic perhaps favoured by Indian staff. Accordingly, Ortiga (2014) suggests that, in the Philippines at least, the prevailing demands of exporting nurses has created an overloaded curriculum which panders to all whims. Consequently, there is therefore an argument that Filipino and Indian nurses are less likely to have as strong an identity as a 'profession' than perhaps Western nurses.

Understanding the cultural background and education of staff may facilitate a diverse group of employees to work together more safely and effectively (Attum et al., 2022). For example, non-Western nurses are not averse to more flexible, independent and accountable learning and both groups of nurses have been noted to respond well to social or group learning and mentoring or role modelling (Magulod, 2019). They have also been noted to value the security and social stability of working in Western countries, where they may be more likely to reap the rewards of a meritocracy (Smith & Gillin, 2021). Irrespective of Filipino and Indian nurses' destination, they unquestionably experience challenges and a degree of discrimination in the workplace (Montayre et al., 2018). Thus while much has been made about cultural competency (NCC, 2018) from the perspective of patients and relatives, there has perhaps been less of an emphasis on ensuring that staff are a key part of that axis, that is, healthcare services that meet the social, cultural and linguistic needs of all—patient, relatives and staff. Similarly, as Abou Hashish (2017) suggests, healthcare organisations also need to invest in strategies to enhance ethical and supportive work environments including job-related benefits such as equitable salaries for all, as these are also likely to impact staff satisfaction and attrition, not just cultural competence.

CULTURAL COMPETENCY INPUTS

The evidence-base on cultural competency and associated interventions has increased exponentially in the past decade (Loftin et al., 2013). Yet despite increasing interest, there remains a number of methodological challenges and unknowns. Cultural competency is often poorly defined (e.g. categorical and nonholistic), that is, the intervention is not tailored appropriately to the content/needs of the training cohort (Rew et al., 2003). Somewhat surprisingly there is also little acknowledgement of 'difference' in most training interventions. Models to enhance cultural competency exist but they are rarely used in training interventions. Moreover, key cultural concepts are often ignored, for example, racism, bias, linguistic competence and while inputs evaluate knowledge, attitudes/beliefs, skills, behaviour and confidence, they rarely evaluate patient satisfaction and outcomes.

Notwithstanding the plethora of cultural competence assessment/measurement scales which may be validated but rarely match (training/educational) content, most cultural competence interventions are usually provided in one setting with one specific group and/or too many vagaries (Perng & Watson, 2012). Additionally, cultural competence interventions generally tend to comprise education and training, mentorship, access and patient information literature, but there is no evidence of general awareness-raising. Nevertheless, the delivery mode and input (time) of existing interventions have notably had no demonstrative impact upon benefit, that is, longer training is not considered more beneficial than shorter interventions.

Rassool (2015) outlines the importance of cultural competency in nursing Islamic patients no matter the setting, while Aboud and Payne in Chapter 16, Mobin-Uddin (2018) and Malik (2012) all highlight how cultural competency is important when Western bio-ethics or biomedicine may clash with Islamic values.

MIGRANT WORKERS

Cultural competence palpably influences healthcare and healthcare interactions across key areas: health-seeking behaviours, symptom interpretation, adherence, satisfaction with care, care experience and attitudes to death and dying. Increasing evidence suggests that cultural incompetence is associated with poor access to healthcare, language/communication barriers, low literacy, negative health consequences, poor quality care and dissatisfaction with care (Truoung et al., 2014). As indicated previously, migrant workers are arguably the foundations on which the Arabian Gulf and Greater Middle East's development is built but this is not without cost.

Migrant workers may live in suboptimal housing conditions and be prone to numerous health conditions (Kumar et al., 2020), yet as Jamil et al. (2021) outline they can be resilient and develop numerous strategies to overcome the daily challenges they face. Migrant workers are undoubtedly worthy of considerably more attention than simply two paragraphs in this chapter. However, what is encouraging is the increasing amount of research that is being undertaken among this section of society (Hamed, 2022; Jamil, 2021) and the growing recognition of the need to attend to migrant workers' health and well-being from a humanitarian perspective.

CARING AND INTIMACY—ISLAM AND FUNDAMENTAL CARE

As discussed in some detail in Chapters 1 and 2, Islam permeates every aspect of a Muslim's life and it is therefore important that healthcare workers better understand peoples' spiritual and cultural values and beliefs to provide safe, effective and quality care. While many healthcare workers will have provided care and treatment to Muslim patients prior to working in the Arabian Gulf and Greater Middle East, it may be that these patients were acculturated Western-oriented Muslims who perhaps adhered to some Islamic practices but not all. Thus while there is diversity in Islam in terms of ethnic and linguistic groups, there will be homogeneity with regard to certain practices, for example, dietary needs, family dynamics, decision-making processes, health risks or beliefs and privacy and modesty (Rassool, 2014).

INTIMACY: PRIVACY, MODESTY, TOUCH AND EYE CONTACT

Ideally, Muslim patients should be cared for by a healthcare worker of the same gender especially in particular specialities like obstetrics and gynaecology (Padela & Rodriguez del Pozo, 2011). Alternatively, a female staff member or a relative can assume the role of chaperone. Good practice should be followed with regard to de-robing, that is, uncover only what is necessary and re-cover at the first opportunity, while any procedure should be fully explained and permission should always be sought in advance. Touch is prohibited between members of the opposite sex except for family members. Thus shaking hands—although considered polite and appropriate in Western societies—is largely inappropriate in this region and the hand may be rapidly withdrawn, often with an apology for doing so. In many Muslim cultures, the left hand is considered unclean as it is likely to be the hand used for cleaning post-toileting although a water hose is generally provided and used for this purpose. Left-handed people would be encouraged to eat with their right hand in particular and to reduce the prospect of offence, tasks such as assisting with feeding, medicine administration and handing cloths, towels, etc, to patients should generally be proffered with the right hand. Notably, several large companies have seen their adverts derided when a left hand has been used to hold a product or food (Ghani & Ahmad, 2015). Where touch is necessary for certain procedures or examinations it is permitted as long as it is valid and the encounter chaperoned.

In many Western countries, eye contact is an important part of nonverbal communication and is thought to occur for approximately one-third of any encounter. In the Arabian Gulf, eye contact may intimate interest, intimacy, affiliation or attention and is largely avoided especially among nonrelated individuals of the opposite sex. Conversely, same sex conversations may use prolonged eye contact to indicate truthfulness. Accordingly, a patient who does not maintain eye contact for any length of time is not likely to be disinterested or rude, but simply observing their modesty (Al-Shahri & Al-Khenaizan, 2005). As indicated elsewhere (see Chapters 2, 16 and 17) the family is central to Islamic life and the family is obligated to care for the sick and visit them on a regular basis.

ABLUTIONS AND HYGIENE

Cleanliness and purification are important daily acts of faith in Islam (Attum et al., 2022). Thus hygiene is important from both a physical and spiritual perspective. For example, Ablutions—a ritual, ceremonial washing of the body or objects to ensure cleanliness prior to religious observance, that is, prayer—are paramount. Similarly, washing is also required after urination or defaecation, menstruation and postnatal bleeding. A full bath is required after seminal discharge and/or sexual intercourse. In addition, any places where grime or dirt may accumulate, for example, nails, armpit hair, nostril hair—should be cleaned with hair removed.

PRAYER

Muslims are required to pray five times a day. Exemptions are made for those who may be unable to do so due to cognitive impairment, menstruation or postnatal discharge. Although prayers are usually undertaken on a prayer mat facing Mecca, they can be performed in bed or seated. Most hospitals in the Arabian Gulf and Middle East will issue the call to prayer through loudspeaker systems.

NUTRITION AND HYDRATION

Muslims must follow a halal diet with halal meaning 'permissable'. Thus certain foods are not permissible such as pork and derivatives, for example, gelatine and any other meat not ritually killed. Notably, some medications contain gelatine or magnesium stearate (stearic acid) and other blood, animal or alcohol derivatives. Halal meat is meat that has been slaughtered in a particular way, for example, via a cut to the jugular vein, carotid artery and windpipe and thereafter, the blood is drained. Other foods such as fish, eggs and vegetarian foods are readily consumed. However, it is important to ensure there is no cross-contamination between

pork or non-halal meats and halal meats and other food. Washing is therefore required pre and post eating. During Ramadan—the holy month of fasting—there may be particular difficulties for patients who are unwell or insulin dependent and it is therefore important for a prefasting assessment to be carried out to consider how best to support the patient. In instances where nutritional support is required, this is considered basic care and not medical treatment, there is an obligation to provide nutrition and hydration for the dying person unless it shortens life (Alsolamy, 2014).

CHILDBIRTH/MATERNITY

In maternity services there are two key practices to be cognisant of:

- Following childbirth a Muslim father may wish to recite a short prayer into the baby's right and then left ear.
- Muslims are required to bury the placenta which is part of the human body and therefore considered sacred and sometimes, the baby's hair is removed 7 days postnatal.

FUNDAMENTAL CARE REVISITED

As indicated at the start of this chapter, nurses provide the vast majority of 'hands-on' care irrespective of the setting and/or nurse–patient ratio. Yet, nursing in the Arabian Gulf and Greater Middle East is still largely viewed as a low-level occupation, similar in some ways to maids. The vagaries of nurse education across the region with low entry qualifications, diverse programmes and standards plus the doctor and their 'orders' predominate, making it a far less autonomous and admired profession than it is arguably considered in Western culture. Various countries across the region have made strides to try and encourage the indigenous population to enter the profession. Nonetheless, it remains a challenge and while here is not the text to discuss the intricacies of these challenges, there are two aspects that are worthy of mention.

First, nursing in the Greater Middle East predates Florence Nightingale, with the first Muslim nurse being Rufaidah Al-Asalmiya in the 8th century. Rufaidah trained nurses and cared for patients outside the Prophet Mohammad's (PBUH) mosque during the time of the Holy Wars and she is also credited with promoting community health. Thus she arguably serves as a distinct role model and pioneer.

Second, an ethnographic study by Dr Sandy Lovering (2008) led to the development of a model which claims to fill the void of previous Western approaches (Leininger, 1995) and attends to Islam as the cornerstone of Muslim's daily lives in a healthcare environment. The Crescent of Care model (COCM) is said to be based on the values and beliefs of Arab Muslim nurses who care for Arab Muslim patients (Lovering, 2012, 2014). This is a useful development and when taken in turn with the promotion of Rufaidah's role in nursing, it helps to build a context and history for prospective nurses in this part of the world. However, given the disproportionate mix of indigenous and expatriate residents and the plethora of ethnicities, religions and cultures who both provide and receive healthcare, the provision of a specific model may be arguably self-limiting. For example, Alharbi and Alhadid (2019) outline Muslim nurses' notions of compassion which are notably not that far removed from those associated with 'western' caring approaches. Western and Eastern approaches arguably have far more commonalities than differences and perhaps nursing globally might be better served with a greater focus on cultural competency per se—across all models, spectrums and cultures.

SUMMARY AND TAKEAWAY POINTS

This chapter reviewed four key aspects relevant to all the chapters presented within this text—communication, caring, diversity and cultural competency:

- Communication is a complex undertaking and should be performative, rather than passive and instructional—especially in a healthcare setting.
- The healthcare working environment in the Arabian Gulf and Greater Middle East is probably the most diverse, challenging and evolving in the world.
- There are distinct differences across high- and low-context cultures that create communication challenges especially in healthcare settings.

- The ward handover or handoff is used to demonstrate the complexities in multicultural communication in such a diverse setting.
- The cultural diversity in healthcare settings in the Arabian Gulf and Greater Middle East demands cultural competency and this requires recognising implicit as well as explicit aspects of communication.
- Migrant workers are a key resource in the region and greater attention should be paid to their healthcare needs.
- Islam permeates an individual's activities of daily living and this needs to be attended to in culturally appropriate ways from intimacy and hygiene to diet, nutrition and prayer.
- Fundamentally, irrespective of culture and ethnicity we have more commonalities than differences and we should use these to build better understanding and applications of cultural competency across all ethnicities.

REFERENCES

Abou Hashish, E. A. (2017). Relationship between ethical work climate and nurses' perception of organizational support, commitment, job satisfaction and turnover intent. *Nursing Ethics*, 24(2), 151–166.

Al-Shahri, M. Z., & Al-Khenaizan, A. (2005). Palliative care for Muslim patients. *J Support Oncol*, 3, 432e436.

Alsolamy, S. (2014). Islamic views on artificial nutrition and hydration in terminally ill patients. *Bioethics*, 28(2), 96–99. https://doi.org/10.1111/j.1467-8519.2012.01996.x.

Alharbi, J., & Al Hadid, L. (2019). Towards an understanding of compassion from an Islamic perspective. *Journal of Clinical Nursing*, 28(7–8), 1354–1358. https://doi.org/10.1111/jocn.14725.

Almutairi, A. F., & McCarthy, A. (2012). A multicultural nursing workforce and cultural perspectives in Saudi Arabia: An overview. *The Health*, 3(3), 71–74.

Australian Commission on Safety and Quality in Health Care, (2008). *A structured evidence-based literature review regarding the effectiveness of improvement interventions in clinical handover*. ACSQHC.

Attum, B., Hafiz, S., Malik, A., & Shamoon, Z. (2022). Cultural competence in the care of Muslim patients and their families: *StatPearls [Internet]*. Treasure Island (FL): StatPearls Publishing. Available at https://www.ncbi.nlm.nih.gov/books/NBK499933/.

Balka, E., Tolar, M., Coates, S., & Whitehouse, S. (2013). Socio-technical issues and challenges in implementing safe patient handovers: Insights from ethnographic case studies. *International Journal of Medical Informatics*, 82, e345–57.

Benwell, B., & McCreaddie, M. (2016). Keeping "small talk" small in health-care encounters: Negotiating the boundaries between on- and off-task talk. *Research on Language and Social Interaction*, *49*(3), 258–271.

Buchan, J., Catton, H., & Shaffer, F.A. (2022). The global workforce and the COVID-19 pandemic: International Centre on Nurse Migration. Available at https://www.intlnursemigration.org/.

Davies, C. (2002). *The Mirth of Nations*. Routledge.

Desmedt, M., Ulenaers, D., Grosemans, J., Hellings, J., & Bergs, J. (2021). Clinical handover and handoff in healthcare: A systematic review of systematic reviews. *International Journal for Quality in Health Care*, *33*(1), 70.

Ghani, E., & Ahmad, B. (2015). Islamic advertising ethics violation and purchase intention. *International Journal of Islamic Marketing and Branding*, *1*(2), 173–198.

Gude, T., Finset, A., Anvik, T., Bærheim, A., Fasmer, O. B., Grimstad, H., & Vaglum, P. (2017). Do medical students and young physicians assess reliably their self-efficacy regarding communication skills? A prospective study from end of medical school until end of internship. *BMC Medical Education*, *17*(1), 107.

Hall, E. T. (1959). *The silent language*. Garden City, NY: Doubleday & Company, Inc.

Hamid, A. A. R. M. (2022). Psychological distress and homesickness among Sudanese migrants in the United Arab Emirates. *Frontiers in Psychology*, *12*, 710115.

Hargie, O. (2019). Skill in theory: Communication as a skilled performance: *The handbook of communication skills* (4th ed.). London: Routledge.

Hull, M. (2016). Medical language proficiency: A discussion of interprofessional language competencies and potential for patient risk. *International Journal of Nursing Studies*, *54*, 158–172.

International Labour Office, (2021). *Global estimates on international migrant workers—results and methodology* (3rd ed.). Geneva: International Labour Office (ILO).

International Organization for Migration, (2020). *World Migration Report*. Switzerland: IOM.

Jamil, R., & Kumar, R. (2021). Culture, structure, and health: Narratives of low-income Bangladeshi migrant workers from the United Arab Emirates. *Health Communication*, *36*(11), 1297–1308.

Kumar, R., & Jamil, R. (2020). Labor, health, and marginalization: A culture-centered analysis of the challenges of male Bangladeshi migrant workers in the Middle East. *Qualitative Health Research*, *30*(11), 1723–1736.

Leininger, M. (1995). *Transcultural nursing: concepts, theories, research and practices*. New York: McGraw-Hill.

Lillrank, P. (2002). The broom and non-routine processes ± a metaphor for understanding variability in organizations. *Knowledge and Process Management*, *9*(3), 1–6.

Koester, J., & Lustig, M. W. (2015). Intercultural communication competence: Theory, measurement, and application. *International Journal of Intercultural Relations*, *48*, 20–21.

Littlejohn, S. W., & Foss, K. A. (2009). Definitions of communication *Encyclopedia of communication theory* (Vol. 1, pp. 296–299). SAGE Publications, Inc.

Loftin, C., Hartin, V., Branson, M., & Reyes, H. (2013). Measures of cultural competence in nurses: An integrative review. *Scientific World Journal*, *2013*, 289101. https://doi.org/10.1155/2013/289101.

Lovering, S. (2014). The crescent of care—a nursing model to guide the care of Muslim patients: *Cultural competence in caring for Muslim patients*. Basingstoke: Palgrave MacMillan.

Lovering, S. (2012). The crescent of care: A nursing model to guide the care of Arab Muslim patients. *Diversity and Equality in Health and Care*, *9*, 171.

Lovering, S. (2008). *Arab Muslim nurses' experiences of the meaning of caring, Doctor of Health Sciences*. Sydney, Australia: University of Sydney, Faculty of Health Sciences.

Magulod, G., Jr. (2019). Learning styles, study habits and academic performance of Filipino University students in applied science courses: Implications for instruction. *Journal of Technology and Science Education, (Sl)*, *9*(2), 184–198. https://doi.org/10.3926/jotse.504.

Malik, M. M. (2012). Islamic bioethics of pain medication: An effective response to mercy argument. *Bangladesh Journal of Bioethics*, *3*(2), 4–15.

Martin, R. A., & Ford, T. E. (2018). *The psychology of humor* (2nd ed.). Elsevier.

Mobin-Uddin, A. (2018). An Islamic perspective: Suffering and meaning in cancer. *Clinical Journal of Oncology Nursing*, *22*(5), 573–575. https://doi.org/10.1188/18.CJON.573-575.

McCreaddie, M., Benwell, B., & Gritti, A. (2021). A qualitative study of National Health Service (NHS) complaint-responses. *BMC Health Services Research*, *21*(1), 696.

McCreaddie, M., Benwell, B., & Gritti, A. (2018). Traumatic journeys: Understanding the rhetoric of patients' complaints. *BMC Health Services Research*, *18*, 551. https://doi.org/10.1186/s12913-018-3339-8.

McCreaddie, M., & Wiggins, S. (2008). The purpose and function of humour in health, healthcare and nursing: A narrative review. *Journal of Advanced Nursing*, *61*(6), 584–595.

McCreaddie, M., & Payne, S. (2012). Humour in healthcare – a risk worth taking. *Health Expectations*, *17*(3), 332–344.

Mobeireek, A. F., Al-Kassimi, F., Al-Zahrani, K., Al-Shimemeri, A., Al-Damegh, S., Al-Amoudi, O., et al. (2008). Information disclosure and decision-making: The Middle East versus the Far East and the West. *Journal of Medical Ethics*, *34*(4), 225–229.

Montayre, J., Montayre, J., & Holroyd, E. (2018). The global Filipino nurse: An integrative review of Filipino nurses' work experiences. *Journal of Nursing Management*, *26*(4), 338–347. https://doi.org/10.1111/jonm.12552.

National Center for Cultural Competence. (2018). Bridging the cultural divide in health care settings: The essential role of cultural broker programs. Available at https://nccc.georgetown.edu/culturalbroker/8_Definitions/index.html. Accessed 16 August 2023.

OECD (Organisation for Economic Co-operation and Development Countries). (2019). Recent trends in international migration of doctors, nurses and medical students. Paris: OECD Publishing. https://doi.org/10.1787/5571ef48-en.

Ortiga, Y. Y. (2014). Professional problems: The burden of producing the "global" Filipino nurse. *Social Science & Medicine*, *115*, 64–71. https://doi.org/10.1016/j.socscimed.2014.06.012.

Padela, A., & Rodriguez del Pozo, P. (2011). Muslim patients and cross-gender interactions in medicine: An Islamic bioethical perspective. *Journal of Medical Ethics*, *37*(1), 40–44.

Parrone, J., Sedrl, D., Donaubauer, C., Phillips, M., & Miller, M. (2008). Charting the 7 C's of cultural change affecting foreign nurses: Competency, communication, consistency, cooperation, customs, conformity and courage. *Journal of Cultural Diversity*, 15(1), 3–6.

Perng, S. -J., & Watson, R. (2012). Construct validation of the Nurse Cultural Competence Scale: A hierarchy of abilities. *Journal of Clinical Nursing*, 21(11–12), 1678–1684.

Rassool, G. H. (2014). Putting cultural competence all together: Some considerations in caring for Muslim patients. In G. H. Rassool (Eds.), *Cultural competence in caring for Muslim patients*. Basingstoke: Palgrave Macmillan.

Rassool, G. H. (2015). Cultural competence in nursing Muslim patients. *Nursing Times*, 111(14), 12–15.

Raeisi, A., Rarani, M. A., & Soltani, F. (2019). Challenges of patient handover process in healthcare services: A systematic review. *Journal of Education and Health Promotion*, 8, 173.

Rew, L., Becker, H., Cookston, J., Khosropour, S., & Martinez, S. (2003). Measuring cultural awareness in nursing students. *Journal of Nursing Education*, 42(6), 249–257.

Shahid, S., & Thomas, S. (2018). Situation, background, assessment, recommendation (SBAR) communication tool for handoff in health care—a narrative review. *Safety in Health*, 4, 7. https://doi.org/10.1186/s40886-018-0073-1.

Smith, D. M., & Gillin, N. (2021). Filipino nurse migration to the UK: Understanding migration choices from an ontological security-seeking perspective. *Social Science & Medicine*, 276, 113881. https://doi.org/10.1016/j.socscimed.2021.113881.

Truong, M., Paradies, Y., & Priest, N. (2014). Interventions to improve cultural competency in healthcare: A systematic review of reviews. *BMC Health Services Research*, 14, 99. https://doi.org/10.1186/1472-6963-14-99.

FURTHER READING

https://hsl.lib.unc.edu/health-literacy/communication-tools/.

https://www.nih.gov/institutes-nih/nih-office-director/office-communications-public-liaison/clear-communication/cultural-respect.

https://ethnomed.org/resource/overview-of-health-care-in-islamic-history-and-experience/.

https://www.mwpsbahrain.com/.

https://www.hse.ie/eng/services/publications/socialinclusion/interculturalguide/islam/care-ill.html.

12 FAMILY MEDICINE

HANI MALIK ■ KHATOON HUSAIN SHUBBAR

CHAPTER OUTLINE

INTRODUCTION

Defining family medicine has been challenged by the overlapping scopes of practice provided by primary care, adding to misconceptions about this specialty among the target patients, other health providers and medical students as well (AAFP, 2021). Whether using terminology such as primary healthcare (PHC), family medicine or general practice, there will always be an associated misinterpretation as to the distinct roles of a relatively new specialty that often intersects with other secondary care specialties. It is often difficult for the public to identify the distinctive role of a primary care physician, being the jack of all trades; this is often underappreciated by colleagues and the public alike.

Family medicine has been defined as 'the medical specialty that manages common and long-term illnesses in children and adults, focusing on overall health and well-being' (Hashim, 2018). Interestingly, the World Organization of Family Doctors (WONCA) has given a unified definition to both general practice and family medicine. The new European definition, which was agreed upon in 2005, is as follows: 'General practice or family medicine is an academic and scientific discipline,

with its own educational content, research, clinical and evidence-based activity, and a clinical specialty orientated to primary care' (WONCA, 2005). The World Health Organization (WHO) defines family medicine as a 'specialty of medicine which is concerned with providing comprehensive care to individuals and families and integrating biomedical, behavioral and social sciences' (WHO, 2003). Following the Declaration of Alma-Ata in 1978, the WHO, with help from global leaders, introduced the Declaration of Astana in 2018; emphasis was placed on the main components of PHC which focus more on a holistic approach as opposed to a disease-centred method. PHC is concerned with people's health needs throughout their lifetime and addresses patients' mental, physical and social well-being. The approach includes health promotion, disease prevention, treatment, rehabilitation and palliative care (WHO, 2021).

An article by Onion and Berrington (1999) compared general practice in the United Kingdom with family practice in the United States. The authors highlighted the vast differences in scope of practice, politics, training, relationships with other medical professionals, responsibilities and even language differences.

Like the United States, the Gulf Cooperation Council (GCC) countries have adopted the family medicine approach to primary care. However, the GCC countries provide PHC services free of charge as a basic citizen's right and need, but with some variation in the scope of services, responsibilities and workflows. These are further reflected by geographical, financial, political, social and some cultural variations. Regardless of the terminology used, in essence, primary care, general practice and family medicine are synonymous entities.

BACKGROUND: FAMILY MEDICINE IN THE GULF COOPERATION COUNCIL

The introduction of the family medicine specialty among the different GCC countries has varied over time. Therefore it is worth exploring the foundations of family practice and associated training programmes in the GCC.

In Bahrain, the first ever medical clinic was founded in 1888, which subsequently evolved into the first non-profitable healthcare institution, the American Mission Hospital in 1893 (Alnasir & Al-Sayyad, 2018). According to the Bahrain Medical Bulletin article by Hunt (1981), the first family medicine residency programme in the Arabian Gulf was created in Bahrain on 1 September 1979. This was the result of years of planning and preparation by representatives from the Ministry of Health and the American University of Beirut. The first cohort of family physicians completed their residency training in 1983 (Alnasir & Al-Sayyad, 2018).

Meanwhile in the Kingdom of Saudi Arabia (KSA), healthcare services were introduced in 1949. PHC as a concept was adopted much later, in 1978. In 1983 it finally became a corner stone in Saudi's healthcare delivery system (Sebai et al., 2001). However, family medicine training started relatively late in KSA compared to neighbouring countries such as Bahrain and Kuwait. In 1980 family practice training finally started in one of KSA's military hospitals as a fellowship programme for postgraduates followed by Arab Board Certification in 1991. Much later, in 1995, a 4-year structured Saudi Board in Family Medicine (SBFM) programme was initiated. In addition to the SBFM, more recently in 2008 a diploma in family medicine was launched as a 14-month structured programme

and upgraded to 24 months in 2014. Despite these initiatives, KSA still struggles with shortages in skilled graduates in this field (Al-Khaldi et al., 2017).

Like many countries in the GCC, most medical practices were introduced through missionary clinics. For example, Oman's first healthcare was delivered in a small clinic in Muttrah back in 1904 (Al Amana Centre, 2021). An official healthcare system, however, was only started much later in 1970 (Al-Azri, 2009). In Oman, family practice training programmes were later established in 1987, aided by the Department of Family and Community Medicine (FAMCO) at the College of Medicine in Sultan Qaboos University (Al-Shafaee, 2009). Later in 1994, a 4-year structured postgraduate training programme was established. Furthermore, the programme was recognised by the UK's Royal College of General Practitioners in 2001.

In Kuwait, it is reported that the history of PHC services started through a small clinic which was established in 1912 (Al-Ansari & El-Enezi, 2001). The family medicine residency programme was established in 1983, which started as a 3-year programme, extending to 4 years in 2001 with hope of implementing a 5-year programme by 2021 (Kuwait Family Medicine Residency Program (KFMRP), 2021). In Qatar, the first Hospital was founded in 1957 which is surprisingly still serving the public (Goodman, 2015). Much later in 1995, a family medicine residency programme was started with the first cohort of physicians completing the training in 1999 (Verjee et al., 2013). Unlike some of the other GCC countries, there was a higher demand for Qatari medicine graduates to enrol into family medicine residency programmes (Verjee et al., 2013). Meanwhile in the United Arab Emirates (UAE), the first healthcare medical centre was established in 1943 in Al Ras area, a locality in Dubai (Dubai Health Authority (DHA), 2021). While the Family Residency Program was initiated in 1987 under the umbrella of Dubai residency training programme, it was regulated by the Arab Board of Medical Specializations (AlSharief et al., 2018).

With the increasing demand on healthcare services and to cope with fast expansion of free public health services, family medicine residency programmes have been given greater attention. According to Osman and Romani (2011), most of the GCC countries have one family medicine residency programme, while KSA and UAE have multiple programmes. Despite the GCC countries starting their respective family medicine eras at differing times, the six countries have now established this specialty and accompanying opportunities for growth and progress in regional healthcare services.

CURRENT PRACTICE

The diversity in scope of services provided in primary healthcare facilities varies among the different GCC countries; regulations are very specific in some and broader in other areas. Many factors may contribute to such diversity including the training provided, expertise, health needs, economical drivers, cultural and social derivatives. Bahrain provides a leading model in PHC practice, which was awarded by the United Nations Public services initiatives in 2017 for providing a full PHC solution as well as improving the availability of early detection for noncommunicable diseases (UN, 2017). PHC in the Kingdom of Bahrain provides a broader scope of services aiming to divert the burden away from secondary and tertiary hospitals by investing and supporting primary healthcare activities. The services include preventive, promotional, therapeutic and rehabilitative services in many different fields. Most healthcare facilities under the umbrella of primary healthcare in Bahrain have the following services: dental services, minor surgical procedures, family medicine, social services, radio imaging, pharmacy, mobile unit community services, physiotherapy services, laboratory services, school health, mental health, sexual health, smoking cessation, women and child health.

Family medicine as a specialty is concerned with providing many specialised services alongside the continuous holistic medical approach to the patients and their families. A family physician provides child health screening, women's health screening, antenatal care, postnatal care and treatment of noncommunicable diseases. Most of the PHC facilities around the GCC countries provide a similar scope of services with variations in workflow and systems. As seen in Table 12.1, the latest statistics and resources display the number of governmental healthcare facilities providing PHC services in the GCC (Federal Competitiveness and Statistics Authority (FCSA) UAE, 2019; Ministry of Health (MOH) Bahrain, 2021; MOH Oman, 2019; MOH Saudi, 2020; Planning and Statistics Authority Qatar, 2019; WHO, 2006, 2008, 2017).

TABLE 12.1

Number of Primary Healthcare Facilities

GCC	Number of Primary Healthcare Facilities	Data Obtaining Year
Bahrain	28	2021
Oman	180	2008
Kuwait	72	2006
Qatar	27	2019
KSA	2261	2020
UAE	149	2019

GCC, Gulf Cooperation Council; *KSA, Kingdom* of Saudi Arabia; *UAE*, United Arab Emirates.

PREVENTATIVE HEALTHCARE

Tackling Chronic Disease: Exercise and Diet

Chronic disease is increasingly becoming a major issue worldwide, complicated by lack of exercise and poor dietary habits. The WHO has reported that 80% of the world's adolescents are not exercising sufficiently (Aljayyousi et al., 2019). Physical inactivity plays a hugely significant role in the high rates of obesity in the gulf region (Musaiger et al., 2011). In the GCC, studies have shown that only 40% and 27% of men and women, respectively, took part in some form of physical activity (Aljayyousi et al., 2019). To counteract this, governments in Qatar and Bahrain have implemented measures such as declaring 14 February as an annual National Sports Day to encourage physical activity (Aljayyousi et al., 2019). The authors surmise that as the main religion in the GCC, Islam encourages physical activity in both adults and children regardless of gender to maintain both spiritual and physical strength. However, environmental and sociocultural factors act as barriers to promote healthy habits. The humid, unforgiving summers in the GCC countries discourage regular exercise (Serour et al., 2007). Moreover, there is a lack of encouragement from parents towards physical activity in their children (Pearson et al., 2020), while lifestyle habits such as watching television and playing computer games have become the norm (Musaiger et al., 2011).

In addition to insufficient physical activity, there has been a paradigm shift in meal patterns and diet consumed by the public in the Middle East. Skipping breakfast, reduced servings of fruit and vegetables and higher consumption of fast food are becoming a trend among school-aged adolescents (Musaiger et al., 2011). Moreover, the authors explain that traditional, healthier GCC diets high in fibre and low in fat are now being displaced by a more convenient 'Western' diet and lifestyle, consisting of saturated fats and sugars coupled with low levels of physical activity.

Noncommunicable conditions result in 2.3 million deaths per year, encompassing 53% of annual mortality rates (Boutayeb et al., 2013). The authors discovered that unfortunately, five GCC countries find themselves in the top 10 list of highest prevalence of diabetes, with diabetes-related deaths ranging from 1% to 12% in the Middle East. To mitigate the problem of 'diabesity' or diabetes associated with obesity (Serour et al., 2007), family physicians need to address two main areas requiring urgent attention: physical inactivity and poor diet. These often overlooked yet interrelated issues have long-term consequences on individuals and health systems in the GCC. Targeting the youth is an important first step. However, communication and education must be contextualised and tailored to the individual while considering crucial environmental, sociocultural and religious perspectives.

Person-centred Care and Self-management

The GCC countries are some of the highest worldwide for risk factors in developing chronic conditions like diabetes or cardiovascular disease; the average prevalence of obesity for a GCC national is at 40% (Khoja et al., 2017). Moreover, patients with multimorbidity as illustrated in Case Study 12.1, often have a passive attitude towards their conditions and medications, either through lack of knowledge or complete dependence on the care provider. As this form of care is unsustainable in tackling noncommunicable disease and multimorbidity in the long term, the traditional doctor–patient relationship requires some constructive scrutiny.

As patient advocates, family physicians are the most suitable cohort to implement a person-centred care (PCC) approach to healthcare. PCC looks to address patient needs by placing them in the centre of the consultation through empowerment and education (Qidwai et al., 2015). The authors suggest that with PCC, family physicians can provide patients with evidence-based choices in simplified, understandable

CASE STUDY 12.1
PATIENT-CENTRED CARE?

A 62-year-old male has been taking medications for his chronic conditions for the past 12 years. He currently has diabetes mellitus, hypertension, hyperlipidaemia and hypothyroidism—all of which are controlled and stable. He attends the local health centre for a routine prescription renewal.

However, when the family physician asks him questions about the medication being taken, he is not able to identify the various medications or dosages and says, 'I trust you doctor, you know best'. The family physician spends the rest of the consultation performing a medication review while using the opportunity to educate the patient about his chronic conditions and the prescribed medications.

language that facilitates shared decision-making and equal partnership in the consultation. Instead of being told what to do by doctors, the patient is encouraged towards making informed decisions to effectively manage multiple conditions (Box 12.1). Interestingly, Qidwai et al.'s (2015) multicountry cross-sectional study of the Eastern Mediterranean region found that 62.6% of physicians favoured a PCC approach, while 53% of patients preferred a mix of PCC and patient-centred approach. The authors discovered that with health promotion and disease prevention as goals, PCC shifts focus onto the individual who is ill, while incorporating their functional, spiritual and psychosocial needs in a truly holistic approach. The main difference is that a patient-centred approach facilitates a functional life while a PCC helps in achieving a meaningful life. Balancing individual patient preferences with appropriate clinical practice requires an investment in training physicians and sufficient consultation time, to not impede progress. With physicians guiding patients as equal partners in a consultation, health systems in the GCC have a potentially effective tool in the fight against the growing prevalence of chronic disease.

APPROPRIATE PRESCRIBING AND ADHERENCE

Antibiotics in Primary Care

Antibiotics have been a game changer in the fight against infectious disease. However, when used inap-

CASE STUDY 12.2
OVERUSE OF ANTIBIOTICS

A 38-year-old worried mother books an urgent appointment for her child suffering from a cough and blocked nose. After the family physician performed a history and physical examination, the mother started demanding antibiotics, specifically Co-amoxiclav. She explains that her child had similar symptoms 6 months ago, and the doctor prescribed Co-amoxiclav for 7 days. She gave her child the dose for 3 days, after which she noticed a marked improvement. She then stopped giving her child the antibiotics and disposed of it.

The family physician explains that the most likely diagnosis is in fact a viral upper respiratory tract infection which would not require nor respond to antibiotics. He also explained the dangers of antibiotic resistance and emergence of 'superbugs' due to inadequate management and prescribing. The mother disagreed with the doctor and left the consultation room disgruntled. She ends up buying antibiotics over the counter at a nearby pharmacy known for lax regulations with prescription medicine.

propriately, complex issues arise. Complications such as antibiotic resistance, adverse events, increased costs and overall poor patient outcomes are increasingly becoming trends due to inappropriate antibiotic usage (Butt et al., 2017). The GCC countries are faced with challenges of antibiotic resistance due to lack of clear, regional policies restricting or monitoring antibiotic use (Enani, 2015). A study in Qatar observed that 45% of patients were prescribed antibiotics for conditions that did not require them; 50% of the cases originated in family practice (Butt et al., 2017). The authors discovered an interesting trend where upper respiratory tract infections accounted for 80% of inappropriate use of antibiotics in primary care (Case Study 12.2). However, the complex issue of appropriate prescribing also incorporates patient agenda and expectations. A study showed that 31.6% of patients would ask for antibiotics during a consultation, especially if they had used antimicrobials in the past, while 49.6% of patients would be dissatisfied if they did not receive treatment (Shaikhan et al., 2018). The authors observed that improper use arises from numerous factors including doctor's knowledge, insufficient information provided to patients, diagnostic ambiguity and patient perceptions of the doctor–patient interaction.

There is a promising opportunity for the GCC countries to promote effective antibiotics usage in primary care. Sharing and consolidating best practice across health centres and ensuring a uniform antimicrobial stewardship programme can pave the way towards preventing antibiotics resistance, associated costs and mitigating long-term healthcare consequences (Enani, 2015). In addition, family physicians need to be steadfast when pressured into prescribing and instead should invest in informative dialogue and patient education about the misuse, associated complications and appropriate indications for antibiotic treatment.

Adherence and Self-medicating

The WHO defines adherence as 'the extent to which a person's behaviour—taking medication, following a diet and/or executing lifestyle changes—corresponds with agreed recommendations from a health care provider' (Chaudri, 2003). In the GCC, various studies have shown a wide range of nonadherence of between 1.4% and 88% (Al Qasem et al., 2011). This is problematic as it means that desired health outcomes for patients in primary care, such as improved quality of life, cannot be effectively achieved. Nonadherence was higher in relatively asymptomatic conditions such as hypertension due to varying misconceptions about the severity of disease. However, there are other common themes as to why patients do not properly take their prescribed medications. Drug side-effects, irregular follow-up, forgetfulness and lack of health education are among the several reported reasons for nonadherence in GCC patients (Al Qasem et al., 2011).

Further complicating poor adherence is the use of complementary and alternative medicine (CAM). The GCC countries have a long tradition of regular CAM use. In KSA, the prevalence of CAM use in diabetic patients is around 30%, while in Bahrain it is shown to be as high as 63%; 43% use it on a daily basis (Khalaf & Whitford, 2010). The authors discovered that natural medicines including garlic, bitter melon, cinnamon and fenugreek are among the most used forms of CAM. However, an unfortunate trend is that patients are not forthcoming about using natural remedies as the main treatment to manage their chronic disease. Sixty-two percent of patients in Bahrain fail to inform their primary care physician of their CAM use

Social Media Opportunities

Social media platforms such as Instagram, Facebook and Twitter are increasingly being used for health promotion and awareness campaigns worldwide. Gulf Cooperation Council (GCC) Facebook users account for 22% of total users in the Arab world, while more than 50% of tweets in the Arab region come from Saudi Arabia and UAE (Zowawi et al., 2015). Health systems in the GCC countries have a real opportunity to launch informative social media campaigns to promote health which can be a true asset to primary care. Person-centred communication is facilitated by arming social media users with regular, updated knowledge and facilitating public discussion around medical conditions or important community health concerns (Menon & George, 2018). A key advantage of social media is the ability to track responses online and use the data to further guide awareness campaigns and tweak marketing strategies (Zowawi et al., 2015). Educational intervention can also be repeated over lengthy periods of time if required. As a result, patients are informed in making better decisions through a person-centred approach. With ease of access, social media provides a golden opportunity to tackle health-related challenges in the GCC.

(Khalaf & Whitford, 2010). Furthermore, this form of self-medication (SM) also includes conventional, prescribed medications.

SM, particularly with antibiotics, is increasingly becoming a complex issue in the GCC. The prevalence of SM is 44.8% in Bahrain and 35.4% in KSA (Khalifeh et al., 2017). One of the main reasons for SM is the easy availability of antibiotics. Such is the case in the UAE, where 44% of patients obtain their antibiotics from the pharmacy without a prescription (Abasaeed et al., 2009). Moreover, in KSA, 95% of antibiotics dispensed by pharmacists without a prescription are done so without patients' explicit request (Alghadeer et al., 2018). Other sources of SM include medications shared from relatives and leftover medication from previous prescriptions and are mainly used to treat mild respiratory tract symptoms (Khalifeh et al., 2017). Furthermore, the authors revealed that noncompliance with initially

prescribed medication, physician overprescribing and lack of knowledge about effective use are all important factors that contribute to SM. As a result, it is of no surprise that countries like KSA and Kuwait have a high prevalence of gram-positive bacteria resistant to conventional antibiotics (Alghadeer et al., 2018). The complex interplay of nonadherence, CAM use and SM poses a significant threat to GCC healthcare delivery. GCC health systems must tackle these issues by collaborating with primary care physicians towards investing time and effort in regular, effective patient education and move towards stricter, national pharmaceutical regulations.

Rethinking Consultation Lengths and the 'Walk-in' Patient

Consultation lengths in primary care vary from country to country around the world. A global study observed a disparity between timings which can be as low as 48 seconds in Bangladesh or a generous 22.5 minutes in Sweden (Irving et al., 2017). A survey from several developed countries has shown that over one-third of physicians in primary care are dissatisfied with time allotted for consultations (Osborn et al., 2015). Furthermore, an alarming statistic shows that more than 50% of the world's population have an average consultation time of 5 minutes or less (Irving et al., 2017).

The GCC countries find themselves somewhere in between Bangladesh and Sweden. For example, appointments at local health centres in Bahrain are registered at 8-minute intervals on weekdays, but every 6 minutes on weekends and public holidays when only a limited number of centres are open. In addition to prebooking through an appointment system, patients can also avail of a 'walk-in' service by arriving to the health centre and seeing a physician if there is an appointment slot available. Often, the 'walk-in' and the prebooked appointments force the already time-pressured physician to juggle between the provided services. In comparison, countries like Bangladesh or Pakistan do not have an appointment system and many physicians can see over 90 patients per day with limited time allotted per consultation (Irving et al., 2017).

Short consultations can diminish the range of primary care services, compromise patient care and add to the physician workload and stress (Irving et al., 2017). Studies have also shown that short consultation times

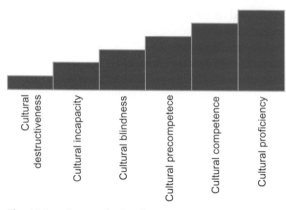

Fig. 12.1 ▪ Stages of cultural competence. (With permission from Bhattacharya, S., Kumar, R., Sharma, N., & Thiyagarajan, A. (2019). Cultural competence in family practice and primary care setting. *Journal of Family Medicine and Primary Care*, 8(1), 1–4.).

result in polypharmacy, overprescribing antibiotics and inadequate communication with patients (Jin et al., 2015). Conversely, longer consultation times are associated with reduced hospital admissions for complications of diabetes, improved quality of life in patients with multiple conditions and effective diagnosis and management of mental health disorders (Irving et al., 2017).

Moreover, there is a strong association between short consultation times and physician burnout as doctors struggle to balance demands with providing adequate care (Soler et al., 2008). One-third of primary care physicians suffer from varying degrees of depression, anxiety and stress in Bahrain (Malik et al., 2017). Comparatively in Saudi Arabia, 28.9% of physicians were reported to have depression, with an important predictor being an increased number of patients seen (Raffah & Alamir, 2013). With the ease of booking appointments through modern technology, perhaps it is worth reconsidering consultation times and the necessity for 'walk-in' services.

CHALLENGES AND OPPORTUNITIES

Cultural and Ethical Considerations

The diverse populations across the GCC countries also extends to healthcare staff. Seventy-eight percent of healthcare staff in KSA are expatriates, while the number is as high as 85% in the UAE (Khoja et al., 2017). Moreover, the authors discovered that only 3% of nurses in the UAE are Emirati. Along with

a large portion of the general population not originating from the GCC, this highlights the importance of cultural competence. Nationals and expatriate healthcare professionals alike need to move towards cultural proficiency as shown in Fig. 12.1. It is important to acknowledge and challenge previously held cultural assumptions and beliefs to provide a respectful, mindful consultation thus improving health outcomes in a vast cross-cultural setting (Watt et al., 2016). With the person-centred approach as previously described, GCC primary care physicians can overcome healthcare disparities and effectively integrate culture into healthcare delivery (Bhattacharya et al., 2019).

The GCC embraces Islam as the main religion, which greatly influences daily behaviour, values and cultural practices. Expatriate staff need to be aware of the religious and cultural nuances that gives the GCC its unique identity. There is often a clash between modern medicine and traditional remedies. For example, cupping is widely used to treat various disorders from headaches to sprains, while Muslims with diabetes often insist on fasting during the holy month of Ramadan and consume honey and also use it in wound dressings (Attum et al., 2021). This can be seen as counterproductive to evidence-based primary healthcare. In addition, with their centralised health systems and vastly diverse populations, the GCC countries are susceptible to ethical dilemmas in primary care. Alkabba et al. (2012) discovered that patients' rights, confidentiality and medical error rank as the top three ethical issues facing healthcare providers in KSA. Case Study 12.3 illustrates a common ethical issue in primary care. On face value this may seem surprising. However in Islam, the family unit in the GCC forms the core of the community (Attum et al., 2021). The authors explain that behaviour and habits are greatly influenced by spouse or first-degree relatives and it is also not uncommon for extended family to have a say in important societal and health-related decisions. Therefore to achieve the best possible outcomes for patients, it is imperative that the primary care physician mindfully navigates through these intricate dynamics that may drastically vary from one consultation to the next.

Mental Health of Physicians

Mental health in the GCC has long been overlooked and as a result is underdiagnosed and undertreated.

Stigma towards mental health confounded by religious beliefs, aetiological perceptions and values add a complex cultural barrier to treatment (Pocock, 2017). However, several GCC countries have taken proactive measures. Kuwait has identified mental health as one of six strategic priorities, while Oman realises the need to improve mental health services and training for primary care physicians (Hickey et al., 2016). The authors observed that Qatar has also recently developed the national mental health strategy, adding promise to a healthcare field requiring urgent attention in the GCC. However, one facet of mental health remains to be addressed: primary care physician mental health.

There have been several mental health reports on family physicians in the GCC. A recent study in Bahrain discovered that 41.2% of primary care physicians suffer from burnout (Al Ubaidi et al., 2020). In Oman, 17.8% of doctors reported emotional exhaustion, while 38.2% exhibited high levels of depersonalisation and 21.5% displayed low levels of personal accomplishments (Al-Hashemi et al., 2019). A Kuwait study revealed significant burnout in primary care doctors, more commonly within non-Kuwaiti physicians and those with lower income (Abdulghafour et al., 2011). Furthermore, a Qatar study in 2018 showed that 16% of family physicians suffer from burnout, a 4% increase from a study conducted in 2011 (Salem et al., 2018). Meanwhile, 42.6% of UAE primary care physicians displayed high scores for emotional exhaustion while 44.1% reported low personal accomplishment (Hussein et al., 2015). Therefore it is not surprising that in the UAE only 25% of trainee doctor applicants considered pursuing a career in primary care (Schiess et al., 2015).

A common theme emerged from these studies. Irrespective of training levels or status, family physicians are marked with indices of occupational burnout. Principal risk factors to developing depersonalisation include increased patient numbers, heavy workload, constraints due to short consultation times and disorganised patient flow (Al Ubaidi et al., 2020). However, if the GCC countries are looking towards progress, the negative consequences of physician burnout to patient care and resulting increased risk of medical errors coupled with decreased patient satisfaction (Al Ubaidi et al., 2020) cannot be ignored. It is imperative that significant measures are taken to counteract this growing mental health epidemic in physicians to protect the interests of all stakeholders involved in healthcare service and delivery.

SUMMARY AND TAKEAWAY POINTS

This chapter raises important points as it relates to family medicine in the Middle East, including:

- The GCC countries have analogous health systems that serve diverse populations requiring culturally competent primary care.
- The GCC countries' westernised and unhealthy dietary practices play a significant long-term role in developing chronic noncommunicable diseases which are further burdening health systems.
- Tapping into religious and cultural values can promote advantageous, preventive practices like adequate physical activity.
- The increasing prevalence of multimorbidity can be an opportune catalyst for self-management and PCC.
- Family physician-led patient education through awareness campaigns and social media is imperative towards correcting misconceptions about

antibiotics, complementary medicine, nonadherence and SM.

■ Mental health issues in primary care physicians pose a significant risk to GCC health systems and patient care, requiring urgent attention and intervention.

REFERENCES

Abasaeed, A., Vlcek, J., Abuelkhair, M., & Kubena, A. (2009). Self-medication with antibiotics by the community of Abu Dhabi Emirate, United Arab Emirates. *Journal of Infection in Developing Countries*, 3(7), 491–497. https://doi.org/10.3855/jidc.466.

Abdulghafour, Y., Bo-hamra, A., Al-Randi, M., Kamel, M., & El-Shazly, M. (2011). Burnout syndrome among physicians working in primary health care centers in Kuwait. *Alexandria Journal of Medicine*, 47(4), 351–357. https://doi.org/10.1016/j.ajme.2011.08.004.

Al Amana Centre. (2021). *History*. Available at https://alamanacentre.org/history/.

Alnasir, F. A., & Al-Sayyad, A. (2018). Bahrain. In Salah, H., & Kidd, M. (Eds.) Family practice in the Eastern Mediterranean region: Universal health coverage and quality primary care. Netherlands: Amsterdam University Press.

Al Qasem, A., Smith, F., & Clifford, S. (2011). Adherence to medication among chronic patients in Middle Eastern countries: Review of studies. *Eastern Mediterranean Health Journal*, 17(4), 356–363.

Al Ubaidi, B., Helal, S., Al-Eid, K., Al-Showaiter, L., AlAsheeri, K., AbdulRasheed, Y., et al. (2020). A study on the prevalence of burnout among primary care physicians on the kingdom of Bahrain. *Journal of the Bahrain Medical Society*, 32(2), 8–16. https://doi.org/10.26715/jbms.32_2020_2_2.

Al-Ansari, H. A., & Al-Enezi, S. (2001). Health sciences libraries in Kuwait: A study of their resources, facilities, and services. *Bulletin of the Medical Library Association*, 89(3), 287–293.

Al-Azri, N. H. (2009). Emergency medicine in Oman: Current status and future challenges. *International Journal of Emergency Medicine*, 11(4), 199–203. https://doi.org/10.1007/s12245-009-0143-6.

Alghadeer, S., Aljuaydi, K., Babelghaith, S., Alhammad, A., & Alarifi, M. N. (2018). Self-medication with antibiotics in Saudi Arabia. *Saudi Pharmaceutical Journal*, 26(5), 719–724. https://doi.org/10.1016/j.jsps.2018.02.018.

Al-Hashemi, T., Al-Huseini, S., Al-Alawi, M., Al-Balushi, N., Al-Senawi, H., Al-Balushi, M., et al. (2019). Burnout syndrome among primary care physicians in Oman. *Oman Medical Journal*, 34(3), 205–211. https://doi.org/10.5001/omj.2019.40.

Aljayyousi, G. F., Abu Munshar, M., Al-Salim, F., & Osman, E. R. (2019). Addressing context to understand physical activity among Muslim university students: The role of gender, family, and culture. *BMC Public Health*, 19(1), 1–12. https://doi.org/10.1186/s12889-019-7670-8.

Alkabba, F., Hussein, G., Albar, A., Bahnassy, A., & Qadi, M. (2012). The major medical ethical challenges facing the public and healthcare providers in Saudi Arabia. *Journal of Family and Community Medicine*, 19(1), 1–6. https://doi.org/10.4103/2230-8229.94003.

Al-Khaldi, Y.M., Al-Ghamdi, E.A., Al-Mogbil, T.I., Al-Khashan, H.I. (2017). Family medicine practice in Saudi Arabia: The current situation and proposed strategic directions plan 2020. *Journal of Family & Community Medicine*, 24(3), 156–163. doi:10.4103/jfcm.JFCM_41_17.

Al-Shafaee, M. (2009). Family medicine practice in Oman: Present and future. *Sultan Qaboos University Medical Journal*, 9(2), 116–118.

AlSharief, W. M., Abdulrahman, M., Khansaheb, H. H., Abdulghafoor, S. A., & Ahmed, A. (2018). Evolution of family medicine residency training program in Dubai health authority: A 24-year review, challenges, and outcomes. *Journal of Family Medicine and Primary Care*, 7(2), 425–429. https://doi.org/10.4103/jfmpc.jfmpc_183_17.

American Academy of Family Physicians (AAFP). (2021). *Primary care*. Available at https://www.aafp.org/about/policies/all/primary-care.html.

Attum, B., Hafiz, S., Malik, A., & Shamoon, Z. (2021). Cultural competence in the care of Muslim patients and their families: *StatPearls [Internet]*. Treasure Island (FL): StatPearls Publishing.

Bhattacharya, S., Kumar, R., Sharma, N., & Thiyagarajan, A. (2019). Cultural competence in family practice and primary care setting. *Journal of Family Medicine and Primary Care*, 8(1), 1. https://doi.org/10.4103/jfmpc.jfmpc_393_18.

Boutayeb, A., Boutayeb, S., & Boutayeb, W. (2013). Multi-morbidity of non communicable diseases and equity in WHO Eastern Mediterranean countries. *International Journal for Equity in Health*, 12(1), 60. https://doi.org/10.1186/1475-9276-12-60.

Butt, A., Navasero, C., Thomas, B., Marri, S., Al Katheeri, H., Al Thani, A., et al. (2017). Antibiotic prescription patterns for upper respiratory tract infections in the outpatient Qatari population in the private sector. *International Journal of Infectious Diseases*, 55, 20–23. https://doi.org/10.1016/j.ijid.2016.12.004.

Chaudri, N. (2003). Adherence to long-term therapies evidence for action. *Annals of Saudi Medicine*, 24(3), 221–222. https://doi.org/10.5144/0256-4947.2004.221.

Dubai Health Authority (DHA). (2021). *Our history*. Available at https://www.dha.gov.ae/en/AboutUs.

Enani, M. (2015). The antimicrobial stewardship program in Gulf Cooperation Council (GCC) states: Insights from a regional survey. *Journal of Infection Prevention*, 17(1), 16–20. https://doi.org/10.1177/1757177415611220.

Federal Competitiveness and Statistics Authority (FCSA) United Arab Emirates (UAE). (2019). *UAE numbers*. Available at https://fcsc.gov.ae/ar-ae/Documents/UAE%20Numbers%20Ar%202019.pdf#search=%D8%A7%D9%84%D8%B5%D8%AD%D8%A9%202019.

Goodman, A. (2015). The development of the Qatar healthcare system: A review of the literature. *International Journal of Clinical Medicine*, 6(3), 177–185. https://doi.org/10.4236/ijcm.2015.63023.

Hashim, M. J. (2018). A definition of family medicine and general practice. *Journal of College of Physicians and Surgeons Pakistan*, 28(1), 76–77. https://doi.org/10.29271/jcpsp.2018.01.76.

Hickey, J. E., Pryjmachuk, S., & Waterman, H. (2016). Mental illness research in the Gulf Cooperation Council: A scoping review. *Health Research Policy and Systems*, *14*(1), 59. https://doi.org/10.1186/s12961-016-0123-2.

Hunt, V. R. (1981). Bahrain's family medicine residency program. *Bahrain Medical Bull*, *3*(2), 60–68.

Hussein, H., Al-Faisal, W., Wasfy, A., Monsef, A., AbdulRahim, M., & El Sawaf, E. (2015). Burnout among primary health care physicians in Dubai health authority Dubai-UAE. *Public Health and Preventive Medicine*, *1*(1), 24–27.

Irving, G., Neves, A. L., Dambha-Miller, H., Oishi, A., Tagashira, H., Verho, A., et al. (2017). International variations in primary care physician consultation time: A systematic review of 67 countries. *BMJ Open*, *7*(10), 1–15. https://doi.org/10.17863/CAM.21761.

Jin, G., Zhao, Y., Chen, C., Wang, W., Du, J., & Lu, X. (2015). The length and content of general practice consultation in two urban districts of Beijing: A preliminary observation study. *PLOS ONE*, *10*(8), 1–10. https://doi.org/10.1371/journal.pone.0135121.

Khalaf, A. J., & Whitford, D. L. (2010). The use of complementary and alternative medicine by patients with diabetes mellitus in Bahrain: A cross-sectional study. *BMC Complementary and Alternative Medicine*, *10*(35), 1–5. https://doi.org/10.1186/1472-6882-10-35.

Khalifeh, M. M., Moore, N. D., & Salameh, P. R. (2017). Self-medication misuse in the Middle East: A systematic literature review. *Pharmacology Research & Perspectives*, *5*(4), 1–13. https://doi.org/10.1002/prp2.323.

Khoja, T., Rawaf, S., Qidwai, W., Rawaf, D., Nanji, K., & Hamad, A. (2017). Health care in Gulf Cooperation Council countries: A review of challenges and opportunities. *Cureus*, *9*(8), e1586. https://doi.org/10.7759/cureus.1586.

Kuwait Family Medicine Residency Program (KFMRP). (2021). *Family medicine: Kuwait family medicine residency program initiated in 1983.* Available at https://kfmrp.com/.

Malik, H., Mandeel, M., Al-Zamil, R., Mohammed, M., Dawood, A., & Hassan, H. (2017). Prevalence of depression, anxiety, and stress among primary care physicians in the kingdom of Bahrain. *Journal of the Bahrain Medical Society*, *29*(3), 19–27. https://doi.org/10.26715/jbms.29.3.2017.39a.

Menon, M., & George, B. (2018). Social media use for patient empowerment in the Gulf Cooperation Council region. *Clinical eHealth*, *1*(1), 21–27. https://doi.org/10.1016/j.ceh.2018.10.002.

Ministry of Health (MOH) Bahrain. (2021). *Health centers.* Available at https://www.moh.gov.bh/HealthInstitution/HealthCenters.

Ministry of Health (MOH) Oman. (2019). *Annual health report 2019.* Available at https://www.moh.gov.om/en/web/statistics/-/-2019.

Ministry of Health (MOH) Saudi Arabi. (2020). *Statistical yearbook 1440H – chapter two.* Available at https://www.moh.gov.sa/en/Ministry/Statistics/book/Pages/default.aspx.

Musaiger, A. O., Bader, Z., Al-Roomi, K., & D'Souza, R. (2011). Dietary and lifestyle habits amongst adolescents in Bahrain. *Food & Nutrition Research*, *55*(1), 7122. https://doi.org/10.3402/fnr.v55i0.7122.

Onion, D. K., & Berrington, R. M. (1999). Comparisons of UK General Practice and US Family Practice. *Journal of the American Board of Family Practice*, *12*(2), 162–172.

Osborn, R., Moulds, D., Schneider, E. C., Doty, M. M., Squires, D., & Sarnak, D. O. (2015). Primary care physicians in ten countries report challenges caring for patients with complex health needs. *Health Affairs*, *34*(12), 2104–2112. https://doi.org/10.1377/hlthaff.2015.1018.

Osman, H., & Romani, M. (2011). Family medicine in Arab countries. *Family Medicine*, *43*(1), 37–42.

Pearson, F., Huangfu, P., Abu-Hijleh, F. M., Awad, S. F., Abu-Raddad, L. J., & Critchley, J. A. (2020). Interventions promoting physical activity among adults and children in the six Gulf Cooperation Council countries: Protocol for a systematic review. *BMJ Open*, *10*(8). https://doi.org/10.1136/bmjopen-2020-037122.

Planning and Statistics Authority (PSA) Qatar. (2019). *Health service statistics.* Available at https://www.psa.gov.qa/en/statistics1/pages/topicslisting.aspx?parent=Social&child=Health.

Pocock, L. (2017). Mental health issues in the Middle East: An overview. *Middle East Journal of Psychiatry and Alzheimers*, *8*(1), 10–15. https://doi.org/10.5742/MEPA.2017.93004.

Qidwai, W., Nanji, K., Khoja, T., Rawaf, S., Kurashi, N., Alnasir, F., Shafaee, M., Shetti, M., Bashir, M., Saad, N. E., Alkaisi, S., Halasa, W., Al-Duwaisan, H., & Al-Ali, A. (2015). Barriers, challenges and way forward for implementation of person centered care model of patient and physician consultation: A survey of patients' perspective from Eastern Mediterranean countries. *Middle East Journal of Family Medicine*, *13*(3), 4–11. https://doi.org/10.5742/MEWFM.2015.92672.

Raffah, E. A., & Alamir, A. M. (2013). Depression among primary health care physicians in Makkah Al-Mukarramah. *American Journal of Research Communication*, *1*(12), 65–82.

Salem, M., Taher, M., Alsaadi, H., Alnema, A., & Al-Abdulla, S. (2018). Prevalence and determinants of burnout among primary healthcare physicians in Qatar. *Middle East Journal of Family Medicine*, *16*(7), 22–28. https://doi.org/10.5742/MEWFM.2018.93474.

Schiess, N., Ibrahim, H., Shaban, S., Perez, M., & Nair, S. (2015). Career choice and primary care in the United Arab Emirates. *Journal of Graduate Medical Education*, *7*(4), 663–666. https://doi.org/10.4300/JGME-D-14-00780.1.

Sebai, Z. A., Milaat, W. A., & Al-Zulaibani, A. A. (2001). Health care services in Saudi Arabia: past, present and future. *Journal of Family and Community Medicine*, *8*(3), 19–23.

Serour, M., Alqhenaei, H., Al-Saqabi, S., Mustafa, A. R., & Ben-Nakhi, A. (2007). Cultural factors and patients' adherence to lifestyle measures. *British Journal of General Practice*, *57*(537), 291–295.

Shaikhan, F., Rawaf, S., Majeed, A., & Hassounah, S. (2018). Knowledge, attitude, perception and practice regarding antimicrobial use in upper respiratory tract infections in Qatar: A systematic review. *Journal of the Royal Society of Medicine Open*, *9*(9). https://doi.org/10.1177/2054270418774971.

Soler, J. K., Yaman, H., Esteva, M., Dobbs, F., Asenova, R. S., & Katic, M. (2008). Burnout in European family doctors: The EGPRN study. *Family Practice*, *25*(4), 245–265. https://doi.org/10.1093/fampra/cmn038.

United Nations (UN). (2017). *Knowledge base of UN public service awards initiatives.* Available at https://publicadministration.un.org/en/Research/Case-Studies/unpsacases/ctl/NominationProfilev2014/mid/1170/id/3903.

Verjee, M., Abdulmalik, M., & Fetters, M. (2013). Family medicine's rapid establishment and early leadership role in Qatar's health care system. *Journal of Healthcare Leadership, 5,* 47–52. https://doi.org/10.2147/JHL.S43715.

Watt, K., Abbott, P., & Reath, J. (2016). Developing cultural competence in general practitioners: An integrative review of the literature. *BMC Family Practice, 17*(1), 158. https://doi.org/10.1186/s12875-016-0560-6.

World Health Organization (WHO). (2003). *Family medicine: report of a regional scientific working group meeting on core curriculum.* Available at https://apps.who.int/iris/bitstream/handle/10665/205046/B3426.pdf?sequence=1&isAllowed=y.

World Health Organization (WHO). (2006). *EMRO – health system profile – Kuwait.* Available at https://rho.emro.who.int/per-country-kwt.

World Health Organization (WHO). (2008). *Oman primary care in action.* Available at https://www.who.int/whr/2008/media_centre/oman.pdf.

World Health Organization (WHO). (2017). *Country cooperation strategy at a glance, Kuwait.* Available at https://apps.who.int/iris/bitstream/handle/10665/136906/ccsbrief_kwt_en.pdf?sequence=1.

World Health Organization (WHO). (2021). *Primary health care.* Available at https://www.who.int/health-topics/primary-health-care#tab=tab_1.

World Organization of Family Doctors (WONCA). (2005). *The European definition of general practice/family medicine.* Available at https://www.woncaeurope.org/page/definition-of-general-practice-family-medicine.

Zowawi, H., Abedalthagafi, M., Mar, F. A., Almalki, T., Kutbi, A. H., Harris-Brown, T., et al. (2015). The potential role of social media platforms in community awareness of antibiotic use in the Gulf Cooperation Council states: Luxury or necessity? *Journal of Medical Internet Research, 17*(10), 1. https://doi.org/10.2196/jmir.3891.

13

PSYCHOLOGICAL SUPPORT

WENDY MADDISON ▪ RAZAN SHAHEEN

CHAPTER OUTLINE

INTRODUCTION

High population growth continues to present a major challenge for the overall provision of healthcare in the Middle East (Abdul Salam et al., 2015; Feuilherade, 2014; Ismail & Hussain, 2018). In addition, conflict, security risks, high unemployment and increasing poverty pose an additional burden for many countries in the region with respect to the provision of mental healthcare and access to services (Merhej, 2019). There is also a recognised shortage of local mental healthcare professionals who are globally oriented yet who can provide appropriate care which is culturally relevant to the context of Arab Islamic sociocultural norms and values (Kain, 2015; Khoja et al., 2017; WHO, 2013, 2018).

For the affluent countries of the Gulf Cooperation Council (GCC) comprising Kuwait, Bahrain, Oman, Qatar, Saudi Arabia and the United Arab Emirates (UAE), psychosocial support has emerged as a priority for local governments (Okasha et al., 2012). With one of the highest population growths in the world, it has been estimated that the demand for psychological services in the GCC countries will rise dramatically in the coming years (Mourshed et al., 2006; Al-Darmaki & Yaaqeib, 2015). National action strategies to address this issue have included integrating mental health into public

health services, training care workers and reaching out into schools. However, overall government healthcare spending remains low, estimated at around 3.8% of the GCC's GDP, below the 10% global average; Saudi Arabia and Bahrain are reported as having the highest expenditure at 3.7% (Khoja et al., 2017) with data remaining scant or unavailable in many Middle Eastern countries. The highest proportion of psychiatrists per capita is reported in Qatar, Bahrain and Kuwait, with indications of rising numbers of psychiatric nurses and social workers in Bahrain, the UAE, Kuwait and Saudi Arabia. However, little data exists on specialist psychosocial therapies and counselling services available in the region, such as addiction and trauma counselling or child psychology, and licensing procedures vary from country to country (Al-Darmaki & Yaaqeib, 2015). In general, there is limited literature published on the provision of mental healthcare services in the Middle East (Alzahrani, 2020; Okasha et al., 2012).

Sociocultural norms and values in the Middle East are based on the tenets of Islam, which inform nearly all aspects of daily life such as education, food, dress, social interactions and healthcare. Religious beliefs can both support mental health but also present a challenge for the treatment of certain conditions as the presentation of particular mental health disorders is intricately braided with the sociocultural background of the individual. Mental health issues are unlike physical illnesses—they are experienced subjectively from the positioning of an individual within his or her own life-world (Smith et al., 2009). A lifeworld consists of lived experiences, relationships and the belief systems that provide a sense of identity and situate a person within their world. As a person's expression of a psychological disorder is therefore understood through the lens of his/her own sociocultural positioning (Hickey et al., 2016), the intricacies of the social–cultural context of the Middle East require unpacking in order to address mental health issues and psychosocial supports available in this particular region.

This chapter will summarise the background to psychosocial support in the Middle East, specifically in the Arabian Gulf countries comprising the GCC. It will address the barriers as well as drivers for local populations to access mental healthcare services as well as provide brief case studies of common therapeutic approaches practiced. The words 'client' and 'patient' are used interchangeably in the chapter to describe the person seeking psychosocial support. The chapter will conclude with recommendations to improve the provision of psychosocial support in the region.

BACKGROUND TO PSYCHOSOCIAL SUPPORT IN THE ARAB WORLD

A 'therapy of the psyche' (Sarhan, 2018) has historically been of medical interest in the Arab world and heralded the establishment of the first psychiatric hospitals in the region. A system of psychological healing evolved in different locations of the Middle East, mostly based on traditional herbal medicine and influenced by Islamic religious practice which over time became a prescribed 'formula' (Al-Krenawi & Graham, 2000). Mental health disorders have traditionally been treated through diverse practices such as mind-body therapy, herbs, diet, meditation, specific prayers, chanting and other religious incantations, with acts of spiritual healing performed by self-proclaimed healers (Alrawi & Fetters, 2012). Such practices are typically scaffolded around local established customs and not based on the tenets of Islam.

The role of traditional and self-proclaimed religious healers can be important in Middle Eastern communities; long established healing methods which include spiritual and religious interventions are still often an integral part of a person's treatment prior to seeking specialised medical or therapeutic assistance (WHO, 2013). WHO (2013) defines traditional medicine as 'the sum total of knowledge, skills and practices based on the theories, beliefs and experiences indigenous to different cultures that are used to maintain health as well as to prevent, diagnose, improve or treat physical and mental illnesses' (p. 1). The philosophy of traditional Arab Islamic medicine focuses on the body and mind as being mutually dependent, which is in tension with Western ideas of the management of mental health, based on the Cartesian dualism of separation of the body and mind. However, there have been challenges to the Western perspective; for example, Engel's (1977) biopsychosocial model of healthcare supports an approach which focuses on the interlinked psychological and social factors that impact biological functioning, and the field of psychoneuroimmunology (Ader, 2001) explores the correlation between the mind and susceptibility to illness, thereby narrowing the gap between Eastern and Western philosophies of mental health.

Arab society is collectivist in nature and family oriented in structure, usually with a male at the head of family decision-making (Badran, 2009). Cultural identity and family dynamics play a major role in therapy experiences, treatment acceptance and efficacy. There are topics that are directly and indirectly discussed within therapeutic settings, such as family rules and sociocultural expectations. Family members would typically be involved in decision-making regarding the health of one of their kin and may even expect to attend consultation sessions with that family member in the role of a 'co-therapist' (El-Islam, 2008). This is an important consideration in inpatient settings where families are actively involved in many steps of the therapeutic process such as medications and length of treatment (Case Study 13.1). Taking a Western perspective of patient or client empowerment in decision-making for his/her own treatment plan without involving family members would be considered an insult (Okasha, 2008) in this cultural context.

Outside of the therapeutic setting, family involvement can greatly influence the success or failure of treatment. Family support in dealing with mental health issues can be empowering and quintessential

CASE STUDY 13.1
AN EXAMPLE OF FAMILY INVOLVEMENT IN PATIENT THERAPY

A female Saudi teenager diagnosed with bulimia nervosa was admitted into inpatient psychiatric care at a private hospital in Bahrain for self-harm. Her treatment plan included an inpatient stay in the hospital for 2 weeks with daily group and/or individual therapy. Medication was a significant part of the treatment plan. The patient had a primary psychologist and psychiatrist coordinating her care.

Upon admission, the patient underwent a psychiatric evaluation. Interviews with the patient's family, both with the patient's presence and absence, were conducted as part of the admission procedure. It was important that there was family consent to admit the teenager for inpatient care as well as the treatment plan, such as discussing the length of stay, psycho-education regarding the diagnosis as well as medication prescribed and an outline of the therapy to be conducted. If the family was not in agreement with a specific part of the treatment plan, it would become a family matter and discussed with the psychiatrist.

For this particular patient, the family did not initially want their daughter to take psychiatric medication; they raised concerns about her being too young, not wanting her to become reliant on medication and were anxious about what people would think if they found out that their daughter was receiving psychiatric treatment. The psychiatrist's role then included educating the patient's family on the aspects of treatment, validating their concerns and working within the realm of their family and cultural dynamics, whilst at the same time gently challenging cultural taboos and ensuring that the family agreed to what was in the best interest of the patient from a healthcare perspective.

Facilitating and fostering healthy communication between the patient and family by teaching them emotion regulation skills was essential as well as maintaining close involvement of the family in the patient's care plan. Attuning and exploring family rules and expectations also became a core function of the patient's healing. Upon discharge from the psychiatric facility, the patient continued to meet with the psychiatrist and psychologist for another 2 months on a bi-weekly basis, supported by her family.

CASE STUDY 13.2
EXAMPLES OF POSITIVE AND NEGATIVE FAMILY INFLUENCE ON TREATMENT PLANS

Two Bahraini clients, both female and married, had presented with obsessive compulsive disorder (OCD). Both had similar presentation and moderate severity of symptoms, such as recurring and unrelenting thoughts and/or urges regarding cleanliness causing significant emotional distress. Patient A could not sleep until she brushed her teeth seven times, believing that if she did not do this, something bad would happen to her family. Patient B would not allow items from the external environment into the house (such as groceries or food delivery) unless everything coming into the house had been thoroughly disinfected. Attempts to ignore or censor these intrusive thoughts and urges only proved successful after performing a ritualistic action, such as showering frequently. Both patients presented the obsessive theme of cleanliness, which was negatively impacting their lives and that of their families and friends around them.

Patient A had access to family support and could return to her family home for a break. Her family was in constant contact with both her and her husband, offering emotional support. The family could understand the current situation as they had previous experience in dealing with her OCD in the past. Patient A found safety in the support of her family and staying in her familiar childhood room in her family home when needed. She found that the severity of her symptoms declined when she stayed with her family. Her treatment involved couple's therapy, individual therapy and medication. She found a significant alleviation of her symptoms after 3 months of intensive treatment.

Patient B, however, lived with her husband and two children. Due to the COVID-19 pandemic at the time, her family did not wish to interact or visit her. Patient B reported feeling isolated and alone during the pandemic and felt that her family did not want to deal with her issues. Feelings of abandonment and being a burden became an added theme to the therapy, in addition to the presenting OCD. Patient B felt stressed by her caretaking responsibilities in her own family, which exasperated her OCD symptoms. She was also seeing a psychiatrist and reported shame in having to take medication. Her treatment included individual therapy and separate support sessions with her husband; he declined to speak in front of her about how he was feeling. As the pandemic continued, she became increasingly hesitant about therapy and ultimately terminated therapy early. Lack of support from others in her life greatly influenced her negative engagement with therapy and the ultimate lack of success in her treatment.

for accessing treatment, intervention and healing. Case Study 13.2 demonstrates treatment outcomes of two different patients, one with a positive family support network and the other without a positive family network.

Issues such as shame, family honour, sex relations, social positioning, modesty and the concepts of 'haram'

CASE STUDY 13.3
LIVING IN AN 'UNAUTHENTIC' WAY

The client in this case study is a 23-year-old Bahraini female living at home with her family. The client's presenting concern at a therapy session was severe anxiety, as evidenced by constant worrying, difficulty controlling the worry, feeling on edge, becoming easily fatigued, irritability and muscle tension. Upon building rapport, the client revealed that she is in a committed relationship with another woman.

The client explained the pressure she felt when lying to her mother and living in an 'unauthentic' way, not acceptable to mainstream Islamic society. She reported that she revealed her sexual orientation and 'came out' to two of her three siblings a couple years ago. Both siblings were kind and accepting. A part of the therapy included processing the anger and disappointment of not living the life the client wanted, due to sociocultural and religious expectations. The client was supported in mourning the loss of not being able to freely inhabit her imagined ideal life. She reported that needing to protect her mother, who was a widow, was more important than being able to live how she wished. The client was afraid that if her mother found out, she would be shocked and become ill.

Processing anxiety using cognitive behavioural therapy (CBT) and STST was helpful for this client, specifically managing expectations within herself and changing strict inflexible family rules to guidelines; this helped the client to find a way to situate herself and operate from a place of authenticity and to rebuild her sense of self-worth and autonomy.

(what is taboo) and 'halal' (what is permitted) according to religious and sociocultural norms are examples of important cultural signifiers to consider in the Arab Islamic world when developing an appropriately contexualised treatment plan (Case Study 13.3). Therapeutic interventions and theories such as Satir Transformational Systemic Therapy (STST), Family Systems Theory and Attachment Theory can be helpful lenses to employ when approaching therapeutic practices in the Middle East.

Sex norms also influence help-seeking behaviour in the Arab world. Within the Arab culture, the definitions of femininity and masculinity have help-seeking expectations rooted within them. The concept of masculinity can be an inhibiting factor which prevents Arab men from seeking psychological support. In the role of a traditional head of the family, Arab males are not expected to show displays of emotion and to 'man up' or 'tough it out' (Alhomaizi et al., 2018). The concept of femininity in the Arab tradition is more

favourable towards help-seeking behaviours; from the patriarchal viewpoint of Arab society, females are considered emotional, therefore weak (Alhomaizi et al., 2018) and need to be cared for. These stereotyped roles and characteristics however often prove burdensome to both males and females. Social and religious norms also constrain what is 'haram' and 'halal' in constructions of alternative identities and genders.

For example, Islam prohibits homosexual practices and there are laws varying from fines to jail sentences to the death penalty as punishment for homosexual acts. The topic of LGBTQ+ continues to be a sensitive topic in the Middle East and there is stigma and shame attached to identifying with this community. The stigma can be internalised (e.g. internalised homophobia) or externalised (e.g. 'outing' someone by non-consensually revealing their identity) and exacerbated by the weight of religious constraints and societal expectations. Expectations, conventions and norms are woven around social institutions such as marriage. Marriage is defined as a union between a male and a female; it is a religious duty and a sacred union (Jaafar-Mohammad & Lehmann, 2011). Sexual activity outside of marriage is 'haram'. Islam prohibits any premarital physical relations in heterosexual relationships, punishable by law. There can also be grave consequences for a family's reputation in the community if a family member is discovered to be in a relationship outside of marriage.

Feelings of shame, guilt, hiding and protecting parents and other family members from the disappointing revelation that a person is homosexual or non-conforming is common. Resentment is often expressed towards the family and society at large, guilt for lying and shame for being different. The goal of therapy in such cases is to work through whatever the client brings up as a concern; not all clients who identify as non-conforming will want to work through their sexuality, but when or if they do, it is imperative for the therapist/counsellor to be unbiased, non-judgemental and aware of the restraints of Arab Islamic values placed on those who do not conform to expected norms.

BARRIERS AND DRIVERS FOR PSYCHOSOCIAL SUPPORT

In a recent systematic review of psychosocial studies in Middle Eastern Arab countries (Al-Sawafi et al.,

2020), more barriers were identified than drivers of help-seeking behaviours. Some of these are evident, such as limited access to psychological support in war-torn countries due to lack of trained mental healthcare practitioners or limited outpatient facilities available in public hospitals or clinics. Others are more nuanced and outlined below.

Firstly, a major barrier to accessing treatment and therapy is the underlying cultural beliefs, norms and practices of clients. If these are not recognised and addressed, clients will not seek or engage in professional mental healthcare support services. A client's preference towards religious or traditional healing may result in non-adherence to a psychosocial intervention (Townsend et al., 2002). In cognitive behavioural therapy (CBT) sessions, for example, the client is guided to analyse thoughts, feelings and behaviours whilst developing rational, self-counselling skills. The client is positioned as exercising active agency during therapy sessions and independently taking decisions as the owner of his/her treatment plan. However, a very different assumption of client positioning is taken when employing traditional healing tools such as prayer or herbal treatments to solve a mental health problem as the client passively depends on faith, religious doctrine and traditional interventions performed by a third party—often a self-proclaimed religious leader or 'imam'. An awareness and understanding of a patient or client's belief system, religious sect and alternative possible treatments related to religion, such as the importance of prayer or meditation, can facilitate discussion between the counsellor or therapist and the patient and his/her family (Case Study 13.1), thereby establishing the necessary rapport for the implementation of a more effective treatment plan (Al Bedah et al., 2013).

The supernatural plays an important role in the explanation of psychological disorders. Evil spirits called 'Jin' can possess the body and the focus of an 'evil eye' on an individual can cause harm, including emotional and physical distress (Ahmad et al., 2016) as well as physical illness. Self-proclaimed religious and traditional healers may suggest treatments ranging from citing specific verses from the Holy Quran to exorcise the 'Jin' or ward off the evil eye, to physically shocking a 'Jin' to exit the body and mind, such as a sudden burn inflicted by a hot instrument to surprise the 'Jin'.

Healthcare practitioners in the region need to be aware of such traditional practices as there can be unintended consequences to a patient's health such as septicaemia arising from an untreated burn as a result of traditional psychosocial healing practices. Time is often lost in such cases before an individual may access the professional treatment required. Having a trusted and reliable self-proclaimed religious leader on call or to refer clients to for specific religious concerns or explanations is a therapeutic recommendation for counsellors or therapists working in the Middle East, as it is preferable to separate religious ideology from psychosocial therapy. Cooperation between mental health professionals and self-proclaimed religious leaders can be helpful in reducing stigma as well as possibly reducing the time and increasing the likelihood of a patient receiving appropriate professional care. It is important to note that religious leaders are not qualified to provide treatment interventions; however, the support from a significant person within the religious community can be helpful towards the goal of getting the patient appropriate and timely professional help.

Stigma is a major barrier to addressing psychological disorders in Arab society. Stigmatisation is the result of negative prejudgement by others based on limited or incorrect assumptions. It results in labelling, prejudice, stereotyping and discrimination, which can lead to low self-esteem and shame, negatively impacting a sense of identity (Zolezzi et al., 2018). There is often stigmatisation of people who seek psychological support outside the cultural boundaries of traditional healers or against advice from family members. Cultural expectations of conformity to religious or cultural norms and the feeling of having failed the family due to mental health illness can weigh heavily, resulting in guilt and further stress. Additionally, many Arab families tend to impose the rule of 'what happens in the family, stays in the family', adding to the feelings experienced of isolation, shame and stigma. Many patients report feeling like they are 'cheating' on their families when going to a therapist; undoing the knot of shame and guilt for sharing family secrets becomes an additional barrier to the therapy.

Arab females, in particular, state that stressors related to family responsibilities and work have increased as a result of the COVID-19 pandemic, leading to a greater incidence of stress being reported

(Arab Youth Survey, 2020) (Case Study 13.2), but this does not necessarily correlate to an increase in the number of females seeking professional help. A recent survey on Arab youth reported that nearly half of the respondents viewed help-seeking behaviours for mental health issues as negative and over half expressed difficulty in accessing mental healthcare services (Arab Youth Survey, 2020). Access issues may be related to the fact that psychological and psychiatric services should typically be hidden and not visible or promoted within the community (Al Adawi et al., 2002). In a study located in Bahrain, Meer et al. (2013) demonstrated that the less experience local GPs in Bahrain had with patients with mental illnesses, the more they believed that treatment should be confined to hospitals, not in health centres or clinics. Such beliefs serve to perpetuate stigma about mental health illness and discourage help-seeking behaviours. The de-stigmatisation of mental health illness must be a priority to ensure access to timely and effective treatment (Ciftci et al., 2013).

Reputation, social status and fear of judgement and stigmatising gossip within communities can also prevent individuals seeking treatment and many will consult with a foreign counsellor rather than a local practitioner who speaks Arabic as they perceive this will maintain their privacy and confidentiality (Scull et al., 2014). In private clinic settings, it is not uncommon to have clients ask their therapist to leave a gap between appointments or have the therapist ensure there is no one in the waiting area in order to reduce the likelihood of running into someone they may know. However, for psychological therapies, in particular the 'talking' therapies, patients or clients speaking Arabic are required to fluently express themselves in the language of the foreign therapist, usually in English, in order to be understood. This raises the topic of the language barrier. As language is intricately bound to culture, difficulties may arise in expression of history by the client and comprehension by the therapist, resulting in an incorrect diagnosis or ineffective treatment plan. Furthermore, many mental healthcare professionals in the GCC region in particular are from overseas, with various training backgrounds and qualifications; thus quality of service may be inconsistent (Al Bedah et al., 2013). Additionally, non-Arab counsellors or therapists who are new to the region may make culturally insensitive suggestions, such as encouraging an unmarried female to live alone and move out of a conflictual environment at home, or to live 'authentically' despite the consequences from a family, religious and cultural perspective (Case Study 13.3). Communication issues can also cause problems when applying a standard diagnostic tool in the Arab world, such as the Diagnostic and Statistical Manual of Mental Disorders, Fifth Edition (DSM-5). Due to possible cultural differences in the expression and interpretation of meaning, it is important that psychometric tests are developed to address the region's specific sociocultural context (Bashmi & Amirkhan, 2018).

The extended family structure of many Arab families can be conducive to providing support to family members suffering from mental health issues, but as treatment becomes a 'family matter' (Okasha, 2008, p. 94) there also is a risk that timely professional assistance may not be sought. Little information exists on successful culturally adapted family interventions (Al-Sawafi et al., 2020). Similarly, religion, and in particular prayer, is an important anchor for positive mental health and adhering to religion can protect an individual from self-harm. Committing certain acts such as suicide are considered 'haram' or taboo and also considered illegal in some countries in the Middle East. In Bahrain for example, the police are called when a suicide attempt is reported and the patient has to complete a police report at the police station after a suicide attempt. This greatly adds to the feelings of guilt, shame and stigma and disempowers a vulnerable person in seeking help. However, being religious has also been positively associated with lower rates of death, anxiety and substance abuse (Hickey et al., 2016), although forced compliance can also cause stress. For example, behaviours that are forbidden and against religious teachings such as alcohol abuse, promiscuity or self-harm may also lead to greater feelings of low self-worth, guilt and depression (Alzahrani, 2020).

An under-researched and at-risk group in the GCC in particular is that of migrant workers. It is estimated that there are over 15 million expatriate workers in the region, with the UAE and Qatar employing more than 90% of its workforce from overseas (Kamrava et al., 2011). Indian nationals, followed by workers from Pakistan, Bangladesh, Philippines and Sri Lanka make up most of this workforce; most are male and are employed as labourers in the construction industry (Kapiszewski, 2006). These workers are often illiterate and poorly paid. They are attracted to work in the afflu-ent GCC countries so they can provide a better life for families often left behind for years, but many end up in very unfavourable conditions and do not know where to go for help. They face serious mental health issues including adjustment disorders, mood disorders, psy-chosis and suicide (Kronfol et al., 2014). Many reports are made in the local press regarding high rates of psy-chosis and suicide amongst this group of workers, but there are few psychosocial interventions available to support this underprivileged group. Although manda-tory health insurance now has to be paid by employers in many GCC countries to cover healthcare costs for workers, this does not always cover access to mental health services and treatment. A larger number of sys-tematic studies are required to understand the grave issues faced by migrant workers and relevant legislation implemented to protect this at-risk group.

SUMMARY AND TAKEAWAY POINTS

To promote help-seeking behaviours for psychoso-cial support and to improve the quality of mental healthcare in the Middle East, the following is rec-ommended:

- Development of a culturally competent and non-stigmatising model of mental healthcare, which takes into account religious and sociocultural values and concerns of local populations and promotes help-seeking behaviours in context.
- Reframing mental health discourse in the Middle East through the creation of spaces for cooperation between mental health professionals and local reli-gious leaders and healers to reduce stigma in seek-ing professional care for mental health issues.
- Implementation of Arabic language models of diagnostic tools and measurements as an alterna-tive to Western models of assessment tools.
- A focus on culturally appropriate services and treatments for effective psychosocial support delivered by culturally competent healthcare professionals who appreciate the importance of traditional beliefs, social roles and lifeworlds of individuals in this geographical and sociocul-tural context and who can refer to these as part of the therapeutic process.

- To draw up national standards and guidelines for a consistent quality of mental healthcare with appropriate levels of funding. This includes a focus on providing increased levels of support for at-risk groups, such as migrant workers.
- To undertake further research into the interplay between psychosocial support and traditional healing methods. Recommendations should be drawn up for different treatment modalities fit for context. Such modalities would consider par-ticular issues confronting the diverse populations of the Arab world and include cultural practices, such as prayer, as part of therapy.

REFERENCES

Abdul Salam, A., Elsegaey, I., Khraif, R., AlMutairi, A., & Aldosari, A. (2015). Components and public health impact of population growth in the Arab world. *PloS ONE*, *10*(5), e0124944. https://doi.org/10.1371/journal.pone.0124944.

Ader, R. (2001). Psychoneuroimmunology. *Current Directions in Psychological Science*, *10*(3), 94–98. https://doi.org/10.1111/1467-8721.00124.

Ahmad, S. A., El-Jabali, A., & Salam, Y. (2016). Mental health and the Muslim world. *Journal of Community Medicine & Health Education*, *6*(445). https://doi.org/10.4172/2161-0711.1000445.

Al Adawi, S., Dorvlo, A. S., Al-Ismaily, S. S., Al-Ghafry, D. A., A-Nloobi, B. Z., Al-Salmi, A., et al. (2002). Perception of and attitude towards mental illness in Oman. *International Journal of Social Psychiatry*, *48*(4), 305–317. https://doi.org/10.1177/002076402128783334.

Al Bedah, A. M., Hussein, A. A., El Olemy, A. T., Khalil, M., & Al Subai, I. (2013). Knowledge and attitudes of the public, primary health care physicians and other health professionals, and policy makers towards religious medical practices. *Majmaah Journal of Health Sciences*, *1*(2), 14–21.

Al-Darmaki, F. & Yaaqeib, S.I. (2015). Psychology and mental health services in the United Arab Emirates. *Psychology International*, (6).

Alhomaizi, D., Alsaidi, S., Moalie, A., Muradwij, N., Borba, C. P., & Lincoln, A. K. (2018). An exploration of the help-Seeking behaviors of Arab-muslims in the US: A socio-ecological approach. *Journal of Muslim Mental Health*, *12*(1). https://doi.org/10.3998/jmmh.10381607.0012.102.

Al-Krenawi, A., & Graham, J. R. (2000). Culturally sensitive social work practice with Arab clients in mental health settings. *Health and Social Work*, *25*(1), 9–22. https://doi.org/10.1093/hsw/25.1.9.

Alrawi, S. N., & Fetters, M. D. (2012). Traditional Arabic and Islamic medicine: A conceptual model for clinicians and researchers. *Global journal of health science*, *4*(3), 164–169. https://doi.org/10.5539/gjhs.v4n3p164.

Al-Sawafi, A., Lovell, K., Renwick, L., & Husain, N. (2020). Psychosocial family interventions for relatives of people living with psychotic disorders in the Arab world: Systematic review. *BMC Psychiatry*, *20*(1), 413. https://doi.org/10.1186/s12888-020-02816-5.

Alzahrani, O. (2020). Depressive disorders in the Arabian Gulf Cooperation Council countries: A literature review. *Journal of International Medical Research*, 48(10). https://doi.org/10.1177/0300060520961917.

Arab Youth Survey (2020). A Voice for Change. ASDA'A BCW. Available at https://arab.org/blog/arab-youth-survey-2020/.

Badran, M. (2009). *Feminism in Islam: Secular and Religious Convergences*. Oxford: Oneworld.

Bashmi, L., & Amirkhan, J. (2018). Constructing an Arabic language version of the Stress Overload Scale (SOS). *Arab Journal of Psychology*, 5, 167–206.

Ciftci, A., Jones, N., & Corrigan, P. W. (2013). Mental health stigma in the Muslim community. *Journal of Muslim Mental Health*, 7(1), 17–32. Available at www.researchgate.net/publication/288623548_Mental_health_stigma_in_the_Muslim_community. Accessed 17 August 2023.

El-Islam, M. F. (2008). Arab culture and mental health care. *Transcultural Psychiatry*, 45(4), 671–682. https://doi.org/10.1177/1363461508100788.

Engel, G. (1977). The need for a new medical model: A challenge for biomedical science. *Science*, 196 126–9.

Feuilherade, P. (2014). GCC healthcare spending surges as demand soars. *Middle East*, 453, 38–39.

Hickey, J. E., Pryjmachuk, S., & Waterman, H. (2016). Mental illness research in the Gulf Cooperation Council: A scoping review. *Health Research Policy and Systems*, 14–59. https://doi.org/10.1186/s12961-016-0123-2.

Ismail, M., & Hussain, S. (2018). Long-term care policies in the Gulf Region: A case study of Oman. *Journal of Aging and Social Policy*, 31(4). https://doi.org/10.1080/08959420.2018.1485392.

Jaafar-Mohammad, I., & Lehmann, C. (2011). Women's rights in Islam regarding marriage and divorce. *Journal of Law and Practice*, 4, 3. Available at http://open.mitchellhamline.edu/lawandpractice/vol4/iss1/3. Accessed 17 August 2023.

Kain, V. J. (2015). Internationalisation of the curriculum in an undergraduate nursing degree. In w GreenC. (2015). Witsed (Eds.), *Critical Perspectives on Internationalising the Curriculum in Disciplines. Global Perspectives on Higher Education* (Vol. 28). Rotterdam: Sense Publishes.

Kamrava, M., Babar, Z., Ahmad, A., Gardner, A., Bristol-Rhys, J., et al. (2011). Migrant labor in the Gulf: Working Group summary report. Center for International and Regional Studies. Available at https://ssrn.com/abstract=2839146. Accessed 20 September 2023.

Kapiszewski, A. (2006). Arab versus Asian migrant workers in the GCC countries, United Nations Expert Group Meeting on International Migration and Development in the Arab Region, Beirut. Available at https://www.un.org/en/development/desa/population/events/pdf/expert/11/P02_Kapiszweski.pdf.

Khoja, T., Rawaf, S., Qidwai, W., Rawaf, D., Nanji, K., & Hamad, A. (2017). Health care in Gulf Cooperation Council countries: A review of challenges and opportunities. *Cureus*, 9(8), e1586. https://doi.org/10.7759/cureus.1586.

Kronfol, Z., Saleh, M., & Al-Ghafry, M. (2014). Mental health issues among migrant workers in Gulf Cooperation Council countries: Literature review and case illustrations. *Asian Journal of Psychiatry*, 10, 109–113.

Meer, S. H., Kamel, C. A., AlFaraj, A. I., & Kamel, E. (2013). Attitude of primary healthcare physicians to mental illness in Bahrain. *The Arab Journal of Psychiatry*, 24(2) 142–7.

Merhej, R. (2019). Stigma on mental illness in the Arab world: Beyond the socio-cultural barriers. *International Journal of Human Rights in Healthcare*, 12(4), 285–298. Available at https://doi.org/10.1108/IJHRH-03-2019-0025.

Mourshed M., Hediger V., & Lambert T. (2006). Gulf Cooperation Council Health Care: Challenges and Opportunities. Chapter 2.1. Available at https://citeseerx.ist.psu.edu/document?repid=rep1&type=pdf&doi=24e92be9322e58156f53e7af9aa148e309ea4e94.

Okasha, A. (2008). The impact of Arab culture on psychiatric ethics. *The Arab Journal of Psychiatry*, 19(2), 81–99. Available at https://arabjournalpsychiatry.com/wp-content/uploads/2015/12/journal_nov_2008_01.pdf. Accessed 2 August 2023.

Okasha, A., Karam, E., & Okasha, T. (2012). Mental health services in the Arab world. *World Psychiatry*, 11(1), 52–54.

Sarhan, W. (2018). The contribution of Arab Islamic civilization to mental health. *The Arab Journal of Psychiatry*, 29(1), 57–66. Available at https://search.emarefa.net/detail/BIM-826429. Accessed 10 August 2023.

Scull, N. C., Khullar, N., Al-Awadhi, N., & Erheim, R. (2014). A qualitative study of the perceptions of mental health care in Kuwait. *International Perspectives in Psychology: Research, Practice, Consultation*, 3(4), 284–299. https://doi.org/10.1037/ipp0000023.

Smith, J. A., Flowers, P., & Larkin, M. (2009). *Interpretative Phenomenological Analysis: Theory, Method and Research*. London: Sage publications.

Townsend, M., Kladder, V., Ayele, H., & Mulligan, T. (2002). Systematic review of clinical trials examining the effects of religion on health. *Southern Medical Journal*, 95(12), 1429–1434.

World Health Organisation (WHO)., (2013).): *Mental Health Action Plan 2013-2020*. Geneva: World Health Organisation.

World Health Organisation (WHO)., (2018). *Mental Health Atlas 2017*. Geneva: World Health Organization. Available at https://www.who.int/publications/i/item/9789241514019.

Zolezzi, M., Alamri, M., Shaar., S., & Rainkie, D. (2018). Stigma associated with mental illness and its treatment in the Arab culture: A systematic review. *International Journal of Social Psychiatry*, 64(6), 597–609. https://doi.org/10.1177/0020764018789200.

Section II KEY HEALTHCARE APPROACHES

SECTION OUTLINE

This section of the text outlines generic approaches as well as a range of issues specific to the region.

14

PHARMACY IN THE ARABIAN GULF AND GREATER MIDDLE EAST

STEPHANIE ANNETT ■ NOON ABUBAKR ADBELRAHMAN KAMIL

INTRODUCTION

In the modern age, globally pharmacy education and practice are undergoing a significant transformation to reflect a more patient-centred, interprofessional approach to practice. Pharmacists are moving beyond dispensing medicines to more advanced integrated medicines management services (Toklu & Hussain, 2013). In the Arab world, advancements in pharmacy practice have been slower than in Europe, Asia and the Americas due to cultural, logistical and legal barriers (Al-Ghananeem et al., 2018). This is less so in the economically developed Arab countries where pharmacy as an academic discipline has enjoyed growth and maturation that resembles other parts of the world (Al-Ghananeem et al., 2018). In contrast, in countries affected by conflict and/or a poor economy, pharmacy practice has stalled or even regressed (Al-Ghananeem et al., 2018). Despite the adversity faced by pharmacy academics and practitioners alike, there is a strong and uniform desire to advance the science and practice of pharmacy in the region collectively (Al-Ghananeem et al., 2018).

PHARMACEUTICAL SUPPLY

There are large differences among Arab countries in terms of demographics and economic indicators. Health systems may be predominately private, such as in Lebanon, or public health systems with general health insurance coverage such as in Kuwait (Hasan et al., 2019). In some countries such as Saudi Arabia and Qatar, patients receive free medication from the public sector but in others such as Jordan or Yemen, patients pay for their medications in both the private and public sectors (Hasan et al., 2019). Most countries procure a mix of original (branded) and generic medicines for their public health sector. Many Arab countries encourage and support their national medication manufacturing by reducing the prices of the locally manufactured generic medications by 20% or more in comparison to the original branded medications (Hasan et al., 2019).

Saudi Arabia is the largest pharmaceutical market in the region and local pharmaceutical manufacturing has grown dramatically with 27 pharmaceutical manufacturing plants registered in 2017. However, local manufacturing is only estimated to cover approximately 20%–25% of the Kingdom's consumption of prescription drugs and most local production is destined for export markets (Alruthia et al., 2018). Jordan has a well-established local pharmaceutical manufacturing sector which has grown rapidly since 1970 (Nazer & Tuffaha, 2017). It covers approximately 25% of the country's requirements and the rest of the medications are imported (Nazer & Tuffaha, 2017).

SUBSTANDARD AND FALSIFIED MEDICINES

Pharmaceuticals are particularly vulnerable to counterfeiting and no country is unaffected by this issue. However, low- and middle-income countries and those in areas of conflict bear the greatest burden. The World Health Organization (WHO) estimates that around 10% of all global pharmaceutical supply is counterfeit and/or substandard, reaching up to 50% of the supply in developing countries and as low as 1% in the developed world (Alghannam et al., 2014). These medicines impact negatively on global health, individual patient safety and may cause death (Mackey & Liang, 2011). Furthermore, contamination of the global drug chain has led to increased antimicrobial resistance in the treatment of malaria, HIV and tuberculosis (Mackey & Liang, 2011). Indeed, there are up to 155,000 childhood deaths annually due to falsified antimalarial drugs in sub-Saharan Africa (Renschler et al., 2015). Substandard and counterfeit medicines also cause macroeconomic burdens worldwide by wasting limited resources, causing loss of productivity and limiting the investment of pharmaceutical companies (Alghannam et al., 2014).

In 2017, WHO Member States designated 'Substandard and Falsified medical products' as the appropriate nomenclature (Box 14.1). This greatly simplifies the previous confusing designation of 'substandard/spurious/falsely labelled/falsified/counterfeit medical products'.

Substandard and falsified (S/F) anti-infective agents, in particular antimalarial drugs, have been studied extensively because of their immediate impact on disease burden and drug resistance (Nayyar et al., 2012). Drugs for treating cardiovascular disease, cancer and other non-communicable conditions are also at risk of falsification, particularly if there is high market demand

BOX 14.1
World Health Organization (2017) Definition

- *Falsified medical products* are those that deliberately or fraudulently misrepresent their identity, composition or source; these products are produced and distributed with criminal intent.
- *Substandard medical products* are issued by national regulatory authorities but fail to meet national or international quality standards or specifications; these products frequently have low active pharmaceutical ingredients or dissolution properties.

and they are sold at less than retail prices (Nayyar et al., 2019). Lifestyle compounds for erectile dysfunction such as sildenafil (Viagra) dominate the falsified drug market (Nayyar et al., 2019). Many of these products are virtually indistinguishable from bona fide compounds (Nayyar et al., 2019). Vaccines are also susceptible to falsifying and this poses significant risks to disease control programmes (Nayyar et al., 2019). Criminals may sell counterfeits at high prices for chronic diseases in developed countries and at cheaper prices for essential medicines to treat communicable diseases in resource-poor countries. In addition, the prevalence of counterfeits in a geographical region varies and is split between urban and rural areas (Mackey & Liang, 2011).

Prevalence in Arabic Countries

A systematic review of the global prevalence of S/F medicines noted there were limited published reports in the Middle East (Alghannam et al,. 2014). An unsettled political situation is a frequent catalyst for S/F medicines and it is widely recognised that falsified medicines in Yemen are a serious problem, although reports differ in their prevalence. The Yemeni government report that S/F medicines account for not more than 10% (Al-Worafi, 2014); however, the Yemen Pharmacists Syndicate estimate that the prevalence is around 60%, with cardiovascular medications, sexual medications, antimalarial products, antiepileptic medications, psychiatric medications and analgesics being the most common (Al-Worafi, 2020).

Saudi Arabia is one of the most economically developed countries within the region and although the data is limited, one report estimates the prevalence of S/F medicines to be around 30%–40% with cardiovascular and sexual health medicines being the most common (Al-Worafi, 2020). Furthermore, a prospective observational study conducted in the arrival terminal at King Abdulaziz International Airport, Jeddah, for 2 weeks during Hajj indicated that 34.4% of medicines were S/F in 2005 and 49.3% were S/F in 2006 (Alsultan, 2010). The majority of the medications were brought from South East Asia, India, Pakistan and African countries (Alsultan, 2010).

Contributing Factors and Potential Solutions

The following factors are core contributors to the prevalence of S/F medicines:

■ **High costs of official medicines or supply cannot meet the demand:**

In Yemen, for example, the pharmaceutical industry cannot meet the demand which leads to some pharmacies not buying medicines from their original manufacturer (Al-Worafi, 2014). In addition, many original medicines are not available in Yemen and are very expensive compared with neighbouring countries such as Saudi Arabia and poverty pushes patients towards the cheaper S/F medicines (Al-Worafi, 2014). The Yemen Community Pharmacy Syndicate have an initiative to launch a local pharmaceutical factory in order to locally make medication at affordable prices to solve the shortage of medication in Yemen and minimise the need for smuggling S/F medications (Al-Worafi, 2020).

■ **Lack of drug regulatory authorities, legislations and strict enforcement:**

Substandard and falsified (S/F) medications flourish in an environment where there is little monitoring of the supply chain, minimal punishment for supplying/selling S/F medicines, a lack of regulation and misuse of advanced technology to produce high-quality packaging to mimic the real medicines. The Saudi Food and Drug Authority (SFDA) initiated the Drug Track and Trace System for pharmaceutical products which aims to adopt a technology for tracking all human registered drugs manufactured in Saudi Arabia and imported from abroad (Al-Worafi, 2020; Alhawassi et al., 2018).

■ **Use of the Internet and mail to deliver and sell medicines, which provides an opportunity for sellers to sell their counterfeit products:**

There is a high risk that patients could unknowingly buy S/F medicines online from organised crime groups, especially in countries with weak legislative laws or enforcement on governing the controls of S/F medicines. In addition, because of extensive intermediaries and suppliers across the globe, online pharmacies and the illegal sale of medicines, it is difficult for law enforcement agencies to control. In the UAE, law enforcement regulations work alongside strategic partners such as customs and the Ministry of Interior and Telecommunications Regulatory Authority (TRA) with the specific aim of preventing the online S/F medicines market (Al-Worafi, 2020).

■ **The complexity of formal pharmaceutical transactions, such as the presence of more than one wholesaler, thereby lengthening the supply chain system and thus increasing the chances of S/F medicine permeation:**

To ensure defence against S/F medicines, the regulatory agencies and pharmaceutical industry need to strengthen national systems globally throughout the supply chain, from manufacturer to bedside. A broad-based strategy is needed across nations, rich and poor to build capacity and extend collaboration (Nayyar et al., 2019).

■ **Lack of public and healthcare professional's awareness of the harmful effects of counterfeit medications:**

Jordan has adopted several strategies to tackle counterfeit medicines through education of the public, healthcare professionals and manufacturers. This included the use of public media campaigns to report suspected S/F medicines, reduce taxes on genuine medicines to make them more affordable and encouraging manufacturers to establish physical and chemical identifiers in their products (Al-Worafi, 2020).

SCOPE OF PRACTICE OF PHARMACIST

The scope of practice for pharmacists is defined by the American Pharmacist Association (APhA) as the 'boundaries within which a pharmacist may practice'. The scope of pharmacy practice in the Arabian Gulf and Greater Middle East is more limited in comparison with the expanded scope of practice in developed countries such as North America and Europe. Information on the scope of pharmacy practice in the region is somewhat patchy; however, several articles have reported experiences in countries including UAE, Qatar and Saudi Arabia (Al-Jedai et al., 2016; Dameh, 2009; Kheir & Fahey, 2011; Kheir et al., 2008; Rayes et al., 2015). In general, pharmacists have no independent or collaborative prescriptive privileges; they cannot order laboratory tests for patients and are not permitted to administer injections, which prevents pharmacists providing immunisations. Like Western countries, hospital pharmacists often have advanced degrees and exercise at a higher level of practice compared with many community pharmacists; however, the same practice boundaries are applied between hospital and community pharmacists (Kheir et al., 2008). There is often no current legislation or formal training for pharmacists to enable them to undertake advanced roles in developed countries. Limiting the scope of practice for pharmacists has a negative impact on patients' clinical and financial outcomes (Tasaka et al., 2016).

A study of the Arabian Gulf community perspectives on pharmacists showed that pharmacists were highly accessible and approximately two-thirds of the Gulf communities surveyed trust the pharmacy profession as a dependable health profession. Among healthcare practitioners and non-healthcare practitioners, approximately three-quarters of participants thought that pharmacists have satisfactory experience and knowledge with which to accommodate patient's needs. However, one-quarter of those surveyed believe that they require more training and education (Alsaeedi et al., 2020).

INTERPROFESSIONAL PHARMACY EDUCATION

The International Pharmaceutical Federation (FIP) reports there are 121 pharmacy programmes in the countries of Arabian Gulf and Greater Middle East. These schools offer Bachelor of Pharmacy (BPharm) and some offer Doctor of Pharmacy (PharmD) degrees. Pharmacy education is undergoing a substantial transformations to advance the practice of pharmacy and improve patient outcomes (Alsharif, 2017; Anderson

et al., 2011) and pharmacists are moving beyond a dispensing model to more advanced services such as comprehensive medication safety systems, collaborative drug therapy management and improving transitions of care (Toklu & Hussain, 2013). This requires competent clinical pharmacists and trained educators (Keown et al., 2014). It also requires strengthening of experiential and interprofessional pharmacy education (IPE) and there is currently a significant gap in new pharmacy graduates' preparation to practice (AbuBlan et al., 2019; Bader et al., 2017).

COMPLEMENTARY AND ALTERNATIVE MEDICINES USE

Complementary and alternative medicine (CAM) is widely reported in many Arab countries in the Middle East (Al-Faris et al., 2008; Ben-Arye et al., 2011; Sawalha, 2007). A study from Saudi Arabia on the knowledge, attitude and practice of CAM showed that about 85% of participants or one of their family members used CAM, and females, housewives and illiterate patients are the most common users of CAM practices. The most commonly used CAM practices were medical herbs (58.89%), prayer (54%), honey and bee products (54%), Hijama (35.71%) or medical massage therapy (22%) (Elolemy & AlBedah, 2012). Patients with cancer in Saudi Arabia used CAM (90.5%), but only 18% of these patients discussed CAM use with their physicians (Jazieh et al., 2012). A study from the UAE involving 145 patients with diabetes reported that the prevalence of CAM use amongst the patients was 21.4%, with most users being female (27.8%). They found that CAM use was more common amongst housewives (28.6%) and the majority (51.6%) used it for the purpose of slowing the progression of diabetes (Alalami et al., 2017).

The most common form of CAM in the UAE was herbal medicine and the main reasons for using CAM were positive previous experiences and the lower perceived prevalence of adverse effects (Mathew et al., 2013). In Qatar, 38.2% of midlife women used CAM in the previous year with herbal remedies and nutritional remedies as the most used CAM, followed by physical methods (Gerber et al., 2014). A study to explore the awareness, patterns of use and attitudes toward natural health products among the public in Kuwait reported 71.4% of the respondents used natural health products.

Herbal remedies were the most used (41.3%) and common reasons for the use of natural health products were to promote and maintain health, to prevent illness and build the immune system (Awad & Al-Shaye 2014).

MEDICATION WASTE AND DISPOSAL

Improper storage and disposal of medications is reported in many of the countries in the region (Hasan et al., 2019) and the main method used for disposal of unused medications is in household waste, which can lead to environmental pollution and public health hazards (Al-Worafi, 2020; Paut Kusturica et al., 2017). In Saudi Arabia, a survey of 300 hospital patients found that 79% disposed of unused and expired medications through household waste and 7% used the toilet or the sink to dispose of their medications (Al-Shareef et al., 2016). Indeed pharmacists in Kuwait were also reported to use public waste disposal systems for unwanted/expired medications (Abahussain et al., 2012).

An assessment of medication waste in Arabian Gulf countries recommended the development of drug collection programmes to redistribute unused medicines to other patients or to donate to humanitarian agencies (Abou-Auda, 2003). It is recommended that drug authorities monitor and supervise the process of medication disposal and arrange and conduct campaigns to increase the public awareness of proper medication storage and disposal.

SELF-MEDICATION WITH ANTIBIOTICS

The practice of self-medication is very common worldwide and although antibiotics are classified as prescription medicines, there are many reports of inappropriate adherence to the dispensing laws in the region (Alghadeer et al., 2018; Almohammed & Bird 2019). For example, many prescription medicines including antibiotics can be obtained over the counter and via websites in Saudi Arabia (Al-Mohamadi et al., 2013; Alshammari et al., 2017).

Penicillin-based antibiotics are commonly used as self-medication in the Middle East and antibiotics are obtained via stored leftover drugs from pharmacies without prescriptions and from friends/relatives (Alhomoud et al., 2017). A study investigating the perception of self-medication among university students in Saudi Arabia found that 31.4% used antibiotics (Saeed et al., 2014). A study of pharmacist's self-medications practice in UAE found that 43% of pharmacists had used antibiotics without a prescription (Sharif et al., 2014). In Kuwait, over one-quarter of 680 participants used antibiotics as self-medication to treat minor ailments such as common colds, sore throats and coughs (Awad & Aboud, 2015).

CASE STUDY 14.1
STRATEGY TO REDUCE THE USE OF ANTIBIOTICS AS SELF-MEDICATION

Historically, in the UAE anyone can enter a pharmacy and purchase antibiotics over the counter without a prescription from a physician. This has resulted in a significant increase in antimicrobial resistance. As a result, the government has legislated that certain antibiotics cannot be dispensed without a physician prescription.

Do you think this is an effective method to control antibiotic use/self-medication?

What other strategies would assist in reducing the use of antibiotics for self-medicating?

- Education campaigns for general public
  - Only obtain antibiotics from a medical doctor who has assessed the symptoms
  - Do not save antibiotics for later use or share leftover antibiotics with others
  - Antibiotics are not pain killers and are ineffective against common viral infections including the common cold and flu
  - Taking inappropriate antibiotics for viral infections will not help you feel better and may cause side effects such as diarrhoea, nausea and skin rashes
  - Ask your pharmacist for other over-the-counter medicines to alleviate symptoms of minor aliments
- Key messages for community pharmacists
  - Ensure antimicrobial dispensing is always with a prescription and educate patients on adherence to the antibiotic course
  - Offer appropriate treatment of minor aliments without antimicrobials using other over-the-counter medications
  - Identify more serious health problems which may require antimicrobials and refer to an appropriate physician
- Government regulatory bodies must have strong regulatory enforcement policies to prohibit the sale of over-the-counter antibiotics at pharmacies

A systematic literature review on self-medication misuse in the Middle East showed that the main reasons for self-medication with antibiotics is the ease of accessing antibiotics and the advice from relatives and community pharmacists (Khalifeh et al., 2017). Among the general public, there is limited understanding of the appropriate use of antibiotics and the risks of antibiotic resistance. Notably, some patients believe that antibiotics can treat the common cold, cough and viral infections, whilst others use antibiotics as analgesics (Alzoubi et al., 2013; Shehadeh et al., 2012).

Self-medication with antibiotics is linked to the antibiotic resistance crisis; therefore, there needs to be a reduction in the use of antibiotics as self-medication. For example, pharmacists should provide comprehensive education and counselling to patients regarding the consequences of using antibiotics as self-medication (Hasan et al., 2016). Case study 14.1 demonstrates one potential strategy to address self-medication.

SUMMARY AND TAKEAWAY POINTS

Overall, the region has slower advancements in pharmacy practice compared with North America and Europe. However, there is a strong and uniform desire to advance the science and practice of pharmacy in the region. Below are some important points to highlight regarding pharmacy in the region:

- There has been a large expansion in clinical pharmacy fellowships and postgraduate qualifications across the region.
- Most countries procure a mix of original (branded) and generic medicines and many countries encourage and support national medication manufacturing, for example, Saudi Arabia and Jordan.
- S/F medicines are prevalent in Arab countries with the poorest regions being the most affected. Efforts to strengthen regulations and laws, international collaboration and enforcement activities are required to reduce the burden.
- The scope of pharmacy practice in the Arabian Gulf and the Greater Middle East is more limited compared with the expanded scope of practice in developed countries such as the USA and Canada.

- Pharmacy education is undergoing advancements to improve patient outcomes.
- People favour CAM use in the Arabian Gulf and the Greater Middle East countries; it is more prevalent in women.
- Inappropriate storage and disposal of medications is frequently reported due to the lack of specific programmes for medication disposal. Medications are disposed of through household waste, toilet and sink.
- Most of the Arabian Gulf and the Greater Middle East countries classify antibiotics as prescription medicines, but the practice of obtaining and using antibiotics without prescription is common. Penicillins are the most commonly used antibiotics for self-medication and antibiotics are frequently used to treat cold, flu and respiratory tract symptoms.

REFERENCES

Abahussain, E., Waheedi, M., & Koshy, S. (2012). Practice, awareness and opinion of pharmacists toward disposal of unwanted medications in Kuwait. *Saudi Pharmaceutical Journal, 20*, 195. https://doi.org/10.1016/J.JSPS.2012.04.001.

Abou-Auda, H. S. (2003). An economic assessment of the extent of medication use and wastage among families in Saudi Arabia and Arabian Gulf countries. *Clinical Therapeutics, 25*, 1276–1292. https://doi.org/10.1016/S0149-2918(03)80083-8.

AbuBlan, R., Nazar, L., Jaddoua, S., & Treish, I. (2019). A hospital-based pharmacy internship program in Jordan. *American Journal of Pharmaceutical Education, 83*, 306–311. https://doi.org/10.5688/AJPE6547.

Alalami, U., Saeed, K. A., Khan, M. A., Alalami, U. A., Saeed, K., & Papandreou, D. (2017). Prevalence and pattern of traditional and complementary alternative medicine use in diabetic patients in Dubai, UAE. *Arab journal of nutrition and exercise, 2*, 118–127. https://doi.org/10.18502/ajne.v2i2.1250.

Al-Faris, E. A., Al-Rowais, N., Mohamed, A. G., Al-Rukban, M. O., Al-Kurdi, A., Al-Noor, M., et al. (2008). Prevalence and pattern of alternative medicine use: The results of a household survey. *Annals of Saudi Medicine, 28*, 4. https://doi.org/10.5144/0256-4947.2008.4.

Al-Ghananeem, A. M., Malcom, D. R., Shammas, S., & Aburjai, T. (2018). A call to action to transform pharmacy education and practice in the Arab world. *American Journal of Pharmaceutical Education, 82*, 1023–1028. https://doi.org/10.5688/AJPE7014.

Alghadeer, S., Aljuaydi, K., Babelghaith, S., Alhammad, A., & Alarifi, M. (2018). Self-medication with antibiotics in Saudi Arabia. *Saudi Pharmaceutical Journal, 26*, 719. https://doi.org/10.1016/J.JSPS.2018.02.018.

Alghannam, A., Aslanpour, Z., Evans, S., & Schifano, F. (2014). A systematic review of counterfeit and substandard medicines in field quality surveys. *Integrated pharmacy research and practiceis*, 3, 71–88. https://doi.org/10.2147/IPRP.S63690.

Alhawassi, T., Abuelizz, H., Almetwazi, M., Mahmoud, M., Alghamdi, A., Alruthia, Y., et al. (2018). Advancing pharmaceuticals and patient safety in Saudi Arabia: A 2030 vision initiative. *Saudi Pharmaceutical Journal, 26*, 71–74. https://doi.org/10.1016/J.JSPS.2017.10.011.

Alhomoud, F., Aljamea, Z., Almahasnah, R., Alkhalifah, K., Basalelah, L., & Alhomoud, F. (2017). Self-medication and self-prescription with antibiotics in the Middle East-do they really happen? A systematic review of the prevalence, possible reasons, and outcomes. *International Journal of Infectious Diseases, 57*, 3–12. https://doi.org/10.1016/J.IJID.2017.01.014.

Al-Jedai, A., Qaisi, S., & Al-meman, A. (2016). Pharmacy practice and the health care system in Saudi Arabia. *The Canadian Journal of Hospital Pharmacy, 69*, 231. https://doi.org/10.4212/CJHP.V69I3.156.

Al-Mohamadi, A., Badr, A., Mahfouz, L., Samargandi, D., & Al Ahdal, A. (2013). Dispensing medications without prescription at Saudi community pharmacy: Extent and perception. *Saudi Pharmaceutical Journal, Jan;21*(1), 13–18. https://doi.org/10.1016/j.jsps.2011.11.003. Epub 2011 Nov 30.

Almohammed, R., & Bird, E. (2019). Public knowledge and behaviours relating to antibiotic use in Gulf Cooperation Council countries: A systematic review. *Journal of Infection and Public Health, 12*, 159–166. https://doi.org/10.1016/J.JIPH.2018.09.002.

Alruthia, Y., Alwhaibi, M., Alotaibi, M., Asiri, S., Alghamdi, B., Almuaythir, G., et al. (2018). Drug shortages in Saudi Arabia: Root causes and recommendations. *Saudi Pharmaceutical Journal, 26*, 947–951. https://doi.org/10.1016/J.JSPS.2018.05.002.

Alsaeedi, W., Alshaikh, H., Almesaifer, A., & Alsamani, O. (2020). Pharmacy profession and practice in Arabian Gulf countries: Challenges and opportunities. *International journal of developmental research, 10*(3), 34329–34334.

Alshammari, T., Alhindi, S., Alrashdi, A., Benmerzouga, I., & Aljofan, M. (2017). Pharmacy malpractice: The rate and prevalence of dispensing high-risk prescription-only medications at community pharmacies in Saudi Arabia. *Saudi Pharmaceutical Journal, 25*, 709–714. https://doi.org/10.1016/J.JSPS.2016.10.001.

Al-Shareef, F., El-Asrar, S., Al-Bakr, L., Al-Amro, M., Alqahtani, F., Aleanizy, F., et al. (2016). Investigating the disposal of expired and unused medication in Riyadh, Saudi Arabia: A cross-sectional study. *International journal of clinical pharmacy, 38*, 822–828. https://doi.org/10.1007/S11096-016-0287-4.

Alsharif, N. (2017). Purposeful global engagement in pharmacy education. *American Journal of Pharmaceutical Education, 81*, 3–5. https://doi.org/10.5688/AJPE6882.

Alsultan, M. (2010). A descriptive study on medications brought by pilgrims during Hajj seasons 2005 and 2006 in Saudi Arabia. *World applied sciences journal, 10*, 1401–1406.

Al-Worafi, Y. (2014). Pharmacy practice and its challenges in Yemen. *The Australasian Medical Journal, 7*, 17. https://doi.org/10.4066/AMJ.2014.1890.

Al-Worafi, Y., 2020. Drug safety in developing countries : achievements and challenges. (1st ed.). Cambridge, MA: Academic Press. pp. 391–447

Alzoubi, K., Al-Azzam, S., Alhusban, A., Mukattash, T., Al-Zubaidy, S., Alomari, N., & Khader, Y. (2013). An audit on the knowledge, beliefs and attitudes about the uses and side-effects of antibiotics among outpatients attending 2 teaching hospitals in Jordan. *Eastern Mediterranean Health Journal, 19*(5), 478–484.

Anderson, C., Brock, T., Bates, I., Rouse, M., Marriott, J., Manasse, H., et al. (2011). Transforming health professional education. *American Journal of Pharmaceutical Education, 75*. https://doi.org/10.5688/AJPE75222.

Awad, A., & Al-Shaye, D. (2014). Public awareness, patterns of use and attitudes toward natural health products in Kuwait: A cross-sectional survey. *BMC Complementary and Alternative Medicine, 14*. https://doi.org/10.1186/1472-6882-14-105.

Awad, A. I., & Aboud, E. A. (2015). Knowledge, attitude and practice towards antibiotic use among the public in Kuwait. *PLoS One, 10*, e0117910. https://doi.org/10.1371/JOURNAL.PONE.0117910.

Bader, L., McGrath, S., Rouse, M., & Anderson, C. (2017). A conceptual framework toward identifying and analyzing challenges to the advancement of pharmacy. *Research in social & administrative pharmacy, 13*, 321–331. https://doi.org/10.1016/J.SAPHARM.2016.03.001.

Ben-Arye, E., Lev, E., & Schiff, E. (2011). Complementary medicine oncology research in the Middle-East: Shifting from traditional to integrative cancer care. *European journal of integrative medicine, 1*, 29–37. https://doi.org/10.1016/J.EUJIM.2011.02.007.

Dameh, M. (2009) Pharmacy in the United Arab Emirates. South Med Rev. 2009 Apr; 2 (1): 15–18. Published online April 16 2009, PMCID:PMC3471164. PMID: 23093873.

Elolemy, A. T., & AlBedah, A. (2012). Public knowledge, attitude and practice of complementary and alternative medicine in Riyadh region, Saudi Arabia. *Oman Medical Journal, 27*, 20. https://doi.org/10.5001/OMJ.2012.04.

Gerber, L., Mamtani, R., Chiu, Y., Bener, A., Murphy, M., Cheema, S., et al. (2014). Use of complementary and alternative medicine among midlife Arab women living in Qatar. *Eastern Mediterranean Health Journal, 20*, 554.

Hasan, S., Farghadani, G., AlHaideri, S. K., Fathy, M., Hasan, S., Farghadani, G., et al. (2016). Pharmacist opportunities to improve public self-medicating practices in the UAE. *Pharmacology & pharmacy, 7*, 459–471. https://doi.org/10.4236/PP.2016.711052.

Hasan, S., Al-Omar, M., AlZubaidy, H., & Al-Worafi, Y. (2019). Use of Medications in Arab Countries. *Handbook of Healthcare in the Arab World*, 3–24.

Jazieh, A., Sudairy, R., Al, Abulkhair, Alaskar, A., Safi, F., Al, Sheblaq, N., et al. (2012). Use of complementary and alternative medicine by patients with cancer in Saudi Arabia. *Journal of Alternative and Complementary Medicine, 18*, 1045–1049. https://doi.org/10.1089/ACM.2011.0266.

Keown, O., Parston, G., Patel, H., Rennie, F., Saoud, F., Kuwari, H., et al. (2014). Lessons from eight countries on diffusing innovation in health care. *Health Affairs. (Millwood), 33*, 1516–1522. https://doi.org/10.1377/HLTHAFF.2014.0382.

Khalifeh, M. M., Moore, N. D., & Salameh, P. R. (2017). Self-medication misuse in the Middle East: A systematic literature review. *Pharmacology Research & Perspectives, 5*, 323. https://doi.org/10.1002/PRP2.323.

Kheir, N., & Fahey, M. (2011). Pharmacy practice in Qatar: Challenges and opportunities. *Southern Med Review*, 4, 92. https://doi.org/10.5655/SMR.V4I2.1007.

Kheir, N., Zaidan, M., Younes, H., Hajj, M., Wilbur, K., & Jewesson, P. (2008). Pharmacy education and practice in 13 Middle Eastern countries. *American Journal of Pharmaceutical Education*, 72. https://doi.org/10.5688/AJ7206133.

Mackey, T., & Liang, B. (2011). The global counterfeit drug trade: Patient safety and public health risks. *Journal of Pharmaceutical Sciences*, 100, 4571–4579. https://doi.org/10.1002/JPS.22679.

Mathew, E., Muttappallymyalil, J., Sreedharan, J., John, L., Mehboob, J., & Mathew, A. (2013). Self-reported use of complementary and alternative medicine among the health care consumers at a tertiary care center in Ajman, United Arab Emirates. *Annals of Medical and Health Sciences Research*, 3, 215. https://doi.org/10.4103/2141-9248.113665.

Nazer, L. H., & Tuffaha, H. (2017). Health care and pharmacy practice in Jordan. *The Canadian Journal of Hospital Pharmacy*, 70, 150. https://doi.org/10.4212/CJHP.V70I2.1649.

Nayyar, G., Breman, J., Newton, P., & Herrington, J. (2012). Poor-quality antimalarial drugs in southeast Asia and sub-Saharan Africa. *The Lancet Infectious Diseases*, 12(6), 488–496. https://doi.org/10.1016/S1473-3099(12)70064-6.

Nayyar, G., Breman, J., Mackey, T., Clark, J., Hajjou, M., Littrell, M., et al. (2019). Falsified and substandard drugs: Stopping the pandemic. *The American Journal of Tropical Medicine and Hygiene*, 100, 1058–1065. https://doi.org/10.4269/AJTMH.18-0981.

Paut Kusturica, M., Tomas, A., & Sabo, A. (2017). Disposal of unused drugs: Knowledge and behavior among people around the world. *Reviews of Environmental Contamination and Toxicology*, 240, 71–104. https://doi.org/10.1007/398_2016_3.

Rayes, I., Hassali, M., & Abduelkarem, A. (2015). The role of pharmacists in developing countries: The current scenario in the United Arab Emirates. *Saudi Pharmaceutical Journal*, 23, 470–474. https://doi.org/10.1016/J.JSPS.2014.02.004.

Renschler, J., Walters, K., Newton, P., & Laxminarayan, R. (2015). Estimated under-five deaths associated with poor-quality antimalarials in sub-Saharan Africa. *The American Journal of Tropical Medicine and Hygiene*, 92, 119–126. https://doi.org/10.4269/AJTMH.14-0725.

Saeed, M., Alkhoshaiban, A., Mohammed Ali Al-Worafi, Y., & Long, C. (2014). Perception of self-medication among university students in Saudi Arabia - Archives of Pharmacy Practice. *Archives of pharmacy practice*, 5, 149–152.

Sawalha, A. (2007). Complementary and alternative medicine (CAM) in Palestine: Use and safety implications. *Journal of Alternative and Complementary Medicine*, 13, 263–269. https://doi.org/10.1089/ACM.2006.6280.

Sharif, S. I., Bugaighis, L., & Sharif, R. S. (2014). Self-medication practice among pharmacists in UAE. *Pharmacol Pharm*, 6, 428–435. https://doi.org/10.4236/pp.2015.69044.

Shehadeh, M., Suaifan, G., Darwish, R., Wazaify, M., Zaru, L., & Alja'fari, S. (2012). Knowledge, attitudes and behavior regarding antibiotics use and misuse among adults in the community of Jordan. A pilot study. *Saudi Pharmaceutical Journal*, 20, 125–133. https://doi.org/10.1016/J.JSPS.2011.11.005.

Tasaka, Y., Yasunaga, D., Tanaka, M., Tanaka, A., Asakawa, T., Horio, I., et al. (2016). Economic and safety benefits of pharmaceutical interventions by community and hospital pharmacists in Japan. *International journal of clinical pharmacy*, 38, 321–329. https://doi.org/10.1007/S11096-015-0245-6.

Toklu, H., & Hussain, A. (2013). The changing face of pharmacy practice and the need for a new model of pharmacy education. *Journal of Young Pharmacists*, 5, 38. https://doi.org/10.1016/J.JYP.2012.09.001.

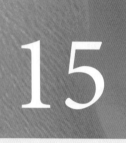

15

PAIN MANAGEMENT

KEITH JOHNSTON

Pain in the body is often a signal of something wrong, which we can cure by remedial measures. Our duty is to find out our own shortcomings and remedy them. If we try to do so in all sincerity of heart, Allah will give us guidance.

Holy Quran (transl.), A. Yousef Ali, 1946, surah 64, ayah 11

CHAPTER OUTLINE

INTRODUCTION

In the West in the 1980s, the 'information era' of modern healthcare emerged (Tompkins et al., 2017). This included the so-called 'pain movement' which was characterised by increasing numbers of informed patient advocate groups and less paternalistic and more assertive doctors (Johnson & Booker 2021). Both patients and doctors agitated for proactive pain management (Campbell 2016) and this culminated in the declaration that pain was the 'fifth vital sign' with the incumbent President of the American Pain Society (APS). During his presidential address to the American Pain Society on 11th November 1996, James Campbell, MD, stated that if pain were assessed with the same zeal as other vital signs are, it would have a much better chance of being treated properly.

Over a decade later, what is widely known as the 'Declaration of Montreal' was presented at the First International Pain Summit stating that access to pain management is a fundamental human right (International Association for the Study of Pain, 2011)

(Box 15.1). Despite statements to the contrary, sadly it appears we remain—yet another decade on—no nearer to addressing the global disparities in the access and provision of pain management globally.

BOX 15.1

The Declaration of Montreal

Article 1: The right of all people to have access to pain management without discrimination.

Article 2: The right of people in pain to have their pain acknowledged and to be informed about how it can be assessed.

Article 3: The right of all people with pain to have access to appropriate assessment and treatment of pain by adequately trained health care professionals.

Brennan, F., Carr, D., & Cousins, M. (2016). Access to pain management: Still very much a human right. *Pain Medicine*, 17(10), 1785–1789.

This chapter is not intended to provide the reader with the fundamentals of pain management, indeed there are many other very good texts available that do the topic justice (e.g., Benzon & Raj, 2022; Macintyre & Schug, 2021). Rather this chapter is intended to present an overview of pain management within the context of the Arabian Gulf and Greater Middle East in comparison with its evolution in Western medicine. However, that said, it is necessary to delineate the subject matter, so let us start with a brief overview of pain and its management.

What is pain? The traditional definition (https://europeanpainfederation.eu/what-is-pain/) is that it is an 'unpleasant sensory and emotional experience associated with, or resembling that associated with, actual or potential tissue damage'. In essence it is the body's way of warning us that damage is being done, or potentially being done, so that we can protect ourselves. Everyone has a different pain threshold and reacts differently to it, so a one-size-fits-all approach to pain does not work. Pain is an entirely subjective experience; therefore, it is important we understand the different kinds of pains, how to assess them properly using various tools and then treat it appropriately in a patient-specific manner.

Pain can be divided into two main categories: acute and chronic. Acute pain is what we associate with tissue damage or injury and it is relieved by treating the causative factor. It is also usually of a relatively short duration. Chronic pain by definition has a much longer duration of action and does not respond to the same treatments as acute pain. Chronic pain requires a very different approach and patients often have to learn how to live with a degree of pain, as this cannot be completely cured.

In order to assess pain and also evaluate whether our treatment of it is being successful, we need to take proper pain histories, locate any aggravating and alleviating factors, associated symptoms and the nature of the pain. Thus, scoring tools are used and can be applied to both adult and paediatric populations. These can be as simple as a numerical scale or visual analogue scale, whilst in children we might decide to use the Faces Pain Scale. For patients with chronic pain, tools such as the McGill Pain Questionnaire are useful.

Once pain has been assessed, it needs to be treated and this requires an individualised treatment plan. In terms of acute pain, this is likely to require treating the underlying cause, e.g., a broken arm or appendicitis. For the vast majority of cases, the patient will require pharmacological intervention, and this can range from something as simple as paracetamol to opioids, depending on the severity and the patient's response. In addition, we also have other families of drugs such as non-steroidal anti-inflammatory drugs (NSAIDs) and nerve-modifying drugs such as pregabalin. These medications may be given via a number of different routes such as oral, intravenous (IV), transdermal or intrathecal, depending on the patient's condition and requirements. All medications have side effects; whatever treatment regime is planned, it is important to be cognisant of side effects at all times to minimise the problems caused by these and to promptly recognise and treat them.

In addition to pharmacological treatment for the patient, healthcare professionals also need to think of a multimodal approach to pain management which may involve many other interventions such as transcutaneous electrical nerve stimulation (TENS), physiotherapy, nerve ablation, psychotherapy and hypnosis.

Understanding pain assessment and treatment in different age groups can be challenging, largely due to communication barriers. These are particularly obvious in both the paediatric and the elderly population as communication may be limited by conditions such as dementia or simply by impaired hearing. In addition, the physiology in patients changes from neonates through to adulthood, thereby affecting their ability to handle different drugs. Moreover, polypharmacy and multiple comorbidities can raise additional challenges, especially in the older population.

PAIN MANAGEMENT IN THE MIDDLE EAST

The countries of the Middle East have an overall population of over 300 million when grouped together and have many distinct differences based on religion, ethnicity, culture, economics, government, population size, education level and available technology and resources. Although healthcare in the Middle East is rapidly progressing, there are many challenges facing pain management as a specialism in the acute, chronic and palliative care settings. Accordingly, there are three main areas that can be identified as potential obstacles to delivering optimum pain management in the region.

Logistical

Many of us take a reliable supply chain for granted and do not think about the many issues that are involved, and compounded by both politico-economic factors and geographical and environmental influences, with this issue being discussed in some detail in Chapter 14.

Governments throughout the Arab Peninsula have varying approaches to the control of opiate drugs, and this is particularly apparent when you reflect on how healthcare is provided via a wide range of sources, such as government hospitals, military hospitals and the private sector, with each of these having different access and restrictions on the availability of medications.

The ability of drugs to reach the hospitals or other healthcare institutions is wholly reliant upon the supply chain. However, medications coming from the West may be held up in customs for some time—for weeks or months—and that poses real difficulties. These delays are compounded by the environmental extremes of temperature faced in this region, making maintenance of the cold chain difficult; this inevitably impacts upon the efficacy of the drugs once they finally reach the patient. Given the short shelf-life of some drugs and the challenges in physically getting them to the patient, there are frequent drug shortages.

In the West, pain management teams, both chronic and acute, are part and parcel of any healthcare establishment, but in the Middle East this specialty is in its infancy. Further, pain management teams or personnel may not be widely or easily available, although they may be present in some tertiary referral centres but lacking in primary care. In addition, the pain management 'team' is unlikely to mimic that available in the West with it being largely unidisciplinary rather than multidisciplinary and consequently, unable to facilitate a range of potential interventions.

The Patient

Patient factors not only affect the need for pain control but also the patient's ability to deal with pain as well as their expectations of pain control. The majority of the indigenous population in this region is Islamic, and they are taught to be steadfast in dealing with any pain and suffering they are confronted with; as such

forbearance of pain and suffering would not only lead to the expiration of sins but would also be rewarded in the afterlife. Accordingly, Islamic patients may not seek treatment until much later or until pain is intractable. This not only leads to further suffering by the patient but is also likely to lead to later presentation of pathology, such as cancer. This later presentation of cancers especially may be further driven by fear of stigmatisation and shame on the family.

Healthcare Professionals

Teaching about pain management has traditionally been very limited in both medical and nursing curricula, leading to a real lack of understanding of pain management, both in terms of assessment and treatment, with the concept of pain as the fifth vital sign largely unheard of. Although this is starting to change, it will take time for education to take effect. The relative absence of pain education has been partially due to the lack of pain specialist doctors, and this, in turn, also limits the pain interventions available to the population.

There is a real fear of addiction in patients, and this is largely due to a lack of understanding of medication and pain management, which leads not only to inadequate prescribing from doctors but also to a reluctance from nurses to give prescribed opioid medication. Moreover, in this region, the variability in hospitals and the limited access to pain management teams leads to limited options in routes of medication administrations. Intramuscular (IM) injection is the most commonly used mode of administration of analgesia, as nursing regulations may limit nurses giving IV drugs and infusion pumps may simply not be available.

Community nursing has not yet developed sufficiently in the region and therefore, the idea of nurses supporting pain management in the community by providing (IM or IV) injections or alternatively managing infusion pumps is not something that is achievable currently.

Pain and the Impact of Culture

It is well understood that pain is composed of highly interactive emotional, cognitive as well as sensory components and bearing this in mind, we can anticipate the obvious effect of culture on both perception and the ability to deal with pain (Maki et al., 2022). The generalisation of the Middle East would be to think of it as a purely Islamic region, but the population is much more diverse than that due to large numbers of migrant workers, with many of the labourers coming from Bangladesh and India, along with many professionals from Western countries. In addition, there is a significant foreign military presence here such as the United States Fifth Fleet who are based in Bahrain. Therefore, a thorough understanding of different culture's perceptions and coping strategies along with appropriate communication is of vital importance in providing optimal pain management.

The Arabic civilisations are founded on a strong history of learning and early scientific development that started around the 7th century at the same time as the Prophet Mohammed's (PBUH) teachings. The first advancement of pain treatment, and best known in the region, came with Ibn Sina (980–1037) who described treatments for 15 kinds of pain in his text, *Canon Medicinae*. Even now, traditional medicine is practiced widely and accepted throughout the Middle East, both in cities as well as rural areas, often under the guise of religious healers or magicians (Kizilhan, 2011). Cupping is widely practiced throughout the Arab region and herbal medicine is commonly used (Aboushanab & AlSanad, 2021). Fasting, which is fundamental to the holy month of Ramadan in Islam, is rapidly gaining popularity in the West as people embrace intermittent fasting. The mainstream acceptance of 'complementary medicine' in the region may be overlooked by expatriate healthcare workers who perhaps fail to realise that the patient may have already consulted a traditional doctor before presenting to hospital. For example, this might be evident in a patient who is admitted for arthroscopy but has already sought blood-letting and cupping of the knee in order to obtain relief from pain. The importance of understanding local practices, how to work with them and educate patients tactfully, without alienating them or losing their trust, needs to be taken onboard in order to optimise compliance with modern medicine. This is not an issue exclusive to the Arab nations but can been seen in any culture where traditional medicine persists, such as the importance of herbalism and ayurvedic medicine within the Indian culture.

Governmental Polices and Legislation

From policies and legislation governing imports on the prescribing of opioids through to the physical availability of drugs at local level, all affect the patient's ability to receive appropriate treatment.

The World Health Organization (WHO) and the International Narcotics Control Board (INCB) provide recommendations on the regulation of narcotics and when these were reviewed across 20 Middle East countries, many were not being met (Al Bahrani & Mehdi, 2018), augmenting the problems of providing a reliable pain management system.

The restriction of opiate prescribing was found to be overly regulated, which leads to severe limitations to such an extent that, in 15 out of the 21 countries reviewed, opioids are only allowed to be prescribed for inpatients or a special permit was required. Even when it comes to prescribing there was found to be limited prescribing amongst doctors and family physicians were excluded from this. The restriction in prescribing privileges led to a further hurdle in the ability to provide quality pain relief as there were no emergency protocols in place for when the doctor entitled to prescribe was not available. Simple factors like overly complex paperwork and bureaucracy provided a further obstacle for prescribing doctors to overcome.

Furthermore, these regulatory issues are compounded by issues at the healthcare providing level (Al Bahrani & Mehdi, 2018). The lack of understanding of opioids and their requirements, along with the response in patients with acute and chronic pain, have been due to failures in the education system. This in turn has led to policies restricting access to opioids due to a lack of understanding about the issues of abuse and addiction. These beliefs are not exclusive to healthcare professionals and can be observed in patients who may be reluctant to accept opioids with concomitant concerns among carers and family members. Such issues extend beyond the acute pain setting and into the area of palliative care and death, with a lack of awareness of the human right to pain relief and a dignified death.

There are different markers for the quality and quantity of pain control. One of the commonly quoted benchmarks is the per capita consumption of opioids. In the Middle East, this is 0.2 to 2.0 mg/capita, hugely contrasting with that for developed countries (50 mg).

The INCB in conjunction with the Middle East Cancer Consortium (MECC) have recommended several aims for pain management in the region including the availability of low-cost opioids which would ensure no one would be excluded on grounds of financial constraints. However, this in itself is not enough as the underlying problem is largely attitudes about pain control. Consequently, the IRNC and MECC have highlighted the need for staff education and development, both at nursing and medical levels, with re-education of doctors to correct personal bias. This is reflected in programs aimed at the re-education of patients as well, especially with the regard to opioids at the time of death and, in relation to addiction.

An example of this can be seen in King Hamad University Hospital in Bahrain and the attached flagship Bahrain Oncology Centre, where they not only have acute and chronic pain services run in the same multidisciplinary manner we see in the West, but they also have an active Palliative Care team and the hospital is currently working to develop homecare services. These initiatives have been developed by both local doctors and nurses working alongside trained pain specialists from abroad, in conjunction with local training in King Faisal Hospital in Riyadh, Saudi Arabia.

Nevertheless, there remains disparities in how pain is managed across the region. For example, a study in Lebanon (Tawil et al., 2018), which has a particularly diverse cultural mix, looked at patient satisfaction with pain management and found that 71.6% of inpatients experienced pain of varying severity and only 24.6% received follow-up in the first 48 hours. Furthermore, a lack of pain score documentation in 54.6% of patients was reported. The major concerns arising from this study are the fundamental failures in undertaking a proper assessment to enable effective delivery of treatment and therefore in delivering high-quality pain relief.

These findings are in stark contrast to another Lebanese study (Nasser et al., 2016) which looked at medical staff's attitudes to pain control with the largest groups of respondents in internal medicine, anaesthesia and surgery. More than half the doctors felt confident in pain management, although this was considerably lower in the more junior doctors. On a positive note, 50% of the doctors had participated in learning activities on pain although government statistics for the same time showed that 99% of the practicing doctors and nurses surveyed required continuing professional development in palliative care. This need

for formal education is illustrated by the fact that the majority of doctors in this survey relied on their own experience rather than international treatment guidelines and many were not aware of their hospital's pain policies and guidelines. A lack of a multidisciplinary approach was also evident.

The recurring message from all studies, no matter which Arab countries they are carried out in, is the need for education of healthcare professionals at all levels. Further, at the government level, there needs to be a rethinking of policies and regulation to make appropriate treatment with opioids more accessible to the patient. The current legislation for managing narcotics is one of the challenges facing healthcare professionals. For example, the legal requirements for prescribing, usage, recording and disposal of narcotics is quite different from Western legislation. Narcotic ampoules must be tracked. The usual dual signage for narcotics is in place, but what is different is each ampoule must be tracked, so every broken or used ampoule must be returned to the pharmacy in order for replacement ampoules to be issued (UAE Federal Law No. 14 1995), (Ministerial Decree No. 888, 2016).

Pain Management in Labour and Delivery: A Middle East Perspective

It was not until the late 70 s and 80 s that birth in Jordan and other Middle Eastern countries moved into hospital settings. Prior to this, giving birth at home was considered normal for Middle Eastern women (Hussein et al., 2020). With a move to the medicalisation of childbirth over the last 40–50 years, the practice of pain management during labour and delivery has not kept pace with Western approaches to obstetric care.

'Historically, research has shown that overall, women from a Middle Eastern compared with a Western background have higher ratings of pain and showed more pain behaviour (during childbirth). This was found especially for Middle Eastern women of a low educational background' (Weisenberg & Caspi, 1989, p. 13). Despite this, over the last 30 years, both expectant mothers and healthcare professionals have a lack of understanding of approaches to pain management.

Research conducted in Saudi Arabia found that 58.7% were unaware of labour pain relief, with 79.8% being unaware of the different forms of labour pain relief available (Alshahrani, 2019). Sadly, the study found that most pregnant women obtained information from friends (57.5%), and only 16.1% of women received information from their healthcare providers (Alshahrani, 2019). The findings of this study would suggest that healthcare providers are not providing sufficient education to pregnant women, or other cultural factors are in play.

A further study in Egypt (Mousa et al., 2018) found that 36.8% of the women surveyed used neither pharmacological nor non-pharmacological pain relief methods during labour. Hospital-related factors were the major barriers against using pain relief methods, as stated by healthcare professionals in the study. While epidural analgesia is widely used and understood in Western obstetric practice, it was found in one Middle East study that approximately 15% of labouring women did not know about epidurals. This study demonstrated the lack of knowledge and understanding of epidurals by women in this region. However, some of the reasons for reluctance in accepting epidural analgesia may have cultural roots.

Pain relief options available to women should be discussed early in pregnancy by doctors and midwives, who understand the cultural societal norms and who are able to give evidence-based information about the choices available (Edwards & Ansari, 2015). Ali Alahmari et al. (2020) reporting on research from Saudi Arabia highlights that most women of childbearing age had limited knowledge about the benefits and complications associated with epidural analgesia.

Overwhelmingly, women in the Middle Eastern countries arguably experience birth as dehumanising and disrespectful with little rapport between women and health professionals with limited support, information and compassion (Hussein et al., 2020). While part of the problem may be the limited use of midwives in the Middle East in the education of pregnant women and pain relief options or cultural differences between healthcare providers and patients, multiple studies across the region all point to strengthening antenatal pain management education.

The Challenges of the Patient with Sickle Cell Disease

Pain management is not just limited to acute pain and cancer pain, but other chronic diseases requiring ongo-ing pain input. In the Middle East, there is the specific challenge of a large number of patients with sickle cell disease (SCD). SCD is well recognised in people of African, Indian, Caribbean and Middle Eastern origin (Case Study 15.1). Originally it was first reported

CASE STUDY 15.1
SICKLE CELL DISEASE

A 25-year-old man with SCD presents to his local accident and emergency department complaining of severe intense stabbing pain in his right leg, along with extreme tiredness, shortness of breath and a headache. He normally attends the sickle cell centre at his local tertiary centre; however, he is currently visiting family. His haemoglobin is normally about 8 g/dL and he suffers from crisis about once every 2 months, and this feels like his normal crisis. Prior to this attack, he had been on a long car journey and has been feeling 'flu-like' symptoms.

When he first felt the pain, he took paracetamol and ibuprofen and drank fluids to improve his hydration status, but the pain got worse.

On presentation to the hospital, the patient had his observations taken which showed saturations of 92%, tachypnoea, tachycardia and elevated blood pressure. The nurse assessing him initially told him he should take paracetamol and drink fluids and it would settle and there was nothing more to do. Eventually after being seen by a doctor, 2 mg of morphine IV was prescribed and after 1 hour the doctor saw him again and gave another 2 mg. He said at this stage no further morphine could be given as he would become addicted. At this point, the patient self-discharged and got his family to drive him home to his regular Sickle Cell Unit.

KEY ISSUES

- Failure to appreciate the severity of the pain and the patient's perception of pain.
- No use of validated scoring tool.
- Failure to appreciate if the patient is on any regular strong analgesia or how much he normally requires to obtain pain control in a crisis.
- The need to keep giving opioids and frequently reassess until pain control is achieved. This will require much larger doses than a patient without SCD due to opioid-induced hyperalgesia, but this does not make the patient an addict—just someone with a lower pain threshold due to repeated opioids.
- Use of opioids in acute settings for pain does not cause addiction.
- SCD crisis is best handled in specialist centres by specialist doctors and nurses who understand the disease and the patient's perspective and have protocols for management of the same.

in Egypt but is common throughout the Middle East region, with a prevalence of up to 5% (El-Hazmi et al., 2011). Pain management is of paramount importance in the management of a sickle cell crisis and ideally is usually managed in specialist sickle cell centres. However, like any other patient, a patient with SCD can present with any other pathology or surgical complaint that requires pain management and may precipitate a crisis. They present a unique challenge due to their tolerance to analgesia (e.g., opioid-induced hyperalgesia) and healthcare staff's lack of understanding of how this affects the management of pain in non-sickle cell crisis situations, such as surgical or traumatic pain. Due to this lack of knowledge, this group of patients is frequently undertreated.

These painful crises are normally due to vaso-occlusive crisis, with the problem being the inflammation associated with this disease worsens with successive attacks and so does the end-organ damage. Effective pain management is the first step in dealing with these crises, but due to the multifactorial aspects of their pain, simple numerical scales used in the general population may not reveal the true picture of the problem. The pharmacological management is complex as simple analgesics such as paracetamol and NSAIDs are insufficient to treat the severe pain and local doctors are concerned that opioids may lead to addiction problems in this population. In Jordan, they have developed a unique multidimensional assessment tool for adolescent patients called the Adolescent Pediatric Pain Tool (APPT) enabling doctors to better assess pain interventions (Abdo et al., 2019). Whilst carrying out this study into the APTT, they discovered that the reason for underusage of opioids was mainly a deficiency in pain management knowledge.

SUMMARY AND TAKEAWAY POINTS

- The provision of pain management in the Middle East shows a wide disparity in quality. This is for a number of reasons which can be divided into the following categories:
  - Governmental/Logistical
  - Healthcare provider
  - Patient/Cultural
- Change needs to start at the top with governmental bureaucracy surrounding opioid supplies and

prescriptions being reviewed to enable appropriate dispensing of drugs.
- The supply chain also needs to be ensured and maintained to guarantee consistency in volume and quality.
- Patients should be able to obtain these drugs no matter how they access the healthcare system. Healthcare providers, both nurses and doctors, require education about pain control, especially in terms of assessment and appropriate dosing.
- Additionally, the number of pain specialist doctors needs to be increased to ensure this is not a luxury restricted to the tertiary referral centres.
- Moreover, the development of multidisciplinary pain management teams still requires encouragement.
- Patients in this region show reticence in presenting to hospital due to cultural and religious values as they believe in suffering.
- There remains a fear among patients about taking strong painkillers with regards to addiction. Patients also present late with their disease which may also limit their treatment options. Thus, education of the patient and their family is important.
- Some hospitals do achieve the level of provision we see in the West and as attitudes and education change, along with government policy, we should eventually see marked improvements in pain management across the Middle East.
- Pain relief for labouring women remains misunderstood or underused and the subject needs further discussion and education with women in the antenatal period to lay out pain options.
- With SCD being more prevalent in the Middle East than other regions, greater understanding of pain management approaches and regimes need to be considered by healthcare professional.

REFERENCES

Abdo, S., Nuseir, K. Q., Altarifi, A. A., Barqawi, M., Ayoub, N. M., & Mukkatash, T. L. (2019). Management of sickle cell disease pain among adolescent and pediatric patients. *Brain Sciences, Aug 9*(8), 182.
Aboushanab, T. S., & AlSanad, S. M. (2021). Cupping Therapy (Hijama) in the Arab World In I. Laher (Eds.), *Handbook of Healthcare in the Arab World*. Cham: Springer. https://doi.org/10.1007/978-3-030-36811-1_176.

Al Bahrani, B. J., & Mehdi, I. (2018). The need for regulatory reforms in the use of opioids for pain management and palliative care in the Middle East. *Gulf Journal of Oncology, 1*(27), 52–59.

Ali Alahmari, S. S., ALmetrek, M., Alzillaee, A. Y., Hassan, W. J., & Ali Alamry, S. M. (2020). Knowledge, attitude, and practice of childbearing women toward epidural anesthesia during normal vaginal delivery in Alsanayeah Primary Health Care in Khamis Mushait. *Journal of Family Medicine and Primary Care, 9*(1), 99–104.

Alshahrani, M. S. (2019). An evaluation of the different types of labor pain relief, preferred methods of pain relief, and effects of social media on awareness and knowledge among pregnant women. A cross-sectional study in the Kingdom of Saudi Arabia. *Saudi Medical Journal, 40*(9), 914–921.

Benzon, H. T., & Raj, S. N. (2022). *Essentials of Pain Medicine and Regional Anesthesia* (4th ed.). Philadelphia: Elsevier.

Campbell, J. N. (2016). The fifth vital sign revisited. *Pain, 157*(1), 3–4.

Edwards, G., & Ansari, T. (2015). A survey of women's views of epidural analgesia in the *Middle East. J Asian midwives, 2*(1), 34–41.

El-Hazmi Mohsen, A. F., Al-Hazmi, A. M., & Warsy, A. S. (2011). Sickle cell disease in Middle East Arab countries. *Indian Journal of Medical Research,* Nov 134(5), 597–610.

Hussein, S., Dahlen, H. G., Ogunsiji, O., & Schmied, V. (2020). Jordanian women's experiences and constructions of labour and birth in different settings, over time and across generations: A qualitative study. *BMC Pregnancy and Childbirth, 20*(1), 357.

International Association for the Study of Pain. (2011). IASP Taxonomy. Available at https://www.iasp-pain.org/AM/Template.cfm?section=Pain_Definitions.

Johnson, A., & Booker, S. Q. (2021). Population-focused approaches for proactive chronic pain management in older adults. *Pain Management Nursing, 22*(6), 694–701.

Kizilhan, J. I. (2011). Understanding and treatment of diffuse aches and pains of patients from tradition-bound cultures. *Europe's Journal of Psychology, 7*(2), 359–373.

Maki, D., Lempp, H., & Critchley, D. (2022). An exploration of experiences and beliefs about low back pain with Arab Muslim patients. *Disability and Rehabilitation, 44*(18), 5171–5183.

Macintyre, P. A., & Schug, S. A. (2021). *Acute Pain Management, A Practical Guide* (5th ed.). Boca Raton: Routledge.

Ministerial Decree No. 888, (2016). *Concerning Rules and Regulations for Prescribing and Dispensing of Narcotic Controlled and Semi Controlled Drugs.* UAE.

Mousa, O., Abdelhafez, A. A., Abdelraheim, A. R., Yousef, A. M., Ghaney, A. A., & El Gelany, S. (2018). Perceptions and practice of labor pain-relief methods among health professionals conducting delivery in Minia Maternity Units in Egypt. *Obstetrics and Gynecology Int.* https://doi.org/10.1155/2018/3060953.

Nasser, S. C., Nassif, J. G., & Saad, A. H. (2016). Physicians' attitudes to clinical pain management and education: Survey from a Middle Eastern country. *Pain Research and Management.* https://doi.org/10.1155/2016/1358593.

Tawil, S., Iskandar, K., & Salameh, P. (2018). Pain management in hospitals: Patients' satisfaction and related barriers. *Pharmacy Pract (Granada), 16*(3), 1268. https://doi.org/10.18549/PharmPract.2018.03.1268.

Tompkins, D., Hobelmann, J. G., & Compton, P. (2017). Providing chronic pain management in the "Fifth Vital Sign" era: Historical and treatment perspectives on a modern-day medical dilemma. *Drug Alcohol Dependency, 173*(Suppl 1), S11–S21. https://doi.org/10.1016/j.drugalcdep.2016.12.002.

UAE. 1995. UAE Federal Law No. 14 of 1995 on the countermeasures against narcotic drugs and psychotropic substances.

Weisenberg, M., & Caspi, Z. (1989). Cultural and educational influences on pain of childbirth. *Journal of Pain and Symptom Management, 4*(1), 13–19.

FURTHER READING

Almalki, M. T., BinBaz, S. S., Alamri, S. A., Alghamdi, H. H., El-Kabbani, A. O., Mulhem, A. A., et al. (2019). Prevalence of chronic pain and high-impact chronic pain in Saudi Arabia. *Saudi Medical Journal, 40*(12), 1256–1266.

Almazrou, S. H., Alsubki, L. A., Alsaigh, N. A., Aldhubaib, W. H., & Ghazwani, S. M. (2021). Assessing the quality of clinical practice guidelines in the Middle East and North Africa (MENA) region: A systematic review. *The Journal of Multidisciplinary Healthcare, 14,* 297–309.

Alsheikh, M. Y., Alshahrani, A., Almutairi, R. D., Althobaiti, H. A., Fathelrahman, A. I., Seoane-Vazquez, E., et al. (2021). Analysis of gabapentinoids abuse-Reports in the Middle East and North Africa region utilizing the Food and Drug Administration adverse event reporting system. *PTB Reports, 7*(1), 5–8.

Ayad, A. E., Ghaly, N., Ragab, R., Majeed, S., Nassar, H., Al Jalabi, A., et al. (2011). Expert Panel Consensus Recommendations for the pharmacological treatment of acute pain in the Middle East Region. *The Journal of International Medical Research, 39*(4), 1123–1141.

British Pain Society: www.britishpainsociety.org.

Egyptian Society of Regional Anaesthesia and Pain Medicine: www.esrapm.com.

European Pain Federation. (2022). What is the definition of pain? Available at https://europeanpainfederation.eu/what-is-pain/. Accessed 1 September 2023.

Centre for Disease Control www.cdc.gov/injury/pdfs/bsc/BSC_Background_Overview_Progress-GL-Update_6_28_cleared_final_D_Dowell-508-fx.pdf.

International Association for the Study of Pain: www.iasp-pain.org.

Kaba, R., & Sooriakumaran, P. (2007). The evolution of the doctor-patient relationship. *International Journal of Surgery (London, England), 5*(1), 57–65.

Silbermann, M. (2012). Availability of pain medication for patients in the Middle East: Status of the problem and the role of the Middle East Cancer Consortium (MECC): Implications for other regions. *Journal of Palliative Care & Medicine, 2*(6), 1–5.

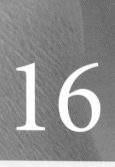

16

END-OF-LIFE CARE

HADYA ABBOUD ABDEL FATTAH ■ SHEILA PAYNE

INTRODUCTION

While some people regard death as a normal part of life, others consider it to be an illness that can be 'cured'. The failure to accept and normalise death means that many people are transferred to hospitals, even very near the end of life, potentially experiencing their last few hours in a lonely and discomforting environment. Death and dying are common in virtually all medical settings. This presents physical and emotional stress for the dying patient, relatives and healthcare professionals (Faronbi et al., 2021; Şahin & Demirkıran, 2021). Currently, only about 14% of people who need palliative care can access it across the world (Dakessian Sailian et al., 2021). Forty million individuals are estimated to need palliative care annually, with 78% of them living in low- and middle-income countries (Dakessian Sailian et al., 2021).

Generally, providing care for patients at the end of life has a number of challenges, especially dealing with physical and psychological concerns in different environments (Muishout et al., 2018). The diversities of recipients and providers in the Middle East create the need to recognise the Arabic and Islamic culture and its social values in order to understand the patient's attitudes to death and dying and to provide the best care at the time of death. Accordingly, this chapter aims to provide guidance on end-of-life and palliative care for healthcare workers, some of whom will be migrant workers in the Middle East, specifically in the Arabian Gulf.

DEFINITIONS OF PALLIATIVE AND END-OF-LIFE CARE

The World Health Organization (WHO, 2002) acknowledges the importance of palliative care and offers a basic definition. Palliative care is now regarded as a core component of universal health coverage (UHC) and has become a key element of quality healthcare, although this has not been translated into practice in all countries

(Knaul et al., 2018). The WHO defined palliative care as 'an approach that improves the quality of life of patients and their families facing the problems associated with life-threatening illness, through the prevention and relief of suffering by means of early identification and impeccable assessment and treatment of pain and other problems, physical, psychosocial and spiritual' (Sepúlveda et al., 2002, p. 94). However, the WHO's definition has some limitations and was criticised by the Lancet Commission (Knaul et al., 2018; see note on Lancet Commission at the end of this section). The authors of the Lancet Commission collaborated with academic leaders from different specialties in science, medicine and global health, to provide recommendations in health policies to improve access to pain management and address health-related suffering. They argued for the need for integrating palliative care in all healthcare settings and in patients' own homes as a mandatory stage to strengthen national healthcare systems. Palliative care is an essential component of comprehensive care for persons with complex chronic or acute, life-threatening health conditions (Knaul et al., 2018). Palliative care also provides an alternative option in such circumstances, as this type of care is primarily focussed on providing relief from the stress and symptoms caused by the dying process, whatever the cause of the death.

End-of-life care offers support in the last part of a patient's life, usually for people who are in the last days, weeks or months of their life (Muishout et al., 2018). End-of-life care attends not just to the physical but also the psychosocial and spiritual concerns of patients and their families and extends into the bereavement period (Gustafson & Lazenby, 2019); considering their values, beliefs and culture to provide them with appropriate comprehensive care (Gamondi et al., 2013; Gustafson & Lazenby, 2019; Radbruch & Payne, 2010). Meanwhile, palliative care focusses on improving the quality of life and quality of care for patients with life-limiting illness and their families through the relief of suffering over a longer period (Harford & Aljawi, 2016). Communication about goals of care, early identification, assessment, treatment of pain and other physical, psychosocial and spiritual problems are the main concerns of palliative care providers. Moreover, palliative care is not just for people nearing the end of their lives. Patients can receive palliative care at the same time as other treatments for particular conditions (Harford & Aljawi, 2016; Muishout et al., 2018).

End-of-life care should help individuals to live as well as possible until they die and to die with dignity. Accordingly, nurses should ask their patients about their wishes and preferences in order to develop a holistic care plan for each patient (Gustafson & Lazenby, 2019). Palliative care is applicable from tertiary hospitals to primary care, delivered by qualified and trained providers (Radbruch & Payne, 2010). People who are approaching the end of life are entitled to high-quality care wherever they are being cared for, including at home, in nursing homes, hospices or hospitals. Helping patients and their relatives realise the nature of their illness and its likely prognosis and trajectory is a crucial aspect of palliative care. Furthermore, palliative care specialists can help patients and their families in determining the appropriate medical care to better align the patient's care goals with those of the healthcare team (Muishout et al., 2018).

Note: The Lancet Commission involved a large group of multidisciplinary international experts who developed an analysis of global access to pain relief and management of health-related suffering.

THE DEVELOPMENT OF PALLIATIVE CARE SERVICES IN THE MIDDLE EAST

In the Middle East, palliative care is relatively new in most countries. Although it is well established in places like Saudi Arabia and Jordan for example, in Yemen and Afghanistan, palliative care is almost unknown. This variation in progress in palliative care development among these countries is largely due to political issues, lack of resources and the lack of professional education and community awareness (Zeinah et al., 2012) (Case Study 16.1). Other reasons include the absence of secure funds and government support, opioid phobia in professionals and the public (Bingley & Clark, 2009), inadequate physical infrastructure, poverty, population density and the geography of the country (Abu-Odah et al., 2020). For example, in Palestine there is very limited provision and they lack most of the basic infrastructure and resources. Palestinian culture is respectful and caring for older people, but most families are unable to take care of their family elders at the end of life when the burden of

CASE STUDY 16.1
CANCER AND FAITH

A 34-year-old Jordanian woman, a mother of three boys and one girl, was diagnosed with breast cancer and referred to the cancer centre for treatment. Unfortunately, the cancer metastasised to the bone, liver, lungs and brain over the course of the next 5 years. Initially, her family chose not to share this information with her in order to maintain her positive attitude but as her condition worsened, they decided to disclose her prognosis. As a devout Muslim, she placed her faith in Allah and wrote letters to all her family members, requesting them to be read after her death. On her brother's wedding day she insisted on missing her chemotherapy session in favour of consuming many painkillers so she could attend the party. The following day, she lapsed into a coma and was initially admitted to ICU. A palliative care room was provided and her family were able to stay with her until she passed away.

She placed her faith in Allah and was able to come to terms with her condition once her prognosis was, eventually, made known to her. She exemplifies the importance of family in decision-making and in the family being visible in providing support at all times.

symptoms is high and consequently most are cared for in hospitals where they usually die (Shawawra & Khleif, 2011). In addition, there are extensive deficiencies in pain management in terminally ill patients with cancer in North Palestine and recommendations on prescribing analgesics fairly without discrimination with regard to the gender and socioeconomic status of patients are required (Ball et al., 2019). Accordingly, developing national and international collaborations, official training and education to professionals, raising public awareness, improving opioid access legislation and healthcare policies as well as secure government or health insurance funding are the suggested solutions to improve palliative care (Ball et al., 2019; Bingley & Clark, 2009; Shawawra & Khleif, 2011; Zeinah et al., 2012).

Globally, 70% of the 9.6 million deaths among cancer patients were recorded in low- and middle-income countries in 2018 (Abu-Odah et al., 2020). The Eastern Mediterranean Region (EMR) anticipates a major increase in cancer and it is expected that there will be 961,000 new cancer cases and 652,000 cancer deaths by 2030 (Fadhil et al., 2017), with the region not being well prepared to manage such cases given insufficient budgets and limited resources (Faronbi

et al., 2021). The EMR, with its 22 countries, has experienced a high level of demand in providing palliative care facilities for cancer patients with a persistent demand to expand access to palliative care services. Furthermore, EMR had the lowest cancer survival rate because most cancer cases are diagnosed at a later stage than, for example, in Europe and the Americas. However, political issues and shortage of resources are the most common factors restricting the progress of palliative care. Moreover, a gap in access to pain relief medicines, lack of national palliative care policies and limited partnerships were the other main barriers to making further improvements to palliative care services in the EMR (Fadhil et al., 2017). This challenge extends to overcoming political influence and providing support to guarantee the sustainability of high-quality palliative care services to patients in low- and middle-income countries (Abu-Odah et al., 2020).

While there are significant challenges in developing palliative care services in EMR, there has been some progress. This region extends from Pakistan in the east to Morocco in the west, with countries that vary in population size, income, Human Development Index (HDI) and health expenditure. For example, in Saudi Arabia, palliative care started at the King Faisal Hospital in the early 1990s, which then increased to 20 institutes led by specialised Saudi trainers. In Qatar, the first palliative care service with 10 beds was established in 2008 (Dakessian Sailian et al., 2021). Since 2010, palliative care in Bahrain is accessible in the Salmanyia Medical Complex (SMC) hospital provided by trained oncology professionals but there has been minimal progress as a result of limited funding (Fadhil et al., 2017). More recently, the Bahrain Oncology Centre, with state-of-the-art facilities attached to the King Hamad University Hospital in Muharraq, was inaugurated in 2019 and continues to develop. The Jordanian WHO Palliative Care Demonstration Project established a professional model of palliative care at King Hussein Cancer Center (KHCC) in 2003 and Al Basheer Hospital (Fadhil et al., 2017). Jordan launched a national strategy for palliative and home care in 2018, endorsed and funded by the government. Further, in 2018, palliative medicine was accredited as a 2-year fellowship programme and a subspecialty board examination, which was accredited by the Jordanian Medical Council (Shamieh et al., 2020).

The United Arab Emirates (UAE) is actively placing great attention and efforts into creating standardised delivery systems within the palliative care structures and is working hard to minimise the suffering of cancer patients. Moreover, it is expecting to further develop palliative care services based upon the WHO recommendations (Al-Alfi, 2015). The WHO country cooperation strategy report stated that UAE is party to the revised International Health Regulations (IHR) that entered into force in 2007. Two authorities, the Ministry of Health for regulating the public health sector and the Emirates health authorities accountable for service delivery at the state level in Dubai and Abu Dhabi, manage the UAE health sector. The UAE Government's 2021 vision is committed to ensuring universal access to world-class healthcare services to fulfil citizens' growing needs and expectations (WHO, 2017). Elsewhere, Kuwait and Tunisia are reported to have a standalone palliative care policy and plan (Fadhil et al., 2017). In addition, there has been a momentous progression in Lebanese palliative care from no palliative care service in 2009 to two non-governmental organisations (NGOs) providing home-based programmes in four hospitals with a national committee (Dakessian Sailian et al., 2021).

TRAINING AND EDUCATIONAL REQUIREMENTS FOR PALLIATIVE CARE IN THE MIDDLE EAST

The nurse's responsibility toward a patient who has almost reached the end of their life is crucial. The nurse's role in palliative care is to provide a certain type of care that focusses on promoting comfort, relief of pain and treating other symptoms by offering support to the patients and the patient's relatives (Gamondi et al., 2013). However, nurses caring for palliative care patients have arguably the most stressful time when compared to other members of the healthcare team as they spend more time interacting with the complex demands of dying patients (Faronbi et al., 2021). Jafari et al. (2015) have noted that nursing students showed negative or neutral attitudes toward caring for dying patients as they had limited previous experience with dying patients in their clinical courses. They argued that direct exposure to terminally ill and dying patients with formal training is expected to affect

students' comfort when treating dying patients positively. Therefore caring for dying patients should be integrated into undergraduate nursing curricula.

Since nurses play a vital role in ensuring quality of care, nursing education plays a crucial role in helping nurses to deal with dying patients both emotionally and physically (Ferri et al., 2021). All palliative care providers should receive training on core competencies of practices via a variety of educational programmes to be able to provide high standards of care to end-of-life patients and their families (Gamondi et al., 2013). Accordingly, health settings need to provide specific education on end-of-life care as part of their continuing professional development strategies for their workers, but many lack proper training on end-of-life care (Dakessian Sailian et al., 2021). Gamondi et al. (2013) discussed the 10 core competencies of palliative care practice in their 'White Paper', which is considered a benchmark for good practice. The key principles of palliative care are working in cooperation as a team, sharing discipline-specific skills with colleagues and having a willingness to learn from each other that could improve the overall outcomes for palliative care patients.

END-OF-LIFE CARE DECISIONS AND TREATMENT OPTIONS IN AN ISLAMIC CULTURE

Many cultural care barriers and gaps have been identified among terminally ill Muslim patients when being treated in hospice care models established for non-Muslim populations (Gustafson & Lazenby, 2019). Palliative care providers come from different clinical backgrounds (Gamondi et al., 2013). Better education and orientation for the standards of culturally competent care are needed to provide Muslim patients at the end of life with safe treatment practices in non-Muslim majority settings. In addition, further research is needed with a particular emphasis on investigating the experiences of terminally ill Muslim patients receiving treatment in Muslim minority settings (Gustafson & Lazenby, 2019).

The Islamic naturalistic belief is that God is the 'owner' of the human body and the manager of his deeds, while individuals should protect their life from any harm and not actively terminate human life (Aramesh, 2009; Padela & Mohiuddin, 2015). Integrating Islamic practices into palliative care is one of the main cultural responsibilities of the healthcare team toward Muslim patients. Providing care with respect and dignity, facing the patient towards Mecca during the dying period, bathing the patient and keeping them physically clean and accommodating religious objects are the most common Islamic practices toward the end of life in Muslim patients.

When it comes to Muslim families, they must be informed about the patient's death right away because they must undertake rapid and traditional funeral rites and this requires considerable effort and preparation. Furthermore, it is of paramount importance to bury the patient's body as soon as possible to ensure the patient's dignity (Gustafson & Lazenby, 2019).

Muslim patients at the palliative care stage require adequate culturally safe care similar to that experienced by other patients, especially when delivered by non-Muslim providers (Harford & Aljawi, 2016). There is considerable diversity with regard to end-of-life issues in the Islamic religion among different subgroups due to local, legal, social and cultural attitudes towards Islamic scholars in general and political norms specifically (Chakraborty et al., 2017). For example, the religious backgrounds of physicians have been noted to influence them in rejecting many treatments that may potentially delay or accelerate the dying process, such as policies on 'Do Not Resuscitate (DNR)' and consequently they may avoid discussing these options with their patients (Seale, 2010). Healthcare providers understand that although Muslim patients follow one religion, they have many subgroups with different views and must deal with them without judgment. Thus Saeed et al. (2015) suggested that 66.8% of Islamic scholars allowed DNR orders while 7.38% did not, with 21.2% saying they had never thought about it.

Although Islam is a religion that encourages its followers to seek medical treatment when they are feeling unwell, it also perceives this as an opportunity to gain good deeds and expiate individual sins to obtain a higher degree in paradise. Moreover, Muslims believe that Allah did not send a sickness on its own, but it comes with natural medication that they must try to find. Therefore Islamic instruction requires the community members to visit the sick and the sick to welcome their guests (Dakessian Sailian et al., 2021).

The impact on perceptions of palliative care, including end-of-life decision-making, has been evaluated in different cultures. The general Islamic view of healthcare supports providing access to unlimited curative therapies to patients (Zargani et al., 2018). Religion is another issue that indicates a cautious approach in evolving policies for end-of-life care and creating up-to-date clinical guidelines addressing many matters through having responses (fatwa's) from respected Islamic authorities. Currently, there are no clear or approved policies of 'Do Not Resuscitate or 'Allow Natural Death' in law that could compromise the health workers' legal situation and license to practice (Al-Alfi, 2015). However, the discontinuation of therapy is accepted if that continuation could harm the patient and will not progress his health based on three reliable physicians' decisions. The Saudi Arabia-based Islamic Fiqh Academy (IFA) in 2015 and other Islamic schools of law supported this opinion. Although Islamic legal and ethical scholars have approved many health practices on end of life, such as the withdrawal of life support or obtaining organs for transplantation from brain dead patients, the rejection of such practices can also be encountered among brain dead patients' families (Khalid et al., 2012; Zargani et al., 2018).

PRACTICAL OPPORTUNITIES AND CHALLENGES IN PROVIDING NURSING CARE NEAR THE END OF LIFE

Middle Eastern families' involvement in the decision-making and end-of-life procedures of the ill person is very common; therefore making sure not to intervene with the patient's family's wishes is essential for healthcare providers. However, sometimes that makes the family members feel ashamed to make decisions on behalf of the patient. Accordingly, nurses in the Middle East understand that their patients are willing to have their own families surrounding them during bedside care and they will feel offended if they are asked to leave the patient alone. Healthcare providers work on building a trusting relationship with Muslim patients and their families through providing space for prayer while facilitating privacy and family gatherings (Harford & Aljawi, 2016). In addition, psychological dignity is accomplished by respecting the patient's emotional response to death as per their own religious-cultural values. Patients are supported through providing privacy and in discussing their needs and treatment progress. In addition, spiritual dignity is observed by integrating the patient's spiritual beliefs and values into their daily care. Thus the end-of-life patient's daily treatment and decision-making should provide them with direct spiritual guidance (Gustafson & Lazenby, 2019; Harford & Aljawi, 2016). Healthcare providers should, therefore, encourage patients to talk about death and dying and other sensitive topics such as the loss of personal dignity (Nils et al., 2020).

Terminally ill patients receiving palliative care may suffer from many common symptoms such as pain and nausea that can be treated by regular medications. However, other intolerable symptoms can be relieved by the use of palliative sedation (Beller et al., 2015; Muishout et al., 2018; Stiel et al., 2018). For example, terminally ill patients in the last days of life may experience psychological and physical distress due to other common symptoms such as delirium, agitation, anxiety, terminal restlessness, dyspnoea, pain and vomiting, which require palliative sedation as a possible solution to relieve the refractory symptoms that are not controlled by other means (Belar et al., 2020).

Palliative sedation is a complex topic and there are differences in how it is used throughout Europe. Physicians have a moral imperative to reduce patients' pain in their final stage of life (Muishout et al., 2018). Healthcare professionals face challenges in dealing with their own thoughts and feelings when treating Muslim patients that are arguably compromised by the absence of fatwas on using palliative sedation. In Islamic legal sources, Prophet Muhammad is of paramount importance: 'Every intoxicant (muskir) is forbidden' (Mustaghfirin, 2019). Islam has strictly prohibited the use of drugs that might affect consciousness. Therefore the ethical dilemma continues that sedation will interfere with the Muslim patient's abilities to perform their mandatory daily five prayers and how to compensate for their prayers after returning to consciousness (Aramesh, 2009; Muishout et al., 2018).

KEY POINTS IN PROVIDING CULTURALLY SENSITIVE PALLIATIVE CARE (CASE STUDY 16.2)

Ultimately, there is a hidden message of hope, meaning that even though diagnosis and evidence might infer

CASE STUDY 16.2
CHRONIC DISEASE MANAGEMENT AND SOCIO-ECONOMIC IMPACTS

Mr X, a 54-year-old Indian man, diagnosed with COPD with a history of hypertension, hyperlipidaemia and hypothyroidism was admitted to the emergency room (ER) complaining of severe shortness of breath, confusion, exhaustion and swelling in both lower limbs. His oxygen saturation level fell markedly and he was put on ventilation in ICU. Mr X was the family wage earner and had a wife and three children as well as providing for his extended family at home. For this reason, although he knew his condition was worsening, he was reluctant to seek help. His increasingly complex healthcare was also expensive. His understandable reluctance to engage with healthcare services made management of his symptoms much more difficult and he sadly passed away without being able to make provision for his family.

KEY ISSUES

- Inaccurate diagnosis and limited resources may result in delays in receiving diagnosis, treatment and palliative care.
- People from migrant groups and, or lower socioeconomic classes, are more likely to be diagnosed at a later stage and therefore have poorer outcomes.
- Cancer and end-of-life care not only involves addressing physical symptoms such as agitation or pain, but also in dealing with important family issues such as money and welfare concerns as well as, of course, spiritual and cultural issues.
- To improve the quality of care for both patients and their families, palliative care should be considered from the time the patient is diagnosed with cancer.
- In palliative care settings, clear and effective communication is essential; therefore key aspects such as disclosure must be handled sensitively. Moreover, the importance of the family in supporting the patient is key.
- Incorporating ethical principles, symptom management, communication and dealing with spiritual and religious issues is essential to improve patient's end-of-life care services.
- Care does not end with death. Following death there may be rituals that need to be observed and these may have to be addressed immediately. Moreover, non-native patients may wish to be repatriated and this is something that requires knowledge, sensitivity and due consideration.

Based on Rattani, S., Dahlke, S., & Cameron, B. (2022). Cancer care in Pakistan: A descriptive case study. *Global Qualitative Nursing Research*, 9, 233339362210809. https://doi.org/10.1177/23333936221080988.

death is near, the future holds something better and unexpected. For example, it is not necessarily true that a person dies immediately after receiving palliative care; in fact, a person may survive and live for many months after receiving such care, in spite of suffering from a terminal illness (Abdulhameed et al., 2011). Nevertheless, this happens only in rare and exceptional cases and is not common. Healthcare providers should always promote hope and faith to all patients in such circumstances.

As Martin Luther King Jr. once said, 'We must accept finite disappointment, but never lose infinite hope'. This light of hope should be given all throughout the patient's care and treatment and likewise to their family members. Moreover, we must ensure the real meaning of palliative care is made known; that is, providing special care to people with life-threatening illnesses, ensuring patients achieve their health goals in their remaining time. Palliative care cannot provide miracles and death is inevitable for all of us. However, the main purpose of palliative care is to ensure a peaceful death with less pain and surrounded by loved ones, ensuring the final memories of the patient are less painful for the patient and their family. All this should be provided to every patient regardless of religion, economic, social, physiological or cultural status (Abdulhameed et al., 2011; Hannawi & Salmi, 2015; Kwon & Choi, 2021; Lovering (2012); Ludin (2018); Radbruch & Payne, 2009).

SUMMARY AND TAKEAWAY POINTS

■ Palliative care is a vital part of healthcare that should be accessible to all patients regardless of their social, cultural and economic background. Hence, the chapter discussed the development of palliative care services in the Middle East, training requirements, end-of-life care decisions and treatment options in Islamic cultures and the practical opportunities and challenges in providing nursing care near the end of life.

■ We provided guidance on end-of-life care for healthcare workers in the Middle East, specifically in the Arabian Gulf. Arab and Islamic countries share a similar background as Arabic is the spoken language and both follow the common tenets of Islam.

■ There are differences with the standards of care in these countries and many of their end-of-life institutions depend on donations.

■ Standards of care also vary depending upon the healthcare workforce and the patient recipients, some of whom may be poor, vulnerable migrants and possibly even refugees. Consequently, such patients may face particular challenges due to language differences, religion, cultural diversity and poverty, making accessing appropriate care difficult.

■ The heterogeneous cultures evident in the region mean that ensuring cultural competence is essential in providing good quality healthcare. Cultural competency therefore is essential with regard to all aspects of 'Muslim' culture as well as attending to the diversity of the majority expatriate workforces (Al-Alfi, 2015).

REFERENCES

Abdulhameed, H., Hammami, M., & Hameed Mohamed, E. (2011). Disclosure of terminal illness to patients and families: Diversity of governing codes in 14 Islamic countries. *Journal of Medical Ethics*, 37(8), 472–475. https://doi.org/10.1136/jme.2010.038497.

Abu-Odah, H., Molassiotis, A., & Liu, J. (2020). Challenges on the provision of palliative care for patients with cancer in low- and middle-income countries: A systematic review of reviews. *BMC Palliative Care*, 19(1), 55. https://doi.org/10.1186/s12904-020-00558-5.

Al-Alfi, N. (2015). Palliative care in the United Arab Emirates: A nurse's perspective. *Journal of Palliative Care and Medicine*, S5, S5–005. https://doi.org/10.4172/2165-7386.1000s5006.

Aramesh, K. (2009). Iran's experience with surrogate motherhood: An Islamic view and ethical concerns. *Journal of Medical Ethics*, 35(5), 320–322. https://doi.org/10.1136/jme.2008.027763.

Ball, S., Mallah, H., Mousa, R., Fadl, N., Musmar, S., & Nugent, K. (2019). Pain severity and adequacy of pain management in terminally ill patients with cancer: An experience from North Palestine. *Indian Journal of Palliative Care*, 25(4), 494. https://doi.org/10.4103/ijpc.ijpc_39_19.

Belar, A., Arantzamendi, M., Payne, S., Preston, N., Rijpstra, M., Hasselaar, J., et al. (2020). How to measure the effects and potential adverse events of palliative sedation? An integrative review. *Palliative Medicine*, 35(2), 295–314. https://doi.org/10.1177/0269216320974264.

Bingley, A., & Clark, D. (2009). A comparative review of palliative care development in six countries represented by the Middle East Cancer Consortium (MECC). *Journal of Pain and Symptom Management*, 37(3), 287–296. https://doi.org/10.1016/j.jpainsymman.2008.02.014.

Beller, E., van Driel, M., McGregor, L., Truong, S., & Mitchell, G. (2015). Palliative pharmacological sedation for terminally ill adults. *Cochrane Database of Systematic Reviews*, 2018(11), CD010206. https://doi.org/10.1002/14651858.cd010206.pub2.

Chakraborty, R., El-Jawahri, A., Litzow, M., Syrjala, K., Parnes, A., & Hashmi, S. (2017). A systematic review of religious beliefs about major end-of-life issues in the five major world religions. *Palliative and Supportive Care*, 15(5), 609–622. https://doi.org/10.1017/s1478951516001061.

Dakessian Sailian, S., Salifu, Y., Saad, R., & Preston, N. (2021). Dignity of patients with palliative needs in the Middle East: An integrative review. *BMC Palliative Care*, 20(1). https://doi.org/10.1186/s12904-021-00791-6.

Fadhil, I., Lyons, G., & Payne, S. (2017). Barriers to, and opportunities for, palliative care development in the Eastern Mediterranean Region. *The Lancet Oncology*, 18(3), e176–e184. https://doi.org/10.1016/s1470-2045(17)30101-8.

Faronbi, J., Akinyoola, O., Faronbi, G., Bello, C., Kuteyi, F., & Olabisi, I. (2021). Nurses' attitude toward caring for dying patients in a Nigerian Teaching Hospital. *SAGE Open Nursing*, 7. https://doi.org/10.1177/23779608211005213. 237796082110052.

Ferri, P., Di Lorenzo, R., Stifani, S., Morotti, E., Vagnini, M., Jiménez Herrera, M. F., et al. (2021). Nursing student attitudes toward dying patient care: A European multicenter cross-sectional study. *Acta Biomed*, 92(S2), e2021018. https://doi.org/10.23750/abm.v92iS2.11403. PMID: 33855982; PMCID: PMC8138802.

Gustafson, C., & Lazenby, M. (2019). Assessing the unique experiences and needs of Muslim oncology patients receiving palliative and end-of-life care: An integrative review. *Journal of Palliative Care*, 34(1), 52–61. https://doi.org/10.1177/0825859718800496.

Gamondi, C., Larkin, P., & Payne, S. A. (2013). Core competencies in palliative care: an EAPC white paper on palliative care education: Part 2. *European Journal of Palliative Care*, 20(3), 140–145. Available at https://www.sicp.it/wp-content/uploads/2018/12/6_EJPC203Gamondi_part2_0.PDF. Accessed 23 August 2023.

Hannawi, S., & Salmi, I. (2015). Health workforce in the United Arab Emirates: Analytic point of view. *The International Journal of Health Planning and Management*, 29(4), 332–341. https://doi.org/10.1002/hpm.2198.

Harford, J., & Aljawi, D. (2016). The need for more and better palliative care for Muslim patients. *Palliative and Supportive Care*, 11(1), 1–4. https://doi.org/10.1017/S1478951512000053.

Jafari, M., Rafiei, H., Nassehi, A., Soleimani, F., Arab, M., & Noormohammadi, M. R. (2015). Caring for dying patients: Attitude of nursing students and effects of education. *Indian J Palliat Care*, 21(2), 192–197. https://doi.org/10.4103/0973-1075.156497.

Khalid, I., Hamad, W., Khalid, T., Kadri, M., & Qushmaq, I. (2012). End-of-life care in Muslim brain-dead patients. *American Journal of Hospice and Palliative Medicine*, 30(5), 413–418. https://doi.org/10.1177/1049909112452625.

Knaul, F. M., Farmer, P. E., Krakauer, E. L., De Lima, L., Bhadelia, A., Jiang Kwete, X., et al. (2018). Alleviating the access abyss in palliative care and pain relief—an imperative of universal health coverage: The Lancet Commission report. *The Lancet*, 391(10128), 1391–1454. https://doi.org/10.1016/S0140-6736(17)32513-8.

Kwon, S., & Choi, S. (2021). Experiences of hospice and palliative nurses in response to the COVID-19 pandemic: A qualitative study. *The Korean Journal of Hospice and Palliative Care*, 24(4), 245–253. https://doi.org/10.14475/jhpc.2021.24.4.245.

Lovering, S. (2012). The crescent of care: A nursing model to guide the care of Arab Muslim patients. *Diversity and Equality in Health and Care*, 9, 171–178. Available at https://www.researchgate.net/publication/265547331. Accessed 1 August 2023.

Ludin, S. (2018). Does good critical thinking equal effective decision-making among critical care nurses? A cross-sectional survey. *Intensive and Critical Care Nursing*, 44, 1–10. https://doi.org/10.1016/j.iccn.2017.06.002.

Muishout, G., van Laarhoven, H., Wiegers, G., & Popp-Baier, U. (2018). Muslim physicians and palliative care: Attitudes towards the use of palliative sedation. *Supportive Care In Cancer*, 26(11), 3701–3710. https://doi.org/10.1007/s00520-018-4229-7.

Mustaghfirin, M. (2019). Marātib al-Wilāyah Min al-Abdāl Wa al-Aqtāb Wa al-Nuqabā' Wa al-Nujabā' 'Inda al-Muhaddithīn. *Refleksi*, 18(2), 201–222. https://doi.org/10.15408/ref.v18i2.13031.

Nils, L., Eggert, S., Lux, K., Werdan, U., & Suhr, R. (2020). Perceptions of clients and their informal caregivers regarding fear of death and dying in home care—a multicenter cross sectional study. *Archives of Palliative Care and Medicine*, 4(01), 2689–9825. https://doi.org/10.29011/2689-9825.000016.

Padela, A., & Mohiuddin, A. (2015). Islamic goals for clinical treatment at the end of life: The concept of accountability before God (Taklīf) remains useful: Response to open peer commentaries on "ethical obligations and clinical goals in end-of-life care: Deriving a quality-of-life construct based on the Islamic concept of accountability before God (Taklīf)". *The American Journal of Bioethics*, 15(1), W1–W8. https://doi.org/10.1080/15265161.2015.983353.

Radbruch, L., & Payne, S. (2009). White paper on standards and norms for hospice and palliative care in Europe: Part 1. *European Journal of Palliative Care*, 16(6), 278–289. https://www.researchgate.net/publication/279547069.

Radbruch, L., & Payne, S. (2010). White Paper on standards and norms for hospice and palliative care in Europe : Part 2. *European Journal of Palliative Care*, 17(1), 22–33. Available at https://www.researchgate.net/publication/279547069. Accessed 3 July 2023.

Stiel, S., Nurnus, M., Ostgathe, C., & Klein, C. (2018). Palliative sedation in Germany: Factors and treatment practices associated with different sedation rate estimates in palliative and hospice care services. *BMC Palliative Care*, 17(1), 2–7. https://doi.org/10.1186/s12904-018-0303-7.

Shamieh, O., Richardson, K., Abdel-Razeq, H., Mansour, A., & Payne, S. (2020). Gaining palliative medicine subspecialty recognition and fellowship accreditation in Jordan. *Journal of Pain and Symptom Management*, 60(5), 1003–1011. https://doi.org/10.1016/j.jpainsymman.2020.05.016.

Saeed, F., Kousar, N., Aleem, S., et al. (2015). End-of-life care beliefs among Muslim physicians. *American Journal of Hospice and Palliative Medicine*, 32(4), 388–392. https://doi.org/10.1177/1049909114522687.

Sepúlveda, C., Marlin, A., Yoshida, T., & Ullrich, A. (2002). Palliative care: The World Health Organization's global perspective. *J Pain Symptom Manage*, 24(2), 91–96. Available at http://www.jpsmjournal.com/article/S0885392402004402/fulltext. Accessed 20 August 2023.

Şahin, M., & Demirkıran, F. (2021). Does death anxiety affect nurses' attitudes about the care of dying patient? A cross-sectional study. *Neuropsychiatric Investigation*, *59*(1), 8–13. https://doi.org/10.5455/nys.20200509104203.

Seale, C. (2010). The role of doctors' religious faith and ethnicity in taking ethically controversial decisions during end-of-life care. *Journal Of Medical Ethics*, *36*(11), 677–682. https://doi.org/10.1136/jme.2010.036194.

Shawawra, M., & Khleif, A. (2011). Palliative care situation in Palestinian Authority. *Journal of Pediatric Hematology/Oncology*, *33*(Supplement 1), S64–S67. https://doi.org/10.1097/mph.0b013e31821223a3.

WHO. (2002). World health report: 2002. Available at https://www.who.int/publications/i/item/9241562072. Accessed 28 September 2023.

WHO. (2017). WHO country cooperation strategy at a glance: United Arab Emirates. Available at https://apps.who.int/iris/handle/10665/136976. Accessed 23 September 2023.

Zeinah, G., Al-Kindi, S., & Hassan, A. (2012). Middle East experience in palliative care. *American Journal of Hospice and Palliative Medicine*, *30*(1), 94–99. https://doi.org/10.1177/1049909112439619.

Zargani, A., Nasiri, M., Hekmat, K., Abbaspour, Z., & Vahabi, S. (2018). A survey on the relationship between religiosity and quality of life in patients with breast cancer: A study in Iranian Muslims. *Asia-Pacific Journal of Oncology Nursing*, *5*(2), 217–222. https://doi.org/10.4103/apjon.apjon_65_17.

FURTHER READING

Cancer Net: http://cancernet.nci.nih.gov/pdq/pdq_supportive_care.shtml.

End-of-Life Physician Education Resource Center (EPERC): http://www.eperc.mcw.edu/.

Health A to Z: www.healthatoz.com/atoz/Palliativecare/pcindex.asp.

Hospice Net: www.hospicenet.org/index.html.

National Hospice and Palliative Care Organization: www.nhpco.org.

WHO. (2007). The world health report 2007: A safer future—global public health security in the 21st century. Available at https://www.who.int/publications/i/item/9789241563444. Accessed 23 September 2023.

17 TECHNOLOGY-ENHANCED LEARNING AND LEADERSHIP

JANE LEANNE GRIFFITHS ▪ JAMES WATERSON

INTRODUCTION

This chapter focusses on nursing leadership and management. It highlights the specific challenges and unique experiences faced by this region in terms of healthcare delivery and healthcare providers. Aside from the problems in managing such a diverse workforce, it also identifies the rapid changes experienced and implemented in a relatively short time frame in comparison to Western countries. These changes have included competency programmes, diversity plans and implementation of technology and informatics to improve patient care and safety.

The nurse leaders of this region face common issues in line with their Western counterparts. These include the dual roles of clinician and leader as well as a focus on economic and administrative efficiencies compared with a fundamental emphasis on patient safety and patient care (Stewart, 2012).

One of the most significant issues facing nursing and midwifery is the cultural perception of nurses in this region. The history of nursing in the Islamic world begins with women such as a Muslim nurse Rufaidah Al-Asalmiya, working with the Prophet Muhammad (peace be upon him) to care for the sick and injured (Al-Osimy, 1994). However, as time progressed the nature of nursing came to be at odds with the local culture. The role and duties of nurses involving after-hours shifts, caring for men (strangers) and working alongside males, led to a low societal perception and a reluctance for Emiratis to choose nursing as a preferred field of study and for their families to support this decision (Kemp & Zhao, 2016). The other component contributing to the adverse perceptions of nursing is also related to the predominantly expatriate workforce. Ninety-six percent of the nursing workforce is sourced from the Asian subcontinent which also supplies the nannies, cooks and cleaners that support the domestic roles in local society. This blurring of roles/nationalities has resulted in nursing staff being viewed as 'second-class citizens' or 'handmaidens', in terms of both treatment and attitude towards them.

The task for any nursing leader in this region is to initially overcome this societal opinion on an individual level and then to develop the nursing workforce into staff who are articulate, critical thinkers and focussed on patient care and safety, which will then ensure they are recognised as essential health professionals at all levels of society.

BACKGROUND

The politics of the region includes differences in geographical names. The 'Persian' or 'Arabian Gulf' borders the region to the north, Saudi Arabia to the south and west and Oman to the east, and it includes Kuwait, Bahrain, Qatar and the United Arab Emirates (UAE). The 1960s saw the discovery of oil and set up the region financially. Each country is ruled by a royal family focussed on the rapid development of infrastructure such as technology, education and the healthcare sector (OECD, 2021).

The total population in the UAE is 9,890,400 (Dubai Online, 2020) of which 88% are expatriate workers with the majority, at 65%, coming from the Asian subcontinent, 18% from the greater Arab countries, 6% from the Philippines and 11% consisting of local Emiratis.

Healthcare is even more focussed on an expatriate workforce. Less than 3% of nurses are Emirati (Al-Rifai, 2003), 96% of expatriate nurses (D'Souza, 2013; El-Haddad, 2006) are recruited from the Philippines, India, Pakistan and other Arab nations such as Jordan, Lebanon and Egypt, while 1% are Western nurses recruited into leadership/management roles from the United States, United Kingdom, Australia, Canada and South Africa.

Healthcare services are a mix of public and private facilities focussed on preventive, elective, emergency, public health and health tourism. Regardless of the facility ownership (public or private), health facilities are regulated by the Government and must meet predetermined policies, procedures and safety regulations. Most healthcare organisations also undergo external review examinations to ensure compliance with international standards (Joint Commission International (JCIA), Australian Council Healthcare Standards (ACHS), International Standards Organisation (ISO), etc.).

Modern healthcare in the region started with the first hospital to be built in the UAE at Al Maktoum in Dubai in 1951. This is a stark comparison with the Western world that started modern healthcare in the 1860s (Sheingold & Hahn, 2014).

The wider and speedy development of the region has forced the rapid development of its healthcare services (Brownie et al., 2015). These advances have drawn attention to specific challenges for nursing leadership in this region.

SPECIFIC CHALLENGES AND INTERVENTIONS

Diversity is probably the most significant challenge faced by healthcare leaders in this region. When discussing diversity most healthcare professionals focus on ensuring that we care for our patients in a culturally competent manner (Bickhoff, 2018). This is important as most nursing staff caring for patients in this region are not Muslims, but their patients are predominantly Muslim. In 2012 a culturally specific model for Arab Muslim populations set within a context of psychosocial, cultural, interpersonal, clinical and spiritual elements of care was developed (Lovering, 2012). This model was designed to teach non-Muslim nursing staff the significance of cultural and spiritual aspects of their patients. This is critical, but to achieve this outcome nursing leaders need to understand thoroughly the actual diversity within our workforce. As discussed previously, the nursing workforce in the region is predominantly expatriate, from India, the Philippines and the greater Arab world. Therefore the clinical, educational and cultural backgrounds of these different nationalities vary from one another significantly.

In 2015 a conference was convened locally in Abu Dhabi to discuss the differences between the three cultures that contribute to the nursing workforce in the region. The purpose was to understand the cultural differences of the nursing staff and the impact this has on communication, education and interactions between themselves and their patients. In the process of teaching both patients and staff effectively, an educator is essentially transmitting their own compiled experiences and distilled information to the learner. This process can, of course, never be effective unless the educator can communicate well and communication can only be effective if one understands their audience. Getting your point of view across, and more importantly, in a way that the learner would comprehend it, depends on how well you can communicate it (Bittar, 2015). It is easier to communicate in an environment where your audience understands your language, your behaviours, your body language and your background culture. This is challenging in a multicultural environment. This is

CASE STUDY 17.1
PERSPECTIVES ON DIFFERENT CULTURES

PERSPECTIVES ON ARABIC CULTURE

Arabs have accumulated rich and diversified cultures that are influenced by many other surrounding cultures. Arabs in general are spirited, which means they are assertive and very expressive, but respond better to considerate forms of communication. They are polite and tend not to 'say no' directly and will often want to speak in private rather than in front of their peers. Arabs are diplomatic and expect you to understand the hidden meaning of their communication but expect to be treated politely. They are very respectful of their educators and elders and are very enthusiastic to be involved in new initiatives. Pride and family is very strong in this culture, which means they will almost never let you know they do not understand what you are saying. This is essential for both nursing leaders and care givers when communicating or teaching staff and patients.

Based on Bittar, W. (2015). Perspectives on education in different cultures. Conference Proceedings, 6th Middle East Nursing Conference, Abu Dhabi.

PERSPECTIVES ON INDIAN CULTURE

Indians in general are outwardly focussed and extrovert in interaction with others. Indians live in time rather than place; they like to contemplate and live in peace with nature. Religion is Indians' first love and they believe in freedom of silence. Learning preferences are passive, they are reluctant to question their teacher or leader. They seek concrete information and are analytic, needing data to aid in reflection—favouring slow, accurate, systematic approaches rather than impulse decisions. They are socially active and work well in groups but are competitive and desire to succeed and seek recognition for action and achievements and moderation. They are more comfortable as 'receivers of knowledge' rather than self-exploring. They respect teachers' and elders' views and are hesitant exploring contradictory views. The preferred learning process is lecture mode with the preferred teaching tool being explanation of concepts and then relating to the applications, with a focus on the use of diagrams, figures, tables, charts, etc.

Based on Anthony, J. (2015). Perspectives on education in different cultures. Conference Proceedings, 6th Middle East Nursing Conference, Abu Dhabi.
    Sharma, A. A. (2009). Learning styles across culture: study on learning style of students pursuing management education in India. *Management & Change, 13*(2), 45–62.

PERSPECTIVES ON FILIPINO CULTURE

The Philippines train 250,000 nurses per year to work/export to a range of overseas countries. Filipinos in general are low in individualism and strong in a collective approach with absolute loyalty to their families and a strong affiliation with their peers. They have a strong respect for their teachers, parents and leaders. Filipinos focus on a hierarchy of decision making and rules and those that are powerful and powerless. They have a basic mistrust of hierarchy but are hesitant to enter into conflict. They are educated in a traditional and formal learning environment with their peers but will participate on an individual basis if the education is informal, incidental or social learning. They prefer to 'watch first' and then undertake 'hands on' learning experiences. They work well in environments that have role models or preceptors. Leaders, managers and trainers need to recognise and acknowledge achievements of students and staff.

Based on Retolin, S. (2015). Perspectives on Education in different cultures. Conference Proceedings, 6th Middle East Nursing Conference, Abu Dhabi.
    Smith, W. (2011). *Exploring the learning experiences of Filipino nurse immigrants new to the U.S. healthcare industry.* Northern Illinois University.

---

also a key requirement for nursing leaders when dealing with their peers, executive teams, staff and patients and relatives.

The differences between the nationalities are both diverse and fascinating. Case Study 17.1 outlines essential differences in three nationalities.

This cultural diversity among nurses and midwives leads to challenges relating to change and career development. Most healthcare leaders have focussed on the development and implementation of guidelines and processes that clearly identify and outline the skills required by the various levels of nurses in different clinical areas. These include pre-employment checks, recruitment interviewing and orientation to the organisation. However, the concept of nondirect care role requirements is used to differentiate the components of a registered nurse's scope of practice that do not relate to the direct delivery of clinical patient care. These nondirect care components include clinical and patient education, clinical and professional leadership and management. These components have become increasingly prominent in the role of registered nurses, particularly with a highly differentiated nursing workforce (assistant nurse, registered nurse mix), greater consumer demands and the increased requirements of healthcare organisations for improvements in efficiency and for measurement and proof of effectiveness.

To address both the nonclinical care components and the cultural diversity among nursing staff, a programme was developed from within the Dubai Health Authority called The Competency Framework—A Triad of Opportunities. The Framework was constructed around three professional streams (domains) considered essential to the professional practice of all registered nurses in the organisation—clinical leadership, management and education. The Competency Framework was also considered to provide clinicians with the opportunity to explore potential career pathways, obtain educational and experiential support to improve their proficiency and to expand their professional portfolios. Within the framework there are 11 competencies generic to each stream and a number of stream-specific competencies—the number and level of competencies required by each staff member is determined by the level of appointment/role within the organisation (Newman, 2012). Case Study 17.2 outlines the competencies developed to assist nursing staff in their career development and to enhance the professional development and perceptions of nursing both within healthcare facilities and the wider society. These change programmes and career ladders can be defined as systems for both reward and recognition of new expertise and skills (Bjork et al., 2007).

The implementation of the fourth industrial revolution has had a direct impact on how we live and work. Technology is significantly affecting healthcare and the use of information and communication is forming the basis of e-health (WHO, 2020). Digital health includes electronic medical records (EMRs), telehealth, smart pharmacy, digital devices, robots and artificial intelligence. These all have a significant impact on both the way nurses work and the care they provide for their patients (Raghunathan & Tomkins, 2019/2020). These changes include allowing patients to be involved in their care and decision making, improving utilisation, ease of access to evidence-based resources and reducing medication and documentation errors (Bichel-Findlay, 2019–2020). It is essential that nurse leaders in this region are at the fore during both the frequently complex, decision-making processes leading to selection of technology and during the implementation processes once the selection has been made. Our nursing workforce is not only culturally diverse, but also technologically diverse. Some of our staff are digital experts (born after 1980) while

CASE STUDY 17.2
COMPETENCY MATRICES FOR THREE NURSING DEVELOPMENT STREAMS
Clinical, Education and Management

These competencies have been developed to assist nursing staff in their career development and to enhance their professional development. Each competency is divided into sections enhancing the theoretical aspect of the competency as well as the practical application of the skill.

MATRIX OF COMPETENCIES
Presenting I
Presenting II
Presenting III
Human Resources II
Performance Management I
Performance Management II
Research I
Research II
Research III
Strategic Planning I
Teaching I
Evaluating and Assessing I
Clinical Leadership I
Clinical Leadership II
Teaching II
Diagnostics, Therapeutics and Clinical Management
Budgeting/Material Management I
Budgeting/Material Management II
Human Resources I
Risk Management

others are digitally immature. However, all are experts in patient care requirements and delivery and therefore must be actively involved in technology implementation. Using the implementation of an EMR to review clinical practice is an effective tool to engage clinical staff. They are the end-users of both policies, procedures and care delivery and they know better than anyone what works and what does not work in their normal roles. Having nursing staff participate in reviews of workflows and processes is very stimulating and ensures the health service has standardised international evidence-based clinical care provision. It also provides a sense of 'ownership' for the new technologies as nursing staff will have, through early and extensive input, a strong and significant impact on the final product. Case Study 17.3 outlines the success of involving clinical staff in the implementation of an EMR.

CASE STUDY 17.3
REDUCTION IN CLINICAL VARIABILITY VIA PROCESS MANAGEMENT REQUIRED FOR EMR ADOPTION

His Highness Sheikh Mohammed bin Rashid Al Maktoum, Vice President and Prime Minister of the UAE and Ruler of Dubai, called on all Dubai Government entities to embrace disruptive innovation as a fundamental mantra of their operations and to seek ways to incorporate its methodologies in all aspects of their work.

To comply with Sheikh Mohammed's directive the Dubai Health Authority contracted a US-based vendor to implement an electronic medical record (EMR) across all government facilities in 2015. At the same time, the Dubai Health Authority (DHA) governing Board of Directors issued a requirement that standardisation of clinical practice based on international evidence was to be implemented across all facilities in DHA. The purpose of this instruction was to ensure patient safety and innovative care became the top priority for all DHA. The decision was made to utilise the implementation of the EMR to facilitate the standardisation of work practices across DHA and to provide the platform for sustainable, efficient and effective healthcare of the future.

The quality and safety literature identifies that 60% of nursing work does not add value to the patient's experience. The purpose of an EMR is to streamline services and provide unprecedented access to information. The DHA made the choice to use lean methodology during the implementation phase of the EMR to ensure:

- Standardisation
- Elimination of waste
- Cost-effective care
- Increase patient safety
- Improve patient satisfaction

DHA is the Government provider of healthcare and regulation for the Emirate of Dubai. Eleven thousand staff work within DHA. It was essential to engage staff from the beginning of the project because once the EMR 'went live' this system would belong to our end-users. Over 500 staff were actively involved in the standardisation process. The end-users understood how our health facilities work and were already frustrated with processes that were duplicated or not effective. This technique ensured staff took responsibility for their own work practices rather than using excuses such as 'it is a decree from higher management' or 'its policy'. Over 500 workflows were revised and 150 policies reviewed.

The system successfully went 'live' in 2017 and since then additional technology has been implemented. These initiatives include home monitoring, AI for retinal scanning, diagnosis for TB, septic shock and blockchain for licensing of healthcare practitioners, materials management and prevention of counterfeit medications.

All 23 applications in the EMR went live in 2017 across all facilities in DHA. One hundred and twenty-eight million existing records were migrated to the EMR. Salama includes a patient portal, which allows patients to access their medical records.

A total of 2.1 million patients are covered in the integrated, effective EMR implemented across DHA. The successful implementation was validated by the achievement of EMRAM and O-EMRAM Stage 6 within 8 weeks of going live across all hospitals, specialty and primary health centres.

TECHNOLOGY AS A POSITIVE DISRUPTOR

The implementation of EMRs across healthcare facilities in the Middle East has allowed for a positive disruption. For example, the 'source of truth' for prescribing, dispensing and administration of medications was formerly found in the physician's pen. Now it is more likely to be found in a centralised formulary and Computerized Provider Ordering Entry (CPOE) systems (Usta et al., 2020). This means that there is a disruption in the formerly rigid social–hierarchical relations within the organisation. Challenging authority or challenging potential errors of senior staff has become easier as the evidence is present at the point of care, for example, in the CPOE, Electronic Medical Administration Record (EMAR) or even the medical device (such as an intravenous pump) itself which has been fixed with limits on prescribing or administration based on the central formulary. Furthermore, technology and budget-impact changes are often now created by departments rather than by individuals, as the integration requirement across systems is wide-ranging and extensive, and even runs through processes not normally associated with clinical care, such as ERP or SAP type set-ups for medication and supply management.

For example, there has been an increase in the role of pharmacy during this last intense period of integration (2017–current), with many senior individuals in pharmacy departments now wearing two hats, as chief pharmacists and as automation and informatics managers. This is not surprising as the ambition for fully integrated healthcare is very much present in the Gulf Cooperation Council (GCC) countries as evidenced by the fact that it is the only region outside of the United States with fully bidirectional interoperable intravenous medication pumps receiving orders directly from the CPOE-EMR (Waterson, 2013). This has also caused tensions between pharmacy and other stakeholders, particularly physicians, and much of this is related to the fact that the best choice of integration *across* the organisation for devices and systems may not necessarily be the best 'specialist' or 'best-in-class' item. This is not to suggest that this process needs to be, or is even commonly, confrontational but the collaborative approach needs to be maintained by leadership and executive sponsorship is always required for these large-scale technology transformations.

Of course, risk management has always been systematic right from the days of James Reason (1997) but what we see with technology, with interoperability and with integration is the ability to stitch every single, disparate part of the system together. In management terms it causes a 'democracy of voices' where data generated from multiple bedsides has more influence within the system than a complex but narrow study or focus undertaken by senior staff.

In the Gulf region data are readily accessible, readable and interpretable and across the region this is really making a change. There is perhaps a greater understanding of the utilisation of data within the region than certainly within many areas of Europe. Furthermore, there is a distinct interest in technology and the uptake of technology, so users are commonly found to be interested in not just *using* advanced healthcare systems, but also *investigating* its functionality and its transparency. In short, highly integrated systems are now being 'interrogated' by its users to ensure that it is operating optimally. Partly, this is also related to the large investments that have been made in integration processes and EMRs, which need to show a clear return on investment (ROI). Large-scale investments and the changing demographics of the region, with an increasingly aged native population and with a shift to chronic disease patterns, have seen a shift from individual organisation-purchasing towards ministry-level Health Technology Assessment Departments producing cost-effective analyses and towards hospital leadership being expected to create at least a budget-impact analysis for purchases, and not uncommonly

a full time-to-ROI estimate. A focus on the best cost–benefit outcomes from a societal perspective has replaced rather more spectacular interventions. The focus on the use of EMR is being explored by most countries in the GCC. Selections have ranged from large well-established health informatics companies to 'locally developed' systems depending on the budget and commitment of differing countries.

In terms of doing business in a HIMSS Level 7 organisation, the rate of adoption of technology is, as alluded to above, absolutely related to the approach taken initially with clinicians. The process has always to be: first, clinician workflow mapping, leading to clinician workflow assisted by technology. This also applies to the specific needs of Gulf patients. Technology has significantly changed the approach to patients at hospital leadership level. This is also related to the availability of big data and to systems that can measure effectively and consistently. For example, there is an ongoing review of the management of patients in the community by large specialist healthcare centres and pharmacies. From this it has become ever more evident that there is a large degree of nonadherence to medication regimes. This has been triangulated by data as simple as (but as massive as!) refill rates of outpatient prescriptions and has led to innovative ways of communicating with the patient through giving fuller access to their own records via apps. As healthcare becomes more of a two-way street access to several healthcare professionals within the organisation can be made directly by the patient without recourse to a doctor's referral—whether this be respiratory care nurses, diabetic nurses or long-term neurological care nurses, psychologists, occupational therapists and physiotherapists.

Since 2020, the Middle East, along with the rest of the world, has been facing the COVID-19 pandemic. If anything, the pandemic has accelerated processes that were already moving along quickly. It has challenged traditional management models where the expectation within highly structured organisations has been that all employees attend the facility with regular shifts, even to the extent of clocking in and clocking out. However, as we have seen during the pandemic, with the desire to reduce footfall within the organisation to reduce transmission risk, there has been an emphasis on working remotely and using technology to achieve this. We have seen pharmacy double-checks undertaken remotely, where a senior pharmacist can virtually make the checks required during key stages of compounding and has the confidence of receiving real-time reports on gravimetric checks from the system, as well the documented visual recording of the entire process undertaken by the pharmacy technician. There is definitely a strong desire within the region to not return to normal patterns of work, particularly when work is out of normal hours. We must remember that many individuals, particularly in the Kingdom of Saudi Arabia, carry a particularly strong family-oriented culture and are therefore reluctant to work outside of hours, particularly when there is a viable technological alternative available. COVID-19 also added to the staffing problems as most nurses working in the GCC come from the Asian subcontinent and went home or stayed at home during the pandemic, thus affecting the number of nurses available.

SUMMARY

Leadership and management of nurses and midwives within this region is both a challenge and a reward. Both the staff and patient cultural diversity and relative 'youth' of the healthcare systems ensure that nursing leaders must be innovative, patient and justify their decisions using international evidence. In most Western health organisations decisions are made based on history or 'we have always done it this way'. This region does not have that history and therefore if leaders ensure nursing voices are heard, amazing changes can be achieved in nursing care and patient safety advances, as well as in technology changes occurring now and in the future. (Seren & Baykal, 2007). The rapid transformation of healthcare due to technology has also formed an awareness in the regions that it has the potential to lead. Examples of this are the medication management interoperability discussed previously and flagship projects such the Dubai Health Authority's big data project to combat sepsis fatalities through the application of a health indicators and variables AI-algorithm. Pride in these achievements is a continually developing norm.

Healthcare cultures are comprised of the norms, values and customs of staff and as nursing leaders it is imperative that we ensure that this regional transformation in nursing is positive and allows for further advances that are recognised internationally.

REFERENCES

Al-Osimy, M. (1994). *Nursing in Saudi Arabia*. Riyadh, Saudi Arabia: King Fahd National Library.

Al-Rifai, F. (2003). *Federal Department of Nursing (FDON), MOH, UAE, Annual Report*. Abu Dhabi: FDON.

Bichel-Findlay, J. (2019–2020). The nursing profession in the digital age. *The Hive* #28.

Bickhoff, L. (2018). Clinical diversity: Variation in skills and experience. *The Hive*, #23, Spring.

Bittar, W. (2015). Perspectives on education in different cultures. Conference Proceedings, 6th Middle East Nursing Conference, Abu Dhabi.

Bjork, I., Hansen, B., Samdel, G., Torstad, S., & Hamilton, G. (2007). Evaluation of clinical ladder participation in Norway. *Journal Nursing Scholarship*, 39(1), 88–94.

Brownie, S. M., Hunter, L. H., Aqtash, S., & Day, G. E. (2015). Establishing policy foundations and regulatory systems to enhance nursing practice in the United Arab Emirates. *Policy, Politics, and Nursing Practice*, 16(1–2), 38–50.

D'Souza, C. (2013). Emirati nurses make up just 3% in UAE. Gulf News. Available at http://gulfnews.com/news/uae/health/emirati-nurses-make-up-just-3-in-uae-1.1161080. Accessed 1 August 2023.

Dubai Online. (2020). UAE Population Statistics.

El-Haddad, M. (2006). Nursing in the United Arab Emirates: An historical background. *International Nursing Review*, 53(4), 284–289. https://doi.org/10.1111/j.1466-7657.2006.00497.x.

Kemp, L., & Zhao, F. (2016). Influences of cultural orientation on Emiratis women's careers. *Personnel Review*, 45(5), 988–1009.

Lovering, S. (2012). The crescent of care: A nursing model to guide the care of Arab Muslim patients. *Diversity and Equality in Health and Care*, 9, 171–178.

OECD. (2021). United Arab Emirates. Available at https://www.oecd.org/countries/unitedarabemirates/.

Newman, S. (2012). *Evaluation of Pilot MCE Competency Programme*. Nursing Department, Rashid Hospital, Dubai Health Authority.

Raghunathan, K., & Tomkins, Z. (2019/2020). Preparing nurses for a digital future. *The Hive* #28.

Reason, J. T. (1997). *Managing the risks of organizational accidents*. Aldershot, UK: Ashgate Publishing Limited.

Seren, S., & Baykal, U. (2007). Relationships between change and organisational culture in hospitals. *Journal of Nursing Scholarship*, 39(2), 191–197.

Sheingold, B., & Hahn, J. (2014). The history of healthcare quality: The first 100 years 1860–1960. *International Journal of Africa Nursing Sciences*, 1, 18–22.

Stewart, L., Holmes, C., & Usher, K. (2012). Reclaiming caring in nursing leadership: A deconstruction of leadership using Habermasian lens. *Collegian*, 19(4), 223–229.

Usta, U., Al-Jaber, R., Mominah, M., Dayem, K., Dabliz, R., Chaker, A., & Ahmad, S. (2020). Ensuring safe and appropriate medication management. Brief report of the 1st Middle East Advisory Board Meeting for Medication Management and Safety. *Omnia Health*, November 2020.

Waterson, J. (2013). Making smart pumps smarter, making IV therapy safer. *British Journal of Nursing*, 22(Sup13), 22–27. https://doi.org/10.12968/bjon.2013.22.Sup13.22.

WHO. (2020). Digital health. https://www.who.int/ehealth/en/.

EPILOGUE
The 'Camel' in the Room…

MAY MCCREADDIE ■ GARY E. DAY ■ JANE LEANNE GRIFFITHS

Before finishing this text we felt it was important, at this juncture, to draw the reader's attention to a really important issue, not just in global healthcare, but one that has considerable implications for healthcare in the Arabian Gulf and Greater Middle East—that of the reducing healthcare workforce.

In most national healthcare workforces, over 50% of healthcare provision is the preserve of nurses (WHO (World Health Organization), 2020). Yet, there has been a persistent and increasing shortfall in the global nursing workforce over the past two decades with low- and middle-income countries mostly bearing the brunt (Buchan et al., 2022). Currently, there is an estimated deficit of 6–13 million nurses expected globally by 2030 (International Council of Nurses, 2023; WHO, 2022) with the Kingdom of Saudi Arabia, for example, estimated to require 33,000 nurses. While the COVID pandemic has impacted nurses in terms of their emotional and physical health, job satisfaction, workload, intention to leave and earlier retirements (Spetz, 2021), it has also shone a light on a festering sore; nurses are a largely depleted and poorly appreciated resource in global terms.

Notwithstanding the challenges of the pandemic and the need for sustainability, there are the increasing demands of medical tourism across the Middle East. Although medical tourism largely involves specialist sub areas such as orthopaedics, neurology, oncology and cardiology (approximately 45%), they nonetheless require considerable resourcing and skills (https://healthcare-digital.com/digital-healthcare/addressing-complex-healthcare-challenges-within-middle-east). In addition, as has been outlined in several chapters, healthcare in the region needs to provide complex care and treatment for the rising numbers of lifestyle-related diseases such as hypertension, diabetes and obesity.

While there has been a persistent drive across the Gulf Cooperation Council (GCC) countries to increase the number of nationals in the workforce, this has met with varying degrees of success (e.g., in UAE, local nurses comprise 4% of the health workforce; Bahrain 61%). In short, the wealthier nations in the region are over-reliant on foreign nationals of varying qualifications, skills and language competencies and they need more resources from what is already a limited global pool. Moreover, other 'supply' countries are increasingly taking steps to attract, retain and prevent nurses migrating (Brush & Sochalski, 2007). This peripatetic, diverse workforce is therefore being stretched across the specialist fields of medical tourism, lifestyle challenges, prevention and provision, late cancer diagnosis and a prevailing lack of specialist palliative and end-of-life care provision. Accordingly, against this global and local context, the challenge of attracting, retaining, appropriately educating and supporting (generic) staff *and* building specialisms that are arguably still in their infancy in the region, (e.g., pain management, end-of-life care) is therefore not insignificant.

This is indeed the 'camel' in the room—and one that cannot be underplayed.

The purpose of this text was to provide an insight into healthcare provision across the Arabian Gulf and Greater Middle East. The challenges facing expatriate healthcare professionals working in the region have been addressed in various chapters. The first chapter on Islamic beliefs and healthcare provides newcomers to this area with a clear understanding of how Islam is central to people's being and that includes healthcare. It is essential for healthcare professionals to understand these cultural aspects in order to provide comprehensive and effective care to their patients. Chapter 11 on communication, caring and diversity focussed on how important communication is when dealing with a diverse, multicultural workforce within healthcare facilities and with a similarly diverse patient population. The text has repeatedly referred to the large expatriate community within the region with the nursing population largely being drawn from across the Asian subcontinents, with a smaller senior nursing workforce coming from the West. Our medical colleagues hail from across the Arabic world, India and Pakistan as well as Eastern Europe. This diverse workforce brings healthcare workers together from differing educational backgrounds as well as a variety of cultures. Accordingly, several chapters explored how expatriate staff can learn to appropriately care for their patients ensuring their religious and cultural needs are addressed.

Chapter 3 on consumer-driven healthcare discussed how the health system is being challenged to develop a consumer focus including the various funding models under development in different countries. This consumer focus needs to be balanced with the existing family culture which may have historically protected patients from 'bad news'.

Chapters 4 and 5 on lifestyle (diabetes and obesity) identified the issues facing the populations of this region when Western culture and food collide and challenge the health of the indigenous population. The increase in fast foods containing high levels of sugar, fats and 'upsized' portions with minimal vegetables together with a more sedentary lifestyle have led to significant increases in obesity and chronic non-communicable diseases such as diabetes, hypertension and cardiovascular disease. These chapters identified the struggle in trying to ensure the population recognises these chronic conditions and the need for ongoing treatment and care.

The focus on women in this text is wholly deliberate as there are a number of hidden disorders faced by women in the region. Unfortunately, social stigma often prevents women from presenting to healthcare facilities for diagnosis and treatment. Discussions around faecal and urinary incontinence and sexual health are considered 'taboo' or too embarrassing for women to address. This results in social isolation and contributes to the depressive illnesses outlined in Chapters 8 and 13. The stigma of mental health illnesses often means patients and their families seek help from friends rather than health professionals. These chapters on mental health and well-being and psychosocial support discussed how families and Islamic beliefs have influenced the care of,

and attitudes to, these illnesses. Both chapters also identified how the traditional treatment of various illnesses can now be dovetailed into current evidence-based practices with religious elders acting as the fulcrum with which to assist patients and their families in better understanding how more modern therapies can help.

Chapter 14 on pharmacy also highlighted some of the issues with medications in the region such as increased, unrecognised usage of complementary and alternative medicines by women and how substandard and falsified medicines are a major issue, particularly in war torn areas and low economic countries where criminals sell substandard or fake drugs. Moreover, over-the-counter purchasing and the use of antibiotics to self-medicate compounds the global problem of antimicrobial resistance.

Men have not been forgotten, with men's health included within Chapter 2 (on the family in healthcare) focussing on the reluctance of men to seek medical aid or health check-ups as this is seen as a 'weakness'. This chapter also discussed marriage and pregnancy, together with children and their genetic problems resulting from consanguineous marriages.

Several chapters explored the difficulties of balancing long-established approaches with international treatment programs. Chapter 12 on family medicine identified the difficulties of physicians trying to engage patients and families in treatment with the time restraints placed upon clinics as well as trying to ensure ongoing patient compliance with treatment. This is another chapter that highlighted the traditional use of complementary therapies/medicine such as cupping and herbal treatments to address chronic diseases.

The challenging chapters on pain management and end-of-life (Chapters 15 and 16, respectively) are relatively new concepts for the region. The speciality of pain management struggles with having few qualified healthcare professionals available and therefore a lack of knowledge in the numerous methods that can manage both acute and chronic pain as well as specific pain such as from labour or sickle cell disease. There remains some reluctance to use narcotics on religious grounds as well as complex laws constraining their use. End-of-life care or palliative care is also in its infancy. Islamic recommendations and laws address this area, but these are open to interpretation on both an individual as well as a country-wide level. However, it is encouraging to see the burgeoning development of palliative care facilities and services as well as the increasing employment and training of palliative care staff in most countries in the region.

Some of the most interesting clinical conditions identified in the region are respiratory illnesses and infections in Chapter 10. The sandy, desert environment together with high levels of smoking and the use of shisha have resulted in high levels of respiratory illnesses, while the millions of travellers passing through the region bring with them infectious diseases often not seen in other parts of the world. The COVID-19 pandemic has highlighted for the world the importance of effectively managing disease spread and perhaps largely because of its history, this region has been very effective in implementing controls in comparison with other countries as discussed in Chapter 9.

The last chapter (Chapter 17) on technology and leadership showcased the future and how it is essential to care for staff who will in turn successfully use some of the most advanced technology. The pandemic has shown us all how effective artificial intelligence and telemedicine can be in improving healthcare.

Finally, the book-end appendix is designed to supply newcomers to the region with 'survival hints'. There are suggestions contained therein that we all wished someone had given each of us before we arrived! It will be different depending on which country you choose to move to but hopefully forewarned is forearmed.

SUMMARY

This text has demonstrated how certain areas of healthcare now being provided in the Middle East are at advanced practice standards. The use of technology, managing infections and addressing both communicable and non-communicable diseases are all such examples. The GCC countries in particular are focussed on providing evidence-based healthcare to their communities and have made significant advances since 2000. It has been a challenge amalgamating culturally historic healthcare with international evidence-based practice. Nevertheless, these advances have been rapidly implemented and have included international accreditation of many hospitals in the region since 2007.

Working in the Middle East offers great rewards and satisfaction for expatriate healthcare workers. The range of clinical cases compared with many Western healthcare systems can be vast. The improvements you can make both clinically and to the healthcare system can also be much more noticeable than in more mature Western healthcare settings. That said, it is important to understand a few key concepts before taking the plunge into working in the Middle East.

First, remember you are a guest in the country. The country invited you because they need your skills and expertise. Treat your host well and they will treat you well in return. Be respectful of the local culture, traditions and norms and see the world through their eyes. If you are not a good guest, there are no unions to advocate for you and you may have your visa cancelled or your employment contract terminated. If you do not have a job, then your stay may be a short one and you may have to leave.

Second, be aware of the mix of cultures and politics in your organisation. Not only do you have to juggle the mix of patient and other healthcare professionals' culture but you also have to manage the interdisciplinary politics. The way you talk with a doctor or a senior nurse in your home country may be very different to the interactions you have in the Middle East. Most of all listen carefully, ensure that your message gets across in a professional manner and always advocate for the patient. If you can do all these things, you will have very fond memories and career highlights in the Middle East.

And last but not least, this region is vast and diverse—a veritable cultural mosaic that provides fantastic opportunities to learn and appreciate nationalities and cultures from across the globe. Make the effort to engage and you will reap the rewards.

REFERENCES

Brush, B. L., & Sochalski, J. (2007). International nurse migration: Lessons from the Philippines. *Policy, politics & nursing practice*, 8(1), 37–46. https://doi.org/10.1177/1527154407301393.

Buchan, J. Catton, H., & Shaffer, F. (2022). The global nursing workforce and the Covid-19 pandemic. ICMN.

International Council of Nurses (ICN). (2023). Recover to rebuild: Investing the nursing workforce for health system effectiveness. Geneva: International Council of Nurses.

Spetz, J. (2021). The Handoff - Episode 51: How COVID-19 has impacted the nursing workforce (trustedhealth.com). March 31.

WHO (World Health Orginzation). (2020). State of the world's nursing: Investing in education, jobs and leadership. Geneva: WHO.

WHO. (2022). *The 2022 Update, Global Health Workforce Statistics*. Geneva: World Health Organization.

APPENDIX
Some Helpful Information and Advice for Those Considering Working in the Region

MAY MCCREADDIE ■ GARY E. DAY ■ JANE LEANNE GRIFFITHS

INTRODUCTION

Healthcare workers migrate for reasons of domestic expectation, financial gain, opportunity for professional development, job satisfaction, or even departure from political instability or oppression. That said, money tends to be the primary reason why the vast majority of migrants choose to work abroad in the Arabian Gulf and Greater Middle East. At home, many nonprofessional workers in particular, may face unemployment or low wages and be unable to support their family. However, although they may appear relatively poorly paid and might be considered cheap labour, it is often overlooked that a position in this region gives migrant workers the opportunity to save and send money home to house and keep their extended families, which they otherwise would not have.

There are different sections of migrant workers from labourers to teachers and doctors who earn varying sums and may or may not have additional benefits such as annual flights to home, health insurance and school fees. Many migrant workers go through significant life events without their family and extended family around them, for example, birth, marriage and funerals. While most families would choose to relocate, this may not be possible on their salary and/or visas/work permits, so the mother and/or father may stay in the region and work while their children stay at home with their extended family. Consequently, some migrant workers may not see their families for years and this will invariably cause a strain on relationships. That said, working abroad is much easier now than it was

in the 1990s, for example, as globalisation has given us numerous means of communication from Facebook to WhatsApp and beyond. It is therefore not uncommon to see unskilled migrant workers (e.g. road sweepers, fast food delivery drivers) go about their business while having a voice call with their wife and children.

The region is a transient place for many and there is likely to be a 'churn' and a regular flux and influx of teachers or other professional workers. These professional workers are likely to be 'western', in their early 20s or towards the end of their retirement, looking to earn and experience a foreign culture for 2–3 years maximum. Conversely, non-western expatriates, for example, Arabs, Indians and Filipinos working in the professions, may stay and work in the region for their whole working life while building houses for family, etc. at home.

Last but not least, some people who work in the region may be seeking to 'escape' difficult situations (e.g. bereavement, divorce) at home and come to try and recharge their batteries. You will meet many different people here with stories to tell and their own aims and aspirations. They may be the young Bangladeshi (Mohammed) who washes your car and who just got married 3 years ago but has only seen his wife once in that time. Or they may be your Sri Lankan cleaner (Theresa) who came to the country 40 years ago with her new husband in a good job only to see him die suddenly from a heart attack and leave her to bring up her two young daughters alone. She took to cleaning, put her daughters through school and saw them marry. Now in her

181

60s, she works hard, attends the Catholic Church and intends to return home soon. Like you, they are simply here to earn a living. Look after them and they will look after you. Be kind. It costs nothing.

PRE-ONBOARDING

There are a number of different things you need to consider prior to working in the region. First, fully check out your potential employer and seek reviews where available. Try and find people who have worked there—what were their experiences? Consider what salary you may be able to earn. This information is not always easy to obtain as employers can be notoriously secretive about who earns what. Coming from a western perspective, I was used to setting salary scales and was shocked to be asked at interview what salary I expected. I was offered X salary and, following some investigation, requested a considerably higher sum, citing experience, qualifications and 'add-on' value—which they subsequently agreed without discussion! Be aware that some organisations—not necessarily local organisations—do not have increments and you may therefore be on the same salary for some time. Be clear about what the salary actually covers. Some salaries may appear attractive only for people to discover they do not include school fees, accommodation allowance or travel. That said, many employers may offer gratuities to entice workers, where employees will be provided with half a month's salary or one month's salary for every full year worked. This can help with relocation which may be expensive.

Check out what support (if any) is provided by your Human Resources Department for onboarding. For example, do they have induction? Is there an occupational health provision? It is important to have appropriate medical insurance. This may be provided as part of the contract and, for example, Bahrain has recently decreed that private employers should provide this for all employees. What does the medical insurance provide and are there any other additional charges? You are probably likely to have to undergo a medical at some point whether pre-boarding or in-country. If you are considering being abroad for some time it may be worthwhile considering having a full medical of your own accord prior to leaving. You should also ensure you have sufficient medications available for several months and these should come with a prescription/letter. Medications vary in the region and you may not be able to obtain the same medications—check availability. It is also important to ensure that you have the relevant vaccinations and certificates to hand.

Flights and Visas

Have you been given sufficient information on flight allowances and what do you require in terms of a visa? How much baggage allowance or freight do you have and what are the arrangements for the end of the contract?

Attestation

It is likely that you will be required to produce your original qualification certificates with appropriate attestation. This means it may be required to be signed by a notary/solicitor/lawyer, by the Foreign, Commonwealth and Development Office (FCDO) UK and then either by the embassy or, once you are in-country, by the Ministry of Health/Labour or similar. This can be relatively expensive and you may have to cover the costs. If you are married, you also need to have your marriage certificate attested.

Families/Schools

What are the local schools like? How much are their school fees? Are there after-school clubs? What about a maid or housekeeper? This kind of information can usually be obtained through local webpages such as https://mumsinbahrain.net or similar https://dubai-mums.com.

Culture

What can I wear, where can I go and what can I do? For example, in the UAE there is a difference between Dubai, Abu Dhabi and Al Ain, with the third being much more conservative. Be respectful at all times, especially in public areas such as malls. If in doubt, cover up, but you will soon work out what is acceptable or not. Be aware of the language barrier and try and learn some Arabic—it goes a long way.

Other

Ensure you bring and/or have access to sufficient cash to last you for at least 2 months as it may take this length of time to set up a bank account.

444 4 4 4 4 4 4444444444444444444444444444444444444444444444444444444444444444444444444444444444444444444444444444444444444444444444444444444444444444444444444444444444444444444444444444444

IN-COUNTRY

It makes good sense to keep a 'cash in hand' fund somewhere in case you lose your bank card or unexpected events happen and the ATMs close, for example, Arab Spring. It is advisable to have at least the cost of a return flight to hand. It is unlikely that you will need to use it, but if an ATM swallows your card and it is a long public holiday, then it makes sense to have some spare cash.

Pets

As someone from the United Kingdom who brought her house rabbits out to Abu Dhabi way back in 2015, I perfectly fit the picture of the archetypal British pet lover. However, pets—especially dogs and cats—are not revered in the same way in this region as they may be elsewhere. Moreover, expats cannot be too sanctimonious about this as they are notorious for dumping pets in the street/villas/apartments when they leave. If you are bringing a pet with you, please check out the local customs and rules. You will find reasonable veterinary practices here but you should check out their qualifications first as some may not be 'vets' but simply have a degree. How will your pet cope with the temperatures? Where can they be exercised safely and are pet food and other supplies easy to obtain? You will require an exporter (UK/elsewhere) and importer (region) to bring your pet(s) into the country safely. Some airlines do not permit pet carriage; others insist pets must be in the hold unless it is a falcon, in which case it is allowed in the cabin! What about pet boarding? Who will look after your pet when you return home for a break or a holiday? There are 'pet groups' in the region on social media where you will be able to obtain all kinds of useful information, specific to your area and pet.

Driving

It will not surprise you to learn that driving can be something of a challenge in this part of the world. You drive on the right-hand side of the road as opposed to the left, but thankfully, the vast majority of cars are automatic. Notably, speed limits are variable. For example, a speed limit may not necessarily be a limit but a general guide and unless you go about 20%–30% above the denoted speed, then you will not be fined. This varies across the region, so please familiarise yourself with the rules of the road. This includes whether you can legally drive using your own country's driving license or whether you need to acquire a local driving license. Cars can be hired easily, but always photograph the car inside and out prior to signing the hire sheet, just in case of any dispute. Be clear about what you need to do if you do have an accident; for example, you may require a police report. Make sure you have satellite navigation or something similar to hand and it is working with sufficient mobile data. It is difficult enough to drive in a new environment without having to work out where you are—especially in the dark.

Finally, I had an accident within the first month of arriving in the UAE when I drove into the back of a Bangladeshi's car who had been somewhat hesitant at a very, very busy roundabout (Tawam Hospital, Al Ain). The police were duly called and brought a female officer who was incredibly polite and spoke perfect English. We went to the police station to report the incident and the staff could not have been more professional in their dealings. Unfortunately, having just received a resident's permit, I should not have been driving on a UK driving license—a fact I was unaware of. Thus the hired car was impounded! I held my hands up to the accident as clearly driving into the back of a car is not the fault of the car in front. Thereafter, I had to go to 'court' and was 'fined' the grand total of 3000 AED (600 GBP). Thus having been driving for over 30 years in the United Kingdom with not even a parking ticket, I now had the (slight exaggeration here) equivalent of a minor criminal record within 1 month of arriving in the UAE! What was slightly amusing was the way the other 'offenders' reacted to being 'in court'; there was coffee and savouries—it was akin to being a rather enjoyable day out with much laughing and 'Insh Allah'.

Alcohol, Drugs, Immoral Behaviour and Social Media

Different areas in the region have different rules regarding the purchase and consumption of alcohol. For example, alcohol licenses are required in some of the UAE states (except Sharjah, which is 'dry') and they have to be authorised by your employer and only allow you to spend a set percentage of your salary on alcohol. You can be arrested in most areas if you are drunk in public. Consequently, you should always exercise caution if you are socialising and drinking alcohol. Similarly, drink-driving is a no-go area, as is any kind of illegal drug consumption. Immoral behaviour covers all manner of indiscretions and you should appraise yourself of the social mores of the area you are going to be living and working in. You should also always exercise care when using social media. Inappropriate comments, pictures, images, swearing, or criticising your employer and/or the government/royal family is patently ill-advised and may contravene publication laws.

Financial Aspects

It is always good practice to keep a note of all your spending for the first 6 months at least. I am Scottish, so I have a note of my spending for the last 7 years(!) It is easy to lose track of spending, especially if you are earning much more than you did previously and are unfamiliar with using a foreign currency. If you are here to 'save money' then please make sure you do; have limits on spending and know what you want to save each month. Consider taking advice on your pension and an investment portfolio, but only with reputable firms and make sure you do not become tied into plans as you may want to be relatively flexible should you have to leave at short notice.

Finally, self-care is very important and you should make sure you look after yourself and your friends and colleagues. Make a social circle, work at it and if you find it is not beneficial, move on. Find a hobby or a club and build yourself a social circle. Try not to stick to expats; make sure you engage with other nationalities and locals. Get into a routine, exercise and eat healthily. Always have a water bottle to hand at all times, especially when driving. Brunches are a great feature of enjoyment in the region, but they should be occasional rather than frequent. Notably, this region is probably one of the safest regions in the world. There are very few places in the world where you could happily go for a walk at two or three in the morning and feel entirely safe.

PREPARING TO LEAVE

Ideally, people should prepare to leave once they arrive. Make sure you know what you are entitled to in terms of salary, gratuities, flight, freight, etc. Have a plan in place should you have to leave suddenly for a family emergency or something similar. Does someone have a spare key for your apartment? What about your pets, if any? Can you access your ready cash and your passport? If your departure is more planned, then be aware that it can take some time to sell furniture and possibly cars, etc. and it is always better to start doing this gradually over the last 6 months. There are usually plenty of social media sites that buy and sell. Where larger items are concerned, it is inadvisable to let possible buyers know when you are leaving as this may strengthen their negotiating hand. Have a 'best price' and try to agree on that in advance. Selling a car, for example, will require you to change over registration and insurance and this takes time. You will need to ensure that any loans or financial obligations are paid in full (e.g. car loan) and likewise any driving offences. Any existing court actions, even for minor offences, may delay your exit and can result in a travel ban. Allow enough time both on arrival and when exiting to connect/disconnect electricity, gas, water, telephone and internet. It goes without saying that planned exits are always much better than unplanned exits and this is something you should always consider from the outset.

Good luck!

INDEX